Forensic Toxicology

Controlled Substances and Dangerous Drugs

Forensic Toxicology
Controlled Substances and Dangerous Drugs

W. T. Lowry and
James C. Garriott

Southwestern Institute of Forensic Sciences
Dallas, Texas

Plenum Press · New York and London

RELEASED
73709

Library of Congress Cataloging in Publication Data

Lowry, William Thomas, 1942-
    Forensic toxicology.

    Bibliography: p.
    Includes index.
    1. Chemistry, Forensic. 2. Drugs. 3. Narcotics, Control of — United States. 4. Drugs
— Laws and legislation — United States. I. Garriott, James C., joint author. II. Title.
HV8073.L75   614'.19   78-26439
ISBN 0-306-40124-X

© 1979 Plenum Press, New York
A Division of Plenum Publishing Corporation
227 West 17th Street, New York, N.Y. 10011

Printed in the United States of America

Preface

With the rapid spread of drug use and abuse in this country over the last decade, events relating to drugs have become increasingly prominent in the court of law as well as in society in general. It is anticipated that throughout the 1980s this problem will continue to be one of the major social problems in the United States. With the complexity of the Federal and state laws and their interrelationships, and with the increasing demand for the expert chemist or toxicologist, or both, in the courtroom, more education for these people relating to drugs must be implemented. The prosecuting and defense attorneys are also in need of accurate toxicological information to adequately handle cases in which drugs play a role.

This book is intended to be a practical as well as an educational book—a resource tool for the active forensic chemist, as well as for the student. It is with the forensic chemist in mind that the material on controlled substances and substances found in cases of drug abuse has been arranged in a systematic order for quick and easy reference. This section includes synonyms, pharmaceutical preparations, biochemistry and/or pharmacognosy, toxicology and/or pharmacology, and how the substance is controlled under Federal law. Under the concept of scientific consideration as compared with the Federal law, this book enables one to deal with some of the major conflicts in the American legal system concerning scientific evidence and how it is presented in a court of law.

The first section of the book discusses the concept of drugs and specifications that pharmaceutical companies must meet and maintain to market a new product. The next section deals with the Federal Controlled Substances Act, including requirements for registration of controlled substances, and the rules and regulations under which a forensic laboratory must handle drug evidence relating to testing. Among the topics discussed are security requirements, including recommendations presented by the Drug Enforcement Administration for handling drug evidence obtained from police seizures, labeling and packaging requirements for controlled substances, record-handling for controlled substances, inventory requirements, prescriptions, and statement of the Act itself, listing drugs included in Schedules I, II, III, IV, and V. Brief discussions on adulterated and misbranded drugs, as well as illicit preparations and their legal status, are included.

The section describing pharmaceutical dosage forms includes packaging types and formulations such as aerosols, capsules, creams, elixirs, emulsions, extracts, fluid extracts, gels, inhalants, injections, jellies, lotions, ointments, pastes, powders, solutions, spirits, suppositories, suspensions, syrups, tablets, tinctures, and waters.

The discussion of excluded and excepted substances under the Controlled Substances Act provides a systematic protocol for handling pharmaceutical preparations encountered in the laboratory, especially when extrapolating Federal law to state laws. Specific exceptions are listed and described.

The discussion termed "dangerous drugs" deals with a broad range of regulations outside the Controlled Substances Act. These include legend drugs, banned drugs, and nonapproved new drugs undergoing clinical trial. Certain over-the-counter drugs, or nonprescription drugs, are listed if they are frequently found in cases of drug abuse or encountered in excepted and excluded substances.

The final section of the text provides an alphabetical listing of all substances listed in the Controlled Substances Act, and other selected dangerous drugs and nonprescription drugs. Each substance is listed by generic name. A listing of other generic names and IUPAC names under the heading "Synonyms" provides the reader with a quick reference to the drug. Included with each substance is a listing of its common trade names and its formulations containing the titled drug. If the pharmaceutical preparation causes deviation of control due to its formulation, it is so stated. Also included for each substance is a discussion of the biochemistry and/or pharmacognosy, and of the toxicology–pharmacology of that substance.

Basically, all information discussed is intended to include the necessary material to provide the scientific expert with information to testify in a court of law; to provide the attorneys with enough information to assist in prosecuting or defending a drug case; and to provide physicians with information on drugs and drug laws to assist in maintaining proper records and prescription practices. Under no circumstances do the authors of this book intend for this to be a legal document. All subject matter is based on legal documents with certain opinions of the authors found throughout.

In general, this book should give the reader an overall working knowledge of how to apply state and Federal laws, how to interrelate these laws, and how to interpret them scientifically when called upon to do so. It is the intent of the authors to bridge the gap between scientific and legal investigations in the fields of controlled substances and dangerous drugs.

We wish to acknowledge some special people who were diligent in their efforts during the preparation of this manuscript. Thanks go to Mrs. Karen Partain, Mrs. Aileen Langston, Mrs. Jan Laird, Miss Laura Seaman, and Mrs. Terri Austin.

Also, we are grateful to Mr. Frank Jackson, Criminal Defense Attorney, Dallas, Texas and Mr. Jim Barklow, Chief Felony Prosecutor, Office of the District Attorney, Dallas County, Texas, for the time they gave in consultation on legal matters set forth in this book.

We are also indebted to the staff of Plenum Publishing Corporation for continuous and skillful advisement during the final stages of preparation of the manuscript. Special appreciation goes to Ms. Nancy Mester, Senior Production Editor, for her patience with us when we failed to meet deadlines.

W. T. Lowry
J. C. Garriott

Dallas

Contents

CONTENTS

1
Introduction

The laws regulating drugs in this country have been categorized listing several general aspects specifically designated to relate to drugs and drug-related products (Gibson, 1976):

1. Drug records for distribution and movement
2. Drug labeling
3. Authorization of persons qualified to work with drugs
4. Practitioner licensing requirements and legal responsibilities
5. Drug quality control
6. Criminal liabilities for noncompliance with drug regulations
7. Commercial marketing regulations

The Federal government regulates drugs categorically as they are legally defined. The criteria for classification are legend drugs, nonlegend drugs (OTCs), investigational new drugs, new drugs, old drugs, veterinary legend drugs, veterinary nonlegend drugs, controlled substances, drugs intended for animal feed purposes, and drugs not intended for use in humans or animals (Gibson, 1976).

For the purpose of this text, the term "dangerous drug" refers to either tranquilizers or legend drugs. Since all tranquilizers not listed as scheduled drugs are either legend drugs or are not registered for approved medicinal use in the United States, they are defined for purposes of simplification as dangerous drugs. Under specific circumstances, many legend drug preparations are frequently abused. These drugs are classified in this text under the legend drug clause of the Controlled Substances Act, which states that the label containing the drug must bear the legend "Caution: Federal law prohibits dispensing without a prescription" or "Caution: Federal law restricts this drug to use by or on the order of a licensed veterinarian."

The Federal Food, Drug, and Cosmetic Act of 1938, as amended in 1962 and 1965, establishes the authority of the government to safeguard the public health against certain potential hazards, and to protect the consumer's interest. The Food and Drug Administration (FDA) is the regulatory agency charged with enforcing these laws. The main provisions of the Act are:

1. Foods, drugs, and cosmetics must be labeled accurately to show all ingredients and their amounts.
2. Drugs deemed unsafe for unsupervised use must not be sold except on prescription.
3. Unsafe drugs must not be marketed at all, even for prescription use.
4. Physicians must be informed fully by the manufacturer regarding toxic potentialities and side effects of prescription drugs.
5. False and misleading claims must not be made either in advertising or in the labeling of drugs.
6. Advertisements and promotional brochures must describe all adverse effects and contraindications.
7. Drugs acting on the central nervous system and subject to abuse must be subject to especially rigorous controls.

The authority of the Federal agencies extends only to drugs shipped in interstate commerce. However, this covers nearly all manufacturers and nearly all drugs. The individual state laws extend similar controls to drugs manufactured and sold entirely within a state. In addition, the states increase control through the licensing of pharmacists, physicians, dentists, and veterinarians.

NEW DRUGS

When a manufacturer has a prospective new drug for the market, a "Notice of Claimed Investigational Exemption for a New Drug" (IND) application must be filed with the FDA. Accurate information concerning the chemical structures of all components, the quantitative composition of the preparation, the sources, and methods of production including quality control procedures must be furnished. All preclinical and any preliminary clinical data already obtained must be included in the application as well as the names and qualifications of the investigators in sufficient detail to permit objective scientific review. The exact labeling of the drug must be disclosed. The names, qualifications, and previous experience of the proposed investigators must be communicated. The proposed investigations must be described in detail, divided into two phases:

Phase 1. A study in a small number of persons to determine the human toxicity, metabolism, absorption, elimination, safe dosage range, and pharmacologic actions.

Phase 2. A full-scale clinical investigation to obtain data that are well controlled.

In all studies, accurate and complete records must be kept. A local institutional review committee, comprised of representatives from the medical prefession, scientists, lawyers, and laymen, must approve and monitor all studies. Informed-consent procedures are explicitly required. During this period, no promotion or commercial distribution is permitted. After 30 days following the filing of an IND application, if the FDA has made no objection, the investigations may proceed. If the application is denied or the FDA requires termination of the investigation after it has begun, appropriate appeal procedures are available. The FDA requires regular reports and is especially interested in the prompt reporting of any adverse reactions attributed to the drug. For drugs with stimulant, depressant, or hallucinogenic action on the central nervous system, the rules set forth in the Controlled Substances Act apply.

After the investigational period, providing the drug appears to merit general distribution, a New Drug Application (NDA) may be filed. This will contain, in greater detail, the basic information called for in the IND application. In addition, it must describe in detail the results of the investigational studies. The results of the clinical trials showing the efficacy as well as the verbatim text of the package insert and certain promotional materials must be submitted. On final approval by the FDA, the drug may be distributed and marketed in accordance with the approved claims, with appropriate warnings and contraindications stated. If the application is for a drug to be sold over-the-counter (OTC), safety for general unsupervised use must be shown. The FDA at any time may require a change in the labeling, in advertising claims, or in the information furnished to physicians, or it may even order the drug withdrawn if evidence is obtained to warrant such action.

Other governmental agencies concerned in the control of drugs include a special agency of the National Institutes of Health, the Division of Biologics Standards. It is responsible for licensing serums, vaccines, and other biologic products, including human blood and its derivatives. Periodic inspection of manufacturing facilities is carried out by agents of the Division. The Federal Trade Commission has general authority to prevent dissemination of false claims with respect to drugs (as with any other commodity) in interstate commerce. Advertising of proprietary drugs comes under its special purview. The Federal Communications Commission monitors advertising on radio and television.

ADVERTISING

Advertising of prescription drugs is directed at physicians. Methods of advertising include package inserts, ads in medical journals, mailings directly to physicians, and personal visits by agents of the manufacturers (detailmen). Package inserts are the small leaflets that are required by law under the full-disclosure regulation to accompany each package of a drug. They are very useful sources of information. The drug's chemical structure, pharmacology, clinical use, toxicities, contraindications, and recommended doses are described in the insert. These inserts are reviewed by the FDA to ensure that they represent a full and accurate disclosure about the drug. Pharmaceutical manufacturers are required to send copies of these inserts to physicians on request. Recently, these inserts have been questioned in court as to whether they are legal documents or merely information (Hirsh, 1977).

ADULTERATED DRUGS

Section 501 of the Controlled Substances Act sets forth the basic description of adulterated drugs. A drug is considered to be adulterated if it purports to be or is represented as a drug that is listed in an official compendium, and its strength, quality, or purity differs from the standards set forth in such compendium. The term "official compendium," as defined in Section 201 of the Controlled Substances Act, means the official *United States Pharmacopeia, Homeopathic Pharmacopeia of The United States, National Formulary*, or any supplement to any of them. The determination as to strength, quality, or purity must be made in accordance with the tests or methods of assay set forth in an official compendium. Whenever tests or methods of assay have not been prescribed in the compendium, or such tests or methods of assay as are prescribed are insufficient for the making of such determination, the fact will be brought to the attention of the appropriate body charged with the revision of the compendium. For scientific–legal purposes, the law is not clear as to whether the laboratory investigating altered or adulterated drugs in criminal offenses must follow methods set forth in the official compendium to the letter, or if the laboratory may use an equivalent method shown to have similar precision.

No drug defined in an official compendium will be classified as being adulterated because it differs from the standard of strength, quality, or purity therefor set forth in such compendium, if its difference in strength, quality, or purity from such standards is plainly stated on its label. Whenever a drug is recognized in both the *United States Pharmacopeia* and the *Homeopathic Pharmacopeia of the United States*, it will be subject to the requirements of the

United States Pharmacopeia unless it is labeled and offered for sale as a homeopathic drug. In the latter case, it will be subject to the provisions of the *Homeopathic Pharmacopeia of the United States* and not to those of the *United States Pharmacopeia.* A homeopathic drug is a drug that is capable of producing in healthy persons symptoms like those of the disease to be treated.

MISBRANDED DRUGS

Section 502 of the Controlled Substances Act sets forth the basic description of misbranded drugs. A drug is correctly branded if its label bears, to the exclusion of any other nonproprietary name (except the applicable systematic chemical name or the chemical formula), the established name of the drug. In addition, if it is fabricated from two or more ingredients, the established name and quantity of each active ingredient must be listed. This includes the quantity, kind, the proportion of any alcohol as well as the established name and quantity or proportion of any bromides, ether, chloroform, acetanilide, acetophenetidin, amidopyrine, antipyrine, atropine, hyoscine, hyoscyamine, arsenic, digitalis glucosides, mercury, ouabain, strophanthin, strychnine, thyroid, or any derivative or preparation of any such substances, contained therein whether active or not. The requirement for stating the quantity of these specific drugs applies only to prescription drugs. For any prescription drug, the established name of such drug or ingredient on the label (and on any labeling on which a name for such drug or ingredient is used) must be printed prominently and in type at least half as large as that used thereon for any proprietary name or designation for such drug or ingredient. If compliance with these requirements is impracticable, exemptions may be established.

The term "established name," with respect to a drug or ingredient thereof, means the applicable official name. If a drug is recognized in the *United States Pharmacopeia* and in the *Homeopathic Pharmacopeia* under different official titles, the official title used in the *United States Pharmacopeia* will apply unless it is labeled and offered for sale as a homeopathic drug. In the latter case, the official title used in the *Homeopathic Pharmacopeia* will apply.

Section 508 of the Controlled Substances Act provides the authority to the Secretary of Health, Education and Welfare to designate an official name for any drug if he determines that such action is necessary or desirable in the interest of usefulness and simplicity. Any official name designated for any drug must be the only official name of that drug used in any official compendium published after such name has been prescribed. In no event, however, will the Secretary establish an official name so as to infringe a valid trademark.

The Secretary will, when necessary, initiate a review of the official names by which drugs are identified in the official *United States Pharmacopeia*, the official *Homeopathic Pharmacopeia of the United States*, and the official *National Formulary*, and all supplements thereto, to determine whether revisions of any of those names is necessary or desirable in the interest of usefulness and simplicity.

Whenever it is determined that (1) any official name is unduly complex or is not useful for any other reason, (2) two or more official names have been applied to a single drug, or to two or more drugs that are identical in chemical structure and pharmacological action and that are substantially identical in strength, quality, and purity, or (3) no official name has been applied to a medically useful drug, the Secretary will notify, in writing, the compiler of each official compendium in which that drug or drugs are identified and request that a single official name be established for such drug or drugs that will have usefulness and simplicity. Whenever a single official name has not been recommended within one hundred and eighty days after such request, or the Secretary determines that any name so recommended is not useful for any reason, he will designate a single official name of such drug or drugs. Such designation will be made as a regulation on public notice and in accordance with the procedure set forth in the Administrative Procedure Act (5 U.S.C. 1003).

After each review, and at such other times as the Secretary may determine to be necessary or desirable, a list of official names will be compiled, published, and publicly distributed. The Secretary, on public notice and in accordance with the procedure set forth in the Administrative Procedure Act (5 U.S.C. 1003), may designate an official name of a drug on receiving a request in writing by any compiler of an official compendium.

DRUG NOMENCLATURE

Every drug has a generic or nonproprietary name. Before a manufacturer receives approval to market a drug, this generic name must be established. The United States Adopted Names Council is a collaborative enterprise of the United States Pharmacopeia (U.S.P.), National Formulary (N.F.), Homeopathic Pharmacopeia of the United States, and Council on Drugs of the American Medical Association. The legalities of generic names are discussed above under the heading "Adulterated Drugs."

Pharmaceutical trade names are registered names given to a product containing one or more drugs (having generic names) as well as possibly other nonmedicinal inert material. Any deviation from the registered properties of the trade preparation will be inconsistent with the trade name. Thus, any reference to the trade name under these conditions would be invalid. A good example of this would be the use of the trade name in filing criminal charges against a person in possession of a drug that was once a "legend drug" but that has been altered (such as powder removed from a capsule). Since the FDA requires the registered markings, etc., to be consistent in all dosage forms, any deviation from the approved dose would classify that dose as an adulterated drug, making the trade name invalid.

2

Pharmaceutical Dosage Forms

AEROSOLS

Pharmaceutical aerosols are packaged under pressure and contain therapeutically active ingredients. They are intended for topical application to the skin as well as local application, including inhalation.

The term "aerosol" has been broadly applied to all self-contained pressurized products, some of which deliver foams or semisolid fluids. For inhalation therapy, the particle size of the delivered medication must be carefully controlled, and the average size should be under 10 μm. Other aerosol sprays may contain particles up to several hundred micrometers in diameter.

The basic components of an aerosol system are the container, the propellant, the concentrate containing the active ingredient(s), the valve, and the actuator. The nature of these components determines such characteristics as particle size and uniformity, delivery rate, wetness and temperatures of the spray, and foam density or fluid viscosity. The component that makes an aerosol unique is the propellant.

Fluoroalkanes are generally used as propellants. A specific fluoroalkane, halothane, has been in common use in most hospitals since 1954 as an inhalation anesthetic. Other fluorocarbon propellants include trichlorofluoromethane (CCl_3F), dichlorodifluoromethane (CCl_2F_2), trichlorotrifluoroethane (CCl_2F—$CClF_2$), dichlorotetrafluoroethane ($CClF_2$—$CClF_2$), and chlorodifluoromethane ($CHClF_2$).

Labeling: Medicinal aerosols should contain at least the following warning information on the label as per Federal regulations:

> "*Warning*—Avoid inhaling. Keep away from eyes or other mucous membranes."

The statement "Avoid inhaling" is not necessary for preparations specifically designed for use by inhalation. The phrase "or other mucous membranes" is not necessary for preparations specifically designed for use on mucous membranes.

> "*Warning*—Contents under pressure. Do not puncture or incinerate container. Do not expose to heat or store at temperatures above 120°F. Keep out of reach of children."

In addition to the aforementioned warnings, the label of a drug packaged in an aerosol container in which the propellant consists in whole or in part of a halocarbon or hydrocarbon should bear the following warning (*U.S. Pharmacopeia*, 1975):

> "*Warning*—Do not inhale directly; deliberate inhalation of content can cause death."

or

> "*Warning*—Use only as directed; intentional misuse by deliberately concentrating and inhaling the contents can be harmful or fatal."

CAPSULES

Capsules are either a hard or a soft, soluble container or "shell" of a suitable form of gelatin. Hard gelatin capsule sizes range from No. 5, the smallest, to No. 000, which is the largest, except for the veterinary sizes. Factory-filled hard capsules are often of distinctive color and shape or are otherwise marked to identify them with the manufacturer.

Hard gelatin capsules are made from special blends of bone and pork skin gelatins of relatively high gel strength. The bone gelatin gives a tough, firm film. Pork skin gelatin contributes plasticity and clarity to the blend. Hard gelatin capsules may also contain colorants, opaquing agents such as titanium dioxide, dispersing agents, hardening agents such as sucrose, and preservatives. They normally contain between 10 and 15% of water.

Soft gelatin capsules are somewhat thicker than hard capsules. They are plasticized by the addition of some polyol, such as glycerin or sorbitol. The shell may contain a preservative to prevent growth of fungi.

Soft gelatin capsules are generally filled with nonaqueous but water-miscible vehicles, such as the liquid polyethylene glycols, as carriers for the drug. Soft gelatin capsules may also be filled with powders or granules (*U.S. Pharmacopeia*, 1975).

CREAMS

Creams are semisolid emulsions of either oil-in-water or water-in-oil type. The term "cream" is most frequently applied to soft, cosmetically acceptable types of preparations (*U.S. Pharmacopeia*, 1975).

ELIXIRS

Elixirs are clear, sweetened, hydroalcoholic liquids intended for oral use. They contain flavoring substances with active medicinal agents. Their primary solvents are alcohol and water, with glycerin, sorbitol, and syrup, which is sometimes added (*U.S. Pharmacopeia*, 1975).

EMULSIONS

An emulsion is a two-phase system in which one liquid is dispersed throughout another liquid. The dispersed liquid is known as the internal or discontinuous phase, while the dispersion medium is known as the external or continuous phase.

Emulsions are stabilized by suitable emulsifying agents or by the use of viscous protective colloids. The emulsifying agent may be anionic, cationic, or nonionic in nature. Substances such as gelatin, acacia, soaps, alkyl sulfates, quaternary ammonium compounds, cholesterol, anhydrous lanolin, fatty acid esters of polyglycols and their polyoxyethylene derivatives, methylcellulose, carboxymethylcellulose solium, and many other substances function as dispersion stabilizers.

All emulsions require an antimicrobial agent. Preservatives commonly used in emulsions include methyl-, ethyl-, propyl-, and butylparabens, benzoic acid, quaternary ammonium compounds, and alcohol (*U.S. Pharmacopeia*, 1975).

EXTRACTS

Extracts are concentrated preparations of drugs obtained from plant or animal sources.

In the manufacture of most extracts, the drugs are extracted by percolation and are made in three forms: semiliquids or liquids of syrupy consistency; plastic masses, known as pilular or solid extracts; and dry powders, known as powdered extracts.

Extracts that must be adjusted to prescribed standards of strength need diluents. Among the diluents are liquid glucose, malt extract, and/or glycerin for pilular extracts; and starch, powdered sucrose, lactose, powdered glycyrrhiza, magnesium carbonate, magnesium oxide, calcium phosphate, or the finely powdered marc remaining after the extraction of the drug (*U.S. Pharmacopeia*, 1975).

GELS AND MAGMAS

Gels are semisolid systems consisting of suspensions of either small inorganic particles or large organic molecules. Where the gel mass consists of floccules of small particles, the gell is classified as a two-phase system and is sometimes called a magma.

Single-phase gels consist of organic macromolecules uniformly distributed throughout a liquid in such a manner that no apparent boundaries exist between the dispersed macromolecules and the liquid (*U.S. Pharmacopeia*, 1975).

INHALATIONS

Inhalations are mixtures of drugs or solutions of drugs administered by the nasal or oral respiratory route for local or systemic effect.

Another group of products, also known as inhalants and sometimes called insufflations, consists of finely powdered or liquid drugs that are carried into the respiratory passages by the use of special devices such as aerosols.

Solutions may be nebulized by use of inert gases. Nebulized solutions may be breathed directly from the nebulizer, or the nebulizer may be attached to a plastic face mask, tent, or intermittent positive-pressure breathing (IPPB) machine.

A special class of inhalations termed "inhalants" consists of drugs or combinations of drugs that, by virtue of their high vapor pressure, can be carried by an air current into the nasal passage where they exert their effect. The container from which the inhalant is administered is known as an inhaler (*U.S. Pharmacopeia*, 1975).

INJECTIONS

The administration of drugs to a patient by injection under or through one or more layers of the skin or mucous membrane is defined as the parenteral route.

Injections may be classiffied in five general categories (Avis, 1975):

1. Solutions (ready for injection)
2. Powders (to be dissolved in solvent just prior to injection)
3. Suspensions (ready for injection)
4. Powders (insoluble—to be suspended in vehicle just prior to injection)
5. Emulsions

Distilled water is generally the most common vehicle used for injections. A number of solvents that are miscible with water have been used as a portion of the vehicle to help increase solubility of the drug. These solvents include ethyl alcohol, polyethylene glycol, and propylene glycol.

Other vehicles used in injection preparations are the nonaqueous vehicles, primarily the fixed oils. These include corn oil, cottonseed oil, peanut oil, and sesame oil. Fixed oils are used particularly as vehicles for certain hormone preparations. Other nonaqueous vehicles are ethyl oleate, isopropylmyristate, and benzylbenzoate. The label on the drug preparation must provide information concerning the vehicle.

The *U.S. Pharmacopeia* states that antimicrobial agents in bacteriostatic or fungistatic concentrations must be added to preparations contained in multiple-dose containers. Among the compounds most frequently employed are phenylmercuric nitrate and thimerosal 0.01%, benzethonium chloride and benzalkonium chloride 0.01%, phenol or cresol 0.5%, chlorobutanol 0.5%, methyl *p*-hydroxybenzoate 0.18% and propyl *p*-hydroxybenzoate 0.20%, and benzyalcohol 0.2% (Avis, 1975).

Buffers, such as citrates, acetates, and phosphates, are used primarily to stabilize a solution against chemical degradation that would occur if the pH changed appreciably.

Antioxidants are frequently required to preserve injection preparations because of the ease with which many drugs are oxidized. The most frequently found antioxidant is 0.1% sodium bisulfite (Avis, 1975).

POWDERS

Powders are mixtures of dry, finely divided drugs and/or chemical substances that may be used for internal or external use.

Stability problems encountered in liquid dosage forms are avoided in powdered dosage forms. Drugs that are unstable in aqueous suspensions or solutions may be prepared in the form of powders. These are mixed by the pharmacist by the addition of a specified quantity of water just prior to dispensing. Because these drugs have limited stability, they are required to have a specified expiration date after constitution and may require storage in a refrigerator.

Oral powders may be dispensed in divided powders premeasured by the pharmacist, or in bulk. Bulk oral powders are limited to relatively nonpotent drugs such as laxatives, antacids, dietary supplements, and certain analgesics that the patient may safely measure by the teaspoonful or capful. Other bulky powders include douche powders, tooth powders, and dusting powders.

Dusting powders are impalpable powders intended for topical application. Dusting powders should be passed through at least a 100-mesh sieve to assure freedom from grit that could irritate traumatized areas (*U.S. Pharmacopeia*, 1975).

SOLUTIONS

Solutions are liquid mixtures that contain one or more soluble chemical substances usually dissolved in water. They are distinguished from injections by the fact that they are not intended for administration by infusion or injection. The solute is usually nonvolatile.

Sterile solutions used as irrigation fluids meet the requirements for injections except those relating to packaging. Their containers may be designed to empty rapidly and could exceed the 1-liter limit imposed on containers for injections (*U.S. Pharmacopeia*, 1975).

SPIRITS

Spirits are alcoholic solutions of volatile substances. Some spirits serve as flavoring agents while other have medicinal value. Spirits require storage in tight, light-resistant containers to prevent loss by evaporation and to limit oxidative changes (*U.S. Pharmacopeia*, 1975).

SUPPOSITORIES

Suppositories are produced in various weights and shapes, adapted for introduction into the rectal, vaginal, or urethral orifice of the human body. They melt, soften, or dissolve at body temperature. A suppository may act as a physical barrier or palliative to the local tissues at the point of introduction or as a carrier of therapeutic agents for systemic or local action. Suppository bases usually employed are cocoa butter, glycerinated gelatin, hydrogenated vegetable oils, mixtures of polyethylene glycols of various molecular weights, and fatty acid esters of polyethylene glycol (*U.S. Pharmacopeia*, 1975).

SUSPENSIONS

Suspensions are preparations of finely divided, undissolved substances dispersed in liquid vehicles. Powders for suspension are preparations of finely powdered drugs intended for suspension in liquid vehicles.

Milks are suspensions of insoluble drugs in a water medium and are distinguished from gels mainly in that the suspended particles are larger.

Some suspensions are sterile and are intended for injection. Suspensions are never injected intravenously or intrathecally.

By its very nature, the particulate matter of a suspension tends to settle slowly from the liquid vehicle in which it is dispersed. Thus, it is important that suspensions be shaken well before each use to ensure a uniform distribution of solid in the vehicle and, thereby, uniform and proper dosage (*U.S. Pharmacopeia*, 1975).

SYRUPS

Syrups are sweetened aqueous liquid preparations containing medicinal or flavoring substances. In addition to sucrose, certain other polyols, such as glycerin or sorbitol, are sometimes used to prevent crystallization of sucrose or to increase the solubility of added ingredients. Syrups may also contain alcohol as a preservative or as a solvent for the flavors, as well as antimicrobial agents to prevent bacterial, yeast, and mold growth.

TABLETS

Tablets are solid dosage forms containing medicinal substances with or without suitable diluents or filler material. The classification of tablets is based on the method of manufacture and is expressed as either molded or compressed tablets.

Molded tablets are prepared by forcing a dampened mixture of the medicinal substance and its diluent (either lactose or sucrose) into die cavities under low pressure. Alcohol is used to dampen the powder. After the mixture is extruded from the mold, it is allowed to dry.

Compressed tablets are prepared by placing a mixture of medicinal substance, diluent, binder, disintegrating agent, and lubricant into a die and compressing the mixture under high pressure. Sometimes included with this mixture are dyes or lakes (dyes absorbed onto aluminum hydroxide), flavor, and/or sweetening agents.

The diluent of filler substance may be lactose, starch, dibasic calcium phosphate, or calcium sulfate. The diluent for chewable tablets may be sucrose, mannitol, or sorbitol.

The binders used in tablet preparation are acacia, gelatin, sucrose, povidone, methylcellulose, carboxymethylcellulose, or hydrolyzed starch pastes. When a dry binding process is used for tablet preparation, microcrystalline cellulose is employed as the binding agent.

Disintegrating agents used in tablet mixtures are chemically modified starches, algenic acid, microcrystalline cellulose, and colloidal silicates. These agents assist in the fragmentation of the tablet after administration.

Lubricants, such as metallic stearates, stearic acid, hydrogenated vegetable oils, and talc, are used to enhance the manufacturing process (*U.S. Pharmacopeia*, 1975).

TINCTURES

Tinctures are medicinal preparations utilizing ethyl alcohol as a solvent (*U.S. Pharmacopeia*, 1975).

3
Classification of Scheduled Substances

The Comprehensive Drug Abuse Prevention and Control Act of 1970 consolidated the provisions of the previous laws into one act. The Act classifies controlled substances in one of five possible categories. The classification is based on the drug's potential for abuse as well as its physiological and psychological effects. The penalties imposed for the various offenses involving these controlled substances are dictated by the schedule under which it is listed.

Drugs that have a potential for abuse are classified according to criteria promulgated by the Act. The Act provides that the Attorney General shall consider the following factors with respect to each drug or substance proposed to be controlled or removed from the schedules:

1. Its actual or relative potential for abuse
2. Scientific evidence of its pharmacological effect if known
3. The state of current scientific knowledge regarding the drug or other substance
4. Its history and current pattern of abuse
5. The scope, duration, and significance of abuse
6. What risk, if any, there is to the public health
7. Its psychic or physiological dependence liability
8. Whether the substance is an immediate precursor of a substance already controlled

SCHEDULES

The criteria set forth above are used as determinative factors in placing a controlled substance within any of the five schedules.

Schedule I

For a drug to be placed in this schedule, the findings must indicate that:

a. The drug or other substance has a high potential for abuse.
b. The drug or other substance has no currently accepted medical use in treatment in the United States.
c. There is a lack of accepted safety for use of the drug or other substance under medical supervision.

The Federal government has defined marijuana as a hallucinogenic substance. This definition may be compared to the definitions used by those states that still define marijuana as a narcotic drug.

Schedule II

For a drug to be placed in this schedule, the findings must indicate that:

a. The drug or other substance has a high potential for abuse.
b. The drug or other substance has a currently accepted medical use in treatment in the United States or a currently accepted medical use with severe restrictions.
c. Abuse of the drug or other substance may lead to severe psychological or physical dependence.

Schedule III

For a drug to be placed in this schedule, the findings must indicate that:

a. The drug or other substance has a potential for abuse less than that of the drugs or other substances in Schedules I and II.
b. The drug or other substance has a currently accepted medical use in treatment in the United States.
c. Abuse of the drug or other substance may lead to moderate or low physical dependence or high psychological dependence.

Schedule IV

To be placed in this schedule, the findings must indicate that:

a. The drug or other substance has a low potential for abuse relative to the drugs or other substances in Schedule III.
b. The drug or other substance has a currently accepted medical use in treatment in the United States.

c. Abuse of the drug or other substance may lead to limited physical dependence or psychological dependence relative to the drugs or other substances in Schedule III.

Schedule V

For a drug to be placed in this schedule, the findings must indicate that:

a. The drug or other substance has a low potential for abuse relative to the drugs or other substances in Schedule IV.
b. The drug or other substance has a currently accepted medical use in treatment in the United States.
c. Abuse of the drug or other substance may lead to limited physical dependence relative to the drugs or other substances in Schedule IV.

The drugs and substances included within this schedule are compounds, mixtures, and preparations containing limited quantities of narcotic drugs and include one or more nonnarcotic active medicinal ingredients so that the mixture or preparation acquires medicinal qualities that are not possessed by the narcotic drug alone.

Regulations Governing Dispensing of Scheduled Substances

Schedule II

No controlled substance in this schedule may be dispensed without the written prescription of a practitioner, except when dispensed directly to an ultimate user by a practitioner other than a pharmacy. However, in emergency situations, drugs in this schedule may be dispensed on oral prescription of a practitioner. This prescription must be reduced promptly to writing by the pharmacy and filed. No prescription for a Schedule II narcotic drug shall be filled after the second day the prescription was issued. No prescription for a drug from this schedule may be refilled.

A controlled substance in this schedule shall be distributed by a registrant to another registrant only pursuant to an order form as set forth by the Federal law.

Schedule III

Except when dispensed directly to an ultimate user by a practitioner, other than a pharmacy, a substance controlled by Schedule III shall not be dispensed without a written or oral prescription of a practitioner. The prescription shall not be filled or refilled more than six months after the date issued. It cannot be refilled more than five times, unless renewed by the practitioner.

A controlled substance in this schedule shall be distributed by a registrant to another registrant only pursuant to an order form as set forth by the Federal law.

Schedule IV

Except when dispensed directly to an ultimate user by a practitioner, other than a pharmacy, a substance controlled by Schedule IV shall not be dispensed without a written or oral prescription of a practitioner. The prescription shall not be filled or refilled more than six months after the date issued. It cannot be refilled more than five times, unless renewed by the practitioner.

A controlled substance in this schedule shall be distributed by a registrant to another registrant only pursuant to an order form as set forth by the Federal law.

FRAUDULENT OFFENSES

Fraudulent offenses are classified as follows:

1. To distribute as a registrant a controlled substance classified in Schedule I or II, except by a registrant to another registrant only pursuant to an order form. The order forms are in compliance with Federal regulations.
2. To use in the course of the manufacture or distribution of a controlled substance a registration number that is fictitious, revoked, suspended, or issued to another person.
3. To acquire or obtain possession of a controlled substance by misrepresentation, fraud, forgery, deception, or subterfuge.
4. To furnish false or fraudulent material information in, or omit any material information from, any application, report, or other document required to be kept or filed by or under the Controlled Substances Act.
5. To make, distribute, or possess any punch, die, plate, stone, or other thing designed to print or imprint any likeness of any of the foregoing on any controlled substance, container, or label thereof so as to render the controlled substance a counterfeit substance.

COMMERCIAL OFFENSES

Commercial offenses are classified as follows:

1. A practitioner knowingly or intentionally distributes or dispenses a controlled substance without proper prescription.
2. A registrant knowingly or intentionally manufactures a controlled substance not authorized by his registration or distributes or dispenses a controlled substance not authorized by his registration to another registrant or other person.
3. To refuse or fail to make, keep, or furnish any record, notification, order form, statement, invoice, or information required under the Controlled Substances Act.
4. To refuse an entry into any premises for any inspection authorized by the Controlled Substances Act.

PRESCRIPTION OF NONSCHEDULED DRUGS

The Federal Drug and Cosmetic Act lists the following criteria for classification as a prescription drug:

1. Any drug in a list of named habit-forming drugs.
2. Any drug that because of its toxicity or other potential for harmful effects, or the method of its use, or the adjunctive measures necessary to its use, is not safe for use except under the supervision of a practitioner licensed by law to administer such a drug.
3. Any substance so named as a prescription drug under the new drug provision of the Act as being a component of an approved new drug application.

The third criterion is basically the classification of substances as legend drugs. Significantly, legend drugs are to be dispensed only on a written prescription written by a practitioner licensed by law to administer such drugs. The law achieves identification of prescription drugs by requiring that the statement "Caution: Federal law prohibits dispensing without prescription" appear on all drugs classified as legend drugs. In addition, if the statement "Caution: Federal law restricts this drug to use by or on the order of a licensed veterinarian, or on his prescription order," then the drug is a veterinary prescription drug and classified as a legend drug.

4

Regulation of Controlled Substances

REQUIREMENTS FOR REGISTRATION

Persons Required to Register (301.21)

Every person who manufactures, distributes, or dispenses any controlled substance or who proposes to engage in such activities shall obtain annually a registration unless exempted by law. Only persons actually engaged in such activities are required to obtain a registration; related or affiliated persons who are not engaged in such activities are not required to be registered.

Separate Registration for Independent Activities (301.22)

The following groups of activities are deemed to be independent of each other:

1. Manufacturing controlled substances.
2. Distributing controlled substances.
3. Dispensing controlled substances listed in Schedules II through V.
4. Conducting research [other than research described in subparagraph (6) of this paragraph] with controlled substances listed in Schedules II through V.
5. Conducting instructional activities with controlled substances listed in Schedules II through V.
6. Conducting clinical research with narcotic drugs listed in Schedules II through V for the purpose of continuing dependence on such drugs

of an addicted person. The sole purpose for such research is in the development of a narcotic addict rehabilitation program. The guidelines are set forth in the "Notice of Claimed Investigational Exemption for a New Drug" approved by the Food and Drug Administration (FDA).

7. Conducting research and instructional activities with controlled substances listed in Schedule I.
8. Conducting chemical analysis with controlled substances listed in any schedule.
9. Importing controlled substances.
10. Exporting controlled substances listed in Schedules I through IV.

Every person who engages in more than one group of independent activities shall obtain a separate registration for each group of activities, except as provided in this paragraph. Any person, when registered to engage in the group of activities, shall be authorized to engage in the coincident activities without obtaining a registration provided that he complies with all requirements and duties prescribed by law for persons registered to engage in such coincident activities.

A person registered to dispense controlled substances listed in Schedules II through V shall be authorized to conduct research [other than research described in subparagraph (6)] and to conduct instructional activities with those substances.

A single registration to engage in any group of independent activities may include one or more controlled substances listed in the schedules authorized in that group of independent activities. A person registered to conduct research with controlled substances listed in Schedule I may do so provided he has filed and had approved a research protocol.

Separate Registrations for Separate Locations (301.23)

A separate registration is required for each principal place of business or professional practice at one general physical location where controlled substances are manufactured, distributed, or dispensed.

Controlled substances are not allowed to be manufactured, distributed, or dispensed in the following locations:

1. A warehouse where controlled substances are stored by, or on behalf of, a registered person. However, it is allowed if the substances are distributed directly from the warehouse to the registered location providing the registered location is different from the location from

which the substances were delivered. It is also allowed if the delivery is to persons not required to register.

2. An office used by agents of a registrant where sales of controlled substances are solicited, made, or supervised, but which neither contains such substances nor serves as a distribution point for filling sales orders.

3. An office used by a practitioner (who is registered at another location) where controlled substances are maintained.

Exemption of Agents and Employees; Affiliated Practitioners (301.24)

The requirement of registration is waived for any agent or employee of a person who is registered to engage in any group of independent activities, providing he is acting in the usual course of his business or employment.

An individual practitioner who is an agent or employee of another practitioner registered to dispense controlled substances may administer and dispense controlled substances provided the individual practitioner is authorized to do so by the jurisdiction in which he practices. However, this individual practitioner may not issue a prescription. Individual practitioners exempt from this section are interns, residents, foreign-trained physicians, physicians on the staff of a Veterans Administration facility, and physicians who are agents or employees of the Health Bureau of the Canal Zone Government. An example of such an individual practitioner would be a pharmacist employed by a pharmacy. He would not need to be registered individually to fill a prescription for controlled substances if the pharmacy is properly registered.

An individual practitioner who is an intern, resident, or foreign-trained physician or physician on the staff of a Veterans Administration facility or physician who is an agent or employee of the Health Bureau of the Canal Zone Government may dispense, administer, and prescribe controlled substances under the registration of the hospital or other institution that is registered and by whom he is employed in lieu of being registered himself, provided that:

1. Such dispensing, administering, or prescribing is done in the usual course of his professional practice.

2. Such individual practitioner is authorized or permitted to do so by the jurisdiction in which he is practicing.

3. The hospital or other institution by whom he is employed has verified that the individual practitioner is so permitted to dispense, administer, or prescribe drugs within the jurisdiction.

4. Such individual practitioner is acting only within the scope of his employment in the hospital or institution.
5. The hospital or other institution authorizes the intern, resident, or foreign-trained physician to dispense or prescribe under the hospital registration and designates a specific internal code number for each practitioner. The code number shall consist of numbers, letters, or a combination thereof and shall be a suffix to the institution's Drug Enforcement Administration (DEA) registration number, preceded by a hyphen.
6. A current list of internal codes and the corresponding individual practitioners is kept by the hospital or other institution and is made available at all times to other registrants and law enforcement agencies on request for the purpose of verifying the authority of the prescribing individual practitioner.

Exemption of Certain Military and Other Personnel (301.25)

The requirement of registration is waived for any official of the United States Army, Navy, Marine Corps, Air Force, Coast Guard, Public Health Service, or Bureau of Prisons who is authorized to prescribe, dispense, or administer, but not to procure or purchase, controlled substances in the course of his official duties. Such officials must follow the general prescription procedures, but, in addition, must state the branch of service or agency (e.g., United States Army, Public Health Service) along with the service identification number of the issuing official in lieu of the registration number required on prescription forms. The service identification number for a Public Health Service employee is his Social Security Number.

If any official exempted by any of the authorizations stated above also engages as a private individual in any activity or group of activities for which registration is required, such official shall obtain a registration for such private activities.

APPLICATIONS FOR REGISTRATION

Time for Application (301.31)

Any person who is required to be registered and who is not may apply for registration at any time. No person required to be registered shall engage in any activity for which registration is required until the application is granted and a Certificate of Registration has been issued by the Director.

Any registered person may apply to be reregistered not more than 60 days before the expiration date of his registration.

At the time any person is first registered, he shall be assigned to one of twelve groups, which shall correspond to the months of the year. The expiration date of the registrations of all persons within any group will be the last day of the month designated for that group. In assigning any person to a group, the DEA may select a group that has an expiration date less than one year from the date such person was registered. If the person is assigned to a group that has an expiration date less than three months from the date on which the person is registered, the registration shall not expire until one year from that expiration date; in all other cases, the registration shall expire on the expiration date first following the date on which the person is registered.

APPLICATION FORMS

Any practitioner, pharmacy, hospital, clinic, or training institution applying for a new registration to dispense controlled substances listed in Schedules II through V must apply on DEA Form 224 (see sample form). For reregistration, however, the application must be made on DEA Form 226.

Any researcher, analytical laboratory, manufacturer, importer, exporter, or distributor applying for a new registration to work with controlled substances listed in Schedules II through V must apply on DEA Form 225 (see sample form). For reregistration, however, the application must be made on DEA Form 227.

Each application must include all information called for in the form. If an item is not applicable to the particular application, it must be indicated in the appropriate place. Each application, attachment, or other document filed as part of an application must be signed by the applicant. If the applicant is an individual, the application must bear the individual's signature. If the applicant is a partnership, all persons in that partnership must sign the application. An officer of a corporation, corporate division, association, trust, or other entity that is an applicant must sign the application form. An applicant may authorize one or more individuals, who would not otherwise be authorized to do so, to sign the application for the applicant. This may be accomplished by filing a power of attorney for each individual with the Registration Branch of the Drug Enforcement Administration. This power of attorney must be signed by both the person authorized to sign applications and the individual being authorized. The power of attorney will be valid until revoked by the applicant.

Applications submitted for filing are dated on receipt. If found to be complete, the application will be accepted. Applications failing to comply with the requirements of this part will not generally be accepted for filing. In the case of minor defects as to completeness, the application may be accepted for filing with a request to the applicant for additional information. A defective application will be returned to the applicant within ten days following its receipt with a statement of the reason for not accepting the application for filing. A defective application may be corrected and resubmitted for filing at any time.

Acceptance of an application for filing does not preclude any subsequent request for additional information and has no bearing on whether the application will be granted.

It may be required for an applicant to submit documents or written statements of fact relevant to the application to determine whether the application should be granted. The failure of the applicant to provide documents or statements within a reasonable time after being requested to do so shall be deemed to be a waiver by the applicant of any opportunity to present such documents or facts for consideration in granting or denying the application.

An application may be amended or withdrawn without permission of the Director at any time before the date on which the applicant receives an order to show cause, or before the date on which a notice of hearing on the application is published. An application may be amended or withdrawn with permission at any time where good cause is shown by the applicant or where the amendment or withdrawal is in the public interest.

After an application has been accepted for filing, the request by the applicant that it be returned or the failure of the applicant to respond to official correspondence regarding the application, when sent by registered or certified mail, return receipt requested, shall be deemed to be a withdrawal of the application.

If, at the time of application for registration of a new pharmacy, the pharmacy has been issued a license from the appropriate state licensing agency, the applicant may include with his application an affidavit as to the existence of the state license.

MODIFICATION, TRANSFER, AND TERMINATION OF REGISTRATION

Any registrant may apply to modify his registration to authorize the handling of additional controlled substances or to change his name or address by submitting a letter of request to the Registration Branch of the DEA. The letter must contain the registrant's name, address, and registration number as printed on the certificate of registration, and the substances and/or schedules to be added to his registration. If the modification is a change of name or address, this information must be included. The letter must be signed by the

(Mar. 197B) — 224   OMB No. 43-RO581   APPLICANT NAME (Last, First, Middle; if an Individual, OR name of Pharmacy, Hospital/Clinic, Teaching Institution)   RETAIN Copy 3. Mail Orig. and 1 copy with FEE to.

NEW
APPLICATION FOR REGISTRATION
UNDER
CONTROLLED SUBSTANCES ACT OF 1970

Please PRINT or TYPE all entries.

UNITED STATES DEPARTMENT OF JUSTICE
DRUG ENFORCEMENT ADMINISTRATION
P.O. Box 28083
CENTRAL STATION
WASHINGTON, D.C. 20005
For INFORMATION, Call: 202 724-1013
See "Privacy Act" Information on reverse

No registration may be issued unless a completed application form has been received (1301.21 CFR 21).

CITY   STATE   ZIP CODE

THIS BLOCK FOR DEA USE ONLY

REGISTRATION CLASSIFICATION: Submit Check or Money Order Payable to the **DRUG ENFORCEMENT ADMINISTRATION** in Amount of $5.00. *DO NOT send CASH or STAMPS.*

FEE MUST ACCOMPANY APPLICATION

1. BUSINESS ACTIVITY: *(Check ☑ ONE only. Read NOTE before completing.)*
A ☐ RETAIL PHARMACY   B ☐ HOSPITAL/CLINIC   C ☐ PRACTITIONER   D ☐ TEACHING INSTITUTION *(Instructional purposes only)*   *Specify DEGREE*

2. DRUG SCHEDULES: *(Check ☑ all applicable schedules in which you intend to handle controlled substances.)*

SCHEDULE II		SCHEDULE III		SCHEDULE IV	SCHEDULE V
1 ☐ NARCOTIC	2 ☐ NONNARCOTIC	3 ☐ NARCOTIC	4 ☐ NONNARCOTIC	5 ☐	6 ☐

3. ☐ **(E)** CHECK THIS BLOCK IF INDIVIDUAL NAMED HEREON IS A FEDERAL, STATE, OR LOCAL OFFICIAL. IF CHECKED, also complete Item 6. ⬆

4. ☐ **(Y)** CHECK HERE IF YOU REQUIRE ORDER FORMS.

5. ALL APPLICANTS MUST ANSWER THE FOLLOWING:

(a) Are you currently authorized to prescribe, distribute, dispense, conduct research, or otherwise handle the controlled substances in the schedules for which you are applying, under the laws of the state or jurisdiction in which you are operating or propose to operate ?   ☐ YES ☐ NO

Current State License Number for the State in which you are applying for Registration _____

(b) Has the applicant been convicted of a felony in connection with controlled substances under state or federal law ?   ☐ YES ☐ NO

(c) Has the applicant ever surrendered a previous CSA registration or had a CSA registration revoked, suspended, or denied ?   ☐ YES ☐ NO

(d) If the applicant is a corporation, association, or partnership; has any officer, partner or stockholder been convicted of a felony in connection with controlled substances under state or federal law ?   ☐ YES ☐ NO

(e) If the applicant is corporation, association, or partnership, has any officer, partner, or stockholder surrendered a previous CSA registration or had a CSA registration revoked, suspended or denied ?   ☐ YES ☐ NO

IF ANSWER TO QUESTIONS (b), (c), (d), or (e) is YES, attach a letter setting forth the circumstances.

SIGN HERE ▶

_____   _____ Date
Signature of applicant or authorized individual

Title (If the applicant is a corporation, institution, or other entity; enter the TITLE of the person signing on behalf of the applicant (I.E.: President, Dean, Procurement Officer, etc....))

_____
Applicants Business Phone Number (Optional)

6. CERTIFICATION OF EXEMPT OFFICIAL *(Complete only if Item 3 is checked)*

ONLY OFFICERS, EMPLOYEES AND AGENCIES OF FEDERAL, STATE, OR LOCAL GOVERNMENTS ARE EXEMPT FROM PAYMENT OF REGISTRATION FEES.

(a) Name of governmental unit by whom applicant is employed or of which agency is a part. *(e.g., U.S. Public Health Service, Iowa Department of Mental Health, Ohio State University, King's County Hospital, Dallas City Clinic, etc...)*

(b) Is the official whose signature appears in Item 5 authorized to obtain from official stock, dispense, administer, conduct research, instructional activities or chemical analyses with controlled substances ?   ☐ YES ☐ NO

(c) Is he authorized to purchase controlled substances ?   ☐ YES ☐ NO

_____   _____ Date
Signature of applicant's certifying superior

_____
Official Title of applicant's certifying superior

WARNING: SECTION 843 (a) (4) OF TITLE 21, UNITED STATES CODE, STATES THAT ANY PERSON WHO KNOWINGLY OR INTENTIONALLY FURNISHES FALSE OR FRAUDULENT INFORMATION IN THIS APPLICATION IS SUBJECT TO IMPRISONMENT FOR NOT MORE THAN FOUR YEARS, A FINE OF NOT MORE THAN $30,000.00 OR BOTH.

NOTE: Registration as a teaching institution authorizes purchase and possession of controlled substances for instructional purposes only. Practitioners, teaching institutions or individuals within teaching institutions desiring to conduct research with any Schedule I substance, must obtain a "Researcher" registration by submitting form DEA - 225 with applicable fee.

MAIL the Original and 1 copy with FEE to the above address. Retain 3rd copy for your records.

● *ATTACH CHECK HERE*

PRIVACY ACT INFORMATION

AUTHORITY: Section 302 and 303 of the Controlled Substances Act of 1970 (PL 91-513)

PURPOSE: To obtain information required to register applicants pursuant to the Controlled Substances Act of 1970 (PL 91-513)

ROUTINE USES: The Controlled Substances Act Registration Records produces special reports as required for statistical analytical purposes. Disclosures of information from this system are made to the following categories of users for the purposes stated:

A. Other Federal law enforcement and regulatory agencies for law enforcement and regulatory purposes

B. State and local law enforcement and regulatory agencies for law enforcement and regulatory purposes

C. Persons registered under the Controlled Substances Act (Public Law 91-513) for the purpose of verifying the registration of customers and practitioners

EFFECT: Failure to complete form will preclude processing of the application.

Form DEA   225   OMB No. 43-R0579

NEW
APPLICATION FOR REGISTRATION
UNDER
CONTROLLED SUBSTANCES ACT OF 1970

(Oct. 1976)

RETAIN Copy 3. Mail Orig. and 1 copy with FEE to

UNITED STATES DEPARTMENT OF JUSTICE
DRUG ENFORCEMENT ADMINISTRATION
P.O. Box 28083
CENTRAL STATION
WASHINGTON, D.C. 20005

For INFORMATION, Call: 202 382-4876

See "Privacy Act" Information on Reverse

THIS BLOCK FOR DEA USE ONLY

ARCOS PARTICIPANT   ☐ Yes ☐ No

READ AND COMPLETE ALL APPLICABLE ITEMS
Print or Type ALL ENTRIES

No registration may be issued unless a completed
application form has been received (1301.21 CFR 21)

BUSINESS NAME *(Last name, First name, Middle initial, if an individual)*

BUSINESS ADDRESS *(Do not use P.O. Box)*

CITY   STATE   ZIP CODE

REGISTRATION CLASSIFICATION: Submit Check or Money Order Payable to: **THE DRUG ENFORCEMENT ADMINISTRATION** in Amount specified for Activity checked below. NO cash or stamps.

1. BUSINESS ACTIVITY: *(Check* ☑ *one only; see NOTES A and B before checking)*

G ☐ RESEARCHER - *Fee $5.00*
H ☐ ANALYTICAL LAB - *Fee $5.00*

E ☐ MANUFACTURER - *Fee $50.00*   F ☐ DISTRIBUTOR - *Fee $25.00*
J ☐ IMPORTER - *Fee $25.00*   K ☐ EXPORTER - *Fee $25.00*

2. DRUG SCHEDULES *(Check* ☑ *all applicable schedules in which you intend to handle controlled substances). Complete Item 9 if applicable.*

1 ☐ SCHEDULE I
2 ☐ SCHEDULE II
3 ☐ SCHEDULE III NARCOTIC
4 ☐ SCHEDULE III NONNARCOTIC
5 ☐ SCHEDULE IV
6 ☐ SCHEDULE V

3. ☐ (E) Check this block if applicant is exempt from payment of Registration Fee. *(If checked, applicant's superior must complete Item 8.)*

4. ☐ (Y) Check here if you require Order Forms.

5. Supply any other current DEA Registration Numbers for any class of business activity at the address shown on this application.

6. **MANUFACTURERS ONLY**
(Item 1E, Business Activity):

Check Schedules & Category applicable in the boxes to the right. *(Definitions on reverse)*

MANUFACTURER CATEGORIES	SCHEDULES				
	I	II	III	III-Non IV	V
A ☐ Bulk, Synthesizer-Extractor					
B ☐ Dosage Form					
C ☐ Repacker-Relabeler					
D ☐ Non-Human Consumption					

7. **ALL APPLICANTS MUST ANSWER THE FOLLOWING:**

(a) Are you currently authorized to manufacture, distribute, dispense, prescribe, conduct research, instructional activities, or chemical analyses with, or otherwise handle the controlled substances in the schedules for which you are applying, under the laws of the state or jurisdiction in which you are operating or propose to operate?   ☐ YES ☐ NO

(b) Has the applicant been convicted of a felony in connection with controlled substances under state or federal law?   ☐ YES ☐ NO

(c) If the applicant is a corporation, association, or partnership, has any officer, partner, or stock-holder been convicted of a felony in connection with controlled substances under state or federal law?   ☐ YES ☐ NO

(d) Has the applicant ever surrendered a previous CSA registration or had a CSA registration revoked, suspended, or denied?   ☐ YES ☐ NO

(e) If the applicant is a corporation, association, or partnership, has an officer, partner, or stock-holder surrendered a previous CSA registration or had a CSA registration revoked, suspended, or denied?   ☐ YES ☐ NO

IF ANSWER TO QUESTIONS (b), (c), (d), or (e) is YES, attach a letter setting forth the circumstances.

● ATTACH CHECK HERE

Applicant's Business Phone Number
(Optional)

SIGN HERE ►

Print or Type Name Here - Sign below

(Signature of applicant or authorized individual)   *(Date)*

Title *(If the applicant is a corporation, institution, or other entity, enter the TITLE of the person signing on behalf of the applicant, e.g., President, Dean, Procurement Officer, etc...)*

8. **CERTIFICATION OF EXEMPTION** *(Complete only if Item 3 is checked)*
ONLY Officers, Employees and Agencies of Federal, State or Local Governments are EXEMPT from Payment of Registration Fees.

(a) Name of governmental unit by whom applicant is employed or of which agency is a part. *(e.g., U.S. Public Health Service, Iowa Department of Mental Health, Ohio State University, King's County Hospital, Dallas City Health Clinic, etc....)*

(b) Is the person whose signature appears in Item 7 authorized to manufacture, distribute, dispense, prescribe, conduct research, instructional activities or chemical analyses with, or otherwise handle, controlled substances?   ☐ YES ☐ NO

(c) Is he authorized to purchase controlled substances?   ☐ YES ☐ NO

Signature of applicant's certifying superior   Date

Official Title of applicant's certifying superior

9. ALL REGISTRANTS with the exception of analytical laboratories must enter in a block below the CODE of the Schedule I substance for which authorization is requested. CODES for Schedules II substances must be entered by all registrants except distributors and analytical laboratories. All manufacturers are required to list any Schedule III and requested to list Schedule IV and V substances which they are currently manufacturing. *(See Code List on information sheet.)* In addition to codes furnished, manufacturer (synthesizer/extractor) applicants MUST furnish a list of those "Basic Classes" of controlled substances in Schedules I and II which they propose to "Manufacture in Bulk". *(For definition of "Basic Class," refer to 21 CFR 1301.02.)*

IF ADDITIONAL SPACE IS REQUIRED, USE SEPARATE SHEET AND RETURN WITH APPLICATION.

WARNING: Section 843 (A) (4), Title 21, United States Code, states that any person who knowingly or intentionally furnishes false or fraudulent information in this application is subject to imprisonment for not more than four years, a fine of not more than $30,000.00, or both.

NOTE A.   Registration as a Manufacturer or Importer conveys distribution privileges only as to those substances manufactured or imported.

NOTE B.   Applicants desiring to conduct research with Schedule I substances must submit 3 copies of a Research Protocol with this application. In the case of a clinical investigation, the applicant must submit 3 copies of a Notice of Claimed Investigational Exemption for a New Drug (IND) to F.D.A. and 3 copies of a certificate of the application of an IND attached to this application. Applicants desiring to conduct research with Schedules II - V substances must submit a separate DEA-225 application.

Retain copy 3 for your records. Mail Orig. and 1 copy with FEE to above address.

DEFINITIONS

1. <u>Bulk, Synthesizer - Extractor</u>: The term bulk manufacture means the production, preparation, propagation, compounding or processing of a drug or other substance, either directly or indirectly or by extraction from substances of natural origin, or independently by means of chemical synthesis or by combination of extraction and chemical synthesis, when the final product is to be used for further manufacture (into dosage forms) or a substance to be used for industrial purposes or for repackaging into non-dosage form units for patient or other uses.

2. <u>Dosage Form Manufacture</u>: Means the production, preparation, compounding or processing of a bulk substance into a form which is to be used without additional production, preparation, compounding or processing by an ultimate user; except that such term does not include the packaging, repackaging, labeling, or relabeling of a drug or other substance, in conformity with applicable State or local law, by a practitioner as an incident to his administration or dispensing of a drug or substance in the course of his professional practice.

3. The term Repackager - Relabeler: Means the packaging or repackaging of a drug or other substance or the labeling or relabeling of its container; except that such term does not include the packaging, repackaging, labeling or relabeling of a drug or other substance, in conformity with applicable State or local law, by a practitioner as an incident to his administration or dispensing of a drug or substance in the course of his professional practice

4. <u>Non-Human Consumption</u>: Means the production, preparation, propogation, compounding or processing of a drug or other substance whether directly or indirectly or by extraction of substances of natural origin or independently by means of chemical synthesis or by a combination of extraction and chemical synthesis, where the final product is not to be used for prevention, treatment or mitigation of diseases, but is to be used for scientific investigation, laboratory analysis, or other non-patient usage.

    A. Industrial Manufacture: Means the use of Controlled Substances in the manufacture of non-drug, non-controlled finished product.

    B. The tagging of a drug or other substance with radioactive material.

PRIVACY ACT INFORMATION

AUTHORITY: Section 302 and 303 of the Controlled Substances Act of 1970 (PL 91-513)

PURPOSE: To obtain information required to register applicants pursuant to the Controlled Substances Act of 1970 (PL 91-513)

ROUTINE USES: The Controlled Substances Act Registration Records produces special reports as required for statistical analytical purposes. Disclosures of information from this system are made to the following categories of users for the purposes stated:

    A. Other Federal law enforcement and regulatory purposes

    B. State and local law enforcement and regulatory agencies for law enforcement and regulatory purposes

    C. Persons registered under the Controlled Substances Act (Public Law 91-513) for the purpose of verifying the registration of customers and practitioners

EFFECT: Failure to complete form will preclude processing of the application.

authorized person initially designated in the original application. If the registrant is seeking to handle additional controlled substances listed in Schedule I for the purpose of research or instructional activities, he must attach three copies of a research protocol describing each research project involving the additional substances, or two copies of a statement describing the nature, extent, and duration of such instructional activities, as appropriate. No fee is required for the modification. The request for modification is handled in the same manner as an application for registration. If the modification in registration is approved, a new certificate will be issued to the registrant. This certificate must be maintained with the old certificate of registration until expiration.

The registration of any person shall terminate if and when such person dies, ceases legal existence, or discontinues business or professional practice. Any registrant who ceases legal existence or discontinues business or professional practice must notify the DEA promptly of such fact.

No registration may be transferred except on specifically designated conditions set forth by written consent of the DEA.

SECURITY REQUIREMENTS

All applicants and registrants must provide effective controls and procedures to guard against theft and diversion of controlled substances. The Controlled Substances Act sets forth security requirements in paragraphs 301.72–301.76 as standards for the physical security controls and operating procedures necessary to prevent diversion.

Substances classified under Schedules I and II must be stored, depending on quantity, in either a secure safe or vault.

A safe is used when small quantities permit. The safe must have an Underwriters' Laboratories Burglary Rating of T-20, E or better, or equivalent. If the safe weighs less than 750 pounds, it must be bolted or cemented to the floor or wall in such a way that it cannot be readily removed. In some cases, it may be necessary to equip the safe with an alarm system that, on unauthorized entry, will transmit a signal directly to an approved control station such as a local police department.

If a vault is used, and was constructed on or before September 1, 1971, it must be substantially constructed with a steel door, combination or key lock, and an alarm system. For a vault constructed after September 1, 1971, the specifications are more detailed.

The walls, floors, and ceilings of the vault must be constructed with at least 8 inches of reinforced concrete or other substantial masonry. The vertical and horizontal reinforcements must be with $\frac{1}{2}$-inch steel rods tied 6 inches on center, or the structural equivalent to such reinforced walls, floors, and ceilings. The door of the vault should contain a multiple-position combination lock or the equivalent, a relocking device or the equivalent, and a steel plate with a thickness of at least $\frac{1}{2}$ inch. If operations require the vault to remain open for frequent access, it should be equipped with a "day-gate" that is self-closing and self-locking, or the equivalent. The walls or perimeter of the vault should be equipped with an alarm that, on unauthorized entry, will transmit a signal directly to an approved control station such as a local police department. The door of the vault should be equipped with contact switches. In addition, it should have complete electrical lacing of the walls, floor, and ceiling, sensitive ultrasonic equipment within the vault, a sensitive sound accumulator system, or some other alarm device that has met the approval of the DEA.

Substances classified under Schedules III, IV, and V may be stored in a safe or vault as described for security requirements for Schedule I and II drugs. However, if drugs that are listed under Schedule I or II are not to be stored, the security requirements may be lessened. Under the latter condition, the drugs may be stored in a building or area located within a building that has walls or perimeter fences sufficiently high and constructed in such a manner as to provide security from burglary. The doors of such an area must be locked during nonworking hours by a multiple-position combination lock or a key lock. This storage area must be equipped with an alarm that, on unauthorized entry, will transmit a signal directly to a central station providing security such as a local police department.

In this area, all controlled substances must be segregated from all other merchandise and kept under constant surveillance during normal business hours. The controlled-substances storage areas must be accessible only to an absolute minimum number of specifically authorized employees. When it is necessary for employee maintenance personnel, nonemployee maintenance personnel, business guests, or visitors to be present in or pass through controlled-substances storage areas, the registrant must provide for adequate observation of the area by an employee specifically authorized in writing.

The security requirements of the forensic laboratory are no less than those required by law. In most cases, additional means of safeguarding controlled substances and dangerous drugs may be required. With the addition of the parameter of "evidence" to these substances, safeguarding against burglary is not enough. The maintenance of the chain of custody is an additional consideration.

There are many safeguards and devices that the forensic laboratory may employ to insure the integrity of the evidence. Each forensic laboratory must consider its work volume, physical location, building design, agency or agencies served, and standard operating procedures when developing additional security measures.

If a drop-box or chute is used for the deposit of evidence in the laboratory after working hours, the box or chute must be tamper-proof. Consideration should be given to installing a cushion at the bottom of the box or chute that will avoid breakage caused by other objects falling on top of fragile objects. Provisions can also be made for individual boxes for each item of evidence deposited. Self-locking doors that provide access to individual lockers or closets of various sizes should be installed. After the evidence is deposited and the outside access doors are closed and locked, the evidence can be removed only from inside the laboratory by unlocking and opening a door opposite the outside access door. The DEA has described this type of security system in detail in the *Guidelines for Narcotic and Dangerous Drug Evidence Handling and Security Procedures.*

When personal laboratory evidence vaults are authorized for and used by forensic scientists assigned to the laboratory, the evidence stored therein should be afforded as much protection as that provided by the laboratory evidence room. Individual vaults should be constructed of steel with safe-type combination-lock pigeonholes for evidence storage.

The type of tiered individual luggage lockers often found in bus depots and air terminals is also acceptable. In no instance, however, should ordinary metal file cabinets be used. The file cabinets are not tamper-proof, and access to one file drawer offers access to the contents of the drawer immediately below and, frequently, to the contents of other drawers as well. When feasible, a relatively secure area (locked room) within the laboratory itself should be designated as the location for placement of the individual evidence vaults.

Consideration should be given to installing a refrigerator within the evidence room for the storage of unstable or perishable items of evidence. Every effort should be made to obtain authority to dispose of refrigerated evidence as expeditiously as possible.

The evidence room should be furnished with sufficient bins and shelves to permit the orderly storage of items in custody. Bins or shelves that can be adjusted to accommodate various-sized packages should be installed whenever possible.

LABELING AND PACKAGING REQUIREMENTS FOR CONTROLLED SUBSTANCES

Definitions (302.02)

Commercial Container

Any bottle, jar, tube, ampule, or other receptacle in which a substance is held for distribution or dispensing to an ultimate user, and in addition, any box or package in which the receptacle is held for distribution or dispensing to an ultimate user. The term "commercial container" does not include any package liner, package insert, or other material kept with or within a commercial container, or any carton, crate, drum, or other package in which commercial containers are stored or are used for shipment of controlled substances.

Label

Any display of written, printed, or graphic matter placed on the commercial container of any controlled substance by any manufacturer of such substance.

Labeling

All labels and other written, printed, or graphic matter on any controlled substance or any of its commercial containers or wrappers. In addition, it includes such material accompanying the controlled substance.

Manufacture

The production, preparation, propagation, compounding, or processing of a drug or other substance or the packaging or repackaging of a controlled substance, or the labeling or relabeling of the commercial container of such substance. However, it does not include the activities of a practitioner who, as an incident activity to his administration or dispensing of the substance in the course of his professional practice, prepares, compounds, packages, or labels such substance. The term also includes the activity of a person who manufactures a drug or other substance under a registration as a manufacturer or under authority of registration as a researcher or chemical analyst.

Symbols (302.03)

Each commercial container of a controlled substance meeting the schedule requirements must have printed on the label the symbol designating the schedule in which such controlled substance is listed. Each such commercial container, if it otherwise has no label, must at least have the symbol.

The following symbols designate the corresponding schedule:

Schedule	Symbol
Schedule I	ℰI or C–I
Schedule II	ℰII or C–II
Schedule III	ℰIII or C–III
Schedule IV	ℰIV or C–IV
Schedule V	ℰV or C–V

The word "schedule" need not be used. No distinction need be made between narcotic and nonnarcotic substances.

The symbol is not required on a carton or wrapper in which a commercial container is held if the symbol is easily legible through the carton or wrapper. Also, the symbol is not required on a commercial container too small or otherwise unable to accommodate a label, if the symbol is printed on the box or package from which the commercial container is removed on being dispensed to an ultimate user. In addition, it is not required on a commercial container containing, or on the labeling of, a controlled substance being utilized in clinical research involving blind and double-blind studies.

Location and Size of Symbol on Label (302.04)

The symbol must be prominently located on the upper right corner of the principal panel of the label and/or the panel of the commercial container normally displayed to dispensers of any controlled substance listed in Schedules I through V. The symbol must be at least two times as large as the largest type otherwise printed on the label.

In lieu of location of the symbol in the corner of the label, the symbol may be overprinted on the label. In this case, the symbol must be printed at least one half the height of the label and in a contrasting color providing clear visibility against the background color.

In all cases, the symbol must be clear and large enough to afford easy identification of the schedule of the controlled substance on inspection without removal from the dispenser's shelf.

Sealing of Controlled Substances (302.07)

On each commercial container of any controlled substance listed in Schedule I or II or of any narcotic controlled substance listed in Schedule III or IV, there must be securely affixed to the stopper, cap, lid, covering, or wrapper of the container a seal to disclose on inspection any tampering or opening of the container.

Package Insert

In 1961, the FDA initiated a regulation that provided for a package insert to be on or with all prescription drug packages. The initial reasoning was the need to present physicians with accurate information regarding a drug's effects, usage, dosage, and safety apart from that listed in the manufacturer's advertising and promotional literature. This full-disclosure regulation requires that labeling on or within the package from which the drug is to be dispensed bear adequate information for its use. Included in this is the information concerning indications, effects, dosages, routes, methods and frequency and duration of administration, relevant hazards, contraindications, side effects, and precautions under which practitioners licensed by law to administer the drug can use the drug safely and for the purpose for which it is intended.

The FDA considers the insert to serve two purposes: It is included to alert the physician to the conditions under which the drug is deemed safe and effective for the designated purpose. It also serves to limit the manufacturer in its claims regarding the drug product. Basically, the FDA considers the package insert as part of the labeling of the drug (Rheinstein, 1976).

This insert has figured in judgments against members of the health care industry and is being used with increasing frequency to determine negligence. However, the physician is not restricted in using the drug only for labeled indications, but may have to defend against a deviation if a lawsuit is brought against him (Mills, 1965; Hirsh, 1977).

RECORDS AND REPORTS OF REGISTRANTS

Definitions (304.02)

Dispenser

An individual practitioner, institutional practitioner, pharmacy, or pharmacist who dispenses a controlled substance.

Individual Practitioner

A physician, dentist, veterinarian, or other individual licensed, registered, or otherwise permitted, by the United States or the jurisdiction in which he practices, to dispense a controlled substance in the course of professional practice. However, it does not include a pharmacist, a pharmacy, or an institutional practitioner.

Institutional Practitioner

A hospital or other institution (other than an individual) licensed, registered, or otherwise permitted, by the United States or the jurisdiction in which it practices, to dispense a controlled substance in the course of professional practice. It does not include a pharmacy.

Pharmacist

Any pharmacist licensed by a state to dispense controlled substances, and including any other person (e.g., pharmacist intern) authorized by a state to dispense controlled substances under the supervision of a pharmacist licensed by such state.

Name

The official name, common or usual name, chemical name, or brand name of a substance.

Readily Retrievable

Certain records that are kept by automatic data-processing systems or other electronic or mechanized record-keeping systems in such a manner that they can be separated from all other records in a reasonable time. It also includes records that are kept on which certain items are asterisked, redlined, or in some other manner visually identifiable apart from other items appearing on the records.

Persons Required to Keep Records and File Reports (304.03)

Each registrant must maintain the records and inventories and file the reports required. Any registrant who is authorized to conduct other activities without being registered must maintain the records and inventories and file the required reports for persons registered to conduct such activities. This latter requirement should not be construed as requiring stocks of controlled substances being used in various activities under one registration to be stored separately, or as requiring that separate records be kept for each activity. The intent is to permit the registrant to keep one set of records that are adapted by the registrant to account for controlled substances used in any activity. Also, the registrant does not have to acquire separate stocks of the same substance to be purchased and stored for separate activities. Otherwise, there is no advantage gained by permitting several activities under one registration. Thus, when a researcher manufactures a controlled item, he must keep a record of the quantity manufactured. When he distributes a quantity of the item, he must use and keep invoices or order forms to document the transfer. When he imports a substance, he keeps as part of his records the documentation required of an importer. However, when substances are used in chemical analysis, a record is not necessary because such a record would not be required of him under a registration to perform chemical analysis. All these records may be maintained in one consolidated record system. Similarly, the researcher may store all his controlled items in one place, and every two years take inventory of all items on hand, regardless of whether the substances were manufactured by him, imported by him, or purchased domestically by him. In addition, the records will reflect whether the substances will be administered to subjects, distributed to other researchers, or destroyed during chemical analysis.

A registered individual practitioner is not required to keep records with respect to narcotic controlled substances listed in Schedules II through V that he prescribes or administers in the lawful course of his professional practice. He must keep records, however, with respect to such substances that he dispenses other than by prescribing or administering. In addition, he is not required to keep records with respect to nonnarcotic controlled substances listed in Schedules II through V that he dispenses in any manner unless he regularly charges his patients, either separately or together with charges for other professional services, for such substances so dispensed (e.g., when he substitutes his services for those of a pharmacist).

Maintenance of Records and Inventories (304.04)

Every inventory and other record required must be kept by the registrant and be available for inspection for at least two years from the date of such inventory or record. However, financial and shipping records (such as invoices and packing slips) may be kept at a central location, rather than at the registered location, if the registrant obtains approval of his central record-keeping system and a permit to keep central records. The permit to keep central records, if approved, will be subject to the following conditions:

1. The permit shall specify the nature of the records to be kept centrally and the exact location where the records will be kept.
2. The registrant agrees to deliver all or any part of such records to the registered location within 48 hours of receipt of a written request for such records. In lieu of required delivery of the records to the registered location, an inspection of the records may be made at the central location on request without a warrant of any kind.

3. The failure of the registrant to perform his agreements under the permit will revoke without further action the permit and all other such permits held by the registrant under other registrations. In the event of a revocation of other permits, the registrant shall, within 30 days after such revocation, comply with the requirements that all records be kept at the registered location.

Each registered manufacturer, distributor, importer, and exporter must maintain inventories and records of controlled substances as follows:

1. Inventories and records of controlled substances listed in Schedules I and II must be maintained separately from all other records of the registrant.
2. Inventories and records of controlled substances listed in Schedules III, IV, and V must be maintained either separately from all other records of the registrant or in such form that the information required is readily retrievable from the ordinary business records of the registrant.

These inventories and records must also be kept by individual practitioners. However, each registered pharmacy must maintain the inventories and records of controlled substances as follows:

1. Inventories and records of all controlled substances listed in Schedules I and II must be maintained separately from all other records of the pharmacy. Prescriptions for such substances must be maintained in a separate prescription file.
2. Inventories and records of controlled substances listed in Schedules III, IV, and V must be maintained either separately from all other records or in such form that the information required is readily retrievable from ordinary business records of the pharmacy. Prescriptions for such substances may be maintained either in a separate prescription file for controlled substances listed in Schedules III, IV, and V only or in such form that they are readily retrievable from the other prescription records of the pharmacy. Prescriptions will be deemed readily retrievable if, at the time they are initially filed, the face of the prescription is stamped in red ink in the lower right corner with the letter "C" no less than 1 inch high and filed either in the prescription file for controlled substances listed in Schedules I and II or in the usual consecutively numbered prescription file for noncontrolled substances.

INVENTORY REQUIREMENTS

Each inventory must contain a complete and accurate record of all controlled substances on hand on the date the inventory is taken. In addition to those controlled substances in stock, the records must include the substances returned by a customer, substances ordered by a customer but not yet invoiced, substances stored in a warehouse on behalf of the registrant, and substances in the possession of employees of the registrant and intended for distribution as complimentary samples.

A separate inventory must be made by a registrant for each registered activity and each registered location. In the event controlled substances are in the possession or under the control of the registrant at a location for which he is not registered, the substances must be included in the inventory of the registered location at which they are subject to control.

A registrant may take an inventory on a date that is within four days of his biennial inventory date providing the Regional Director of the DEA is notified in advance. The inventory may be taken as of either the opening of business or the close of business on the inventory date. However, this fact must be noted in the inventory records. This inventory may be maintained in a written, typewritten, or printed form. If an inventory is taken by use of an oral recording device, it must be promptly transcribed.

The initial inventory date begins when the registrant first engages in the manufacture, distribution, or dispensing of controlled substances. In the event the registrant commences business with no controlled substances on hand, this fact must be recorded as the initial inventory.

Following this date, the registrant must take a new inventory of all stocks of controlled substances every two years. The biennial inventory may be taken on the day of the year on which the initial inventory was taken or on the registrant's regular general physical inventory date, if any, that is nearest to and does not vary by more than six months from the biennial date that would otherwise apply. The registrant may also elect to take inventory on any other fixed date that does not vary by more than six months from the biennial date that would otherwise apply. If the registrant elects to take the biennial inventory on his regular general physical inventory date or another fixed date, he must notify the DEA of this election and of the date on which the biennial inventory will be taken.

When a drug is added to any schedule of controlled substances, the registrant is required to take an inventory of all stocks of the substance on hand. This inventory must be taken on the effective date the drug becomes a scheduled substance. Thereafter, the substance is included in each regularly scheduled inventory.

Inventories of Manufacturers (304.15)

Each person registered or authorized to manufacture controlled substances must include the following information in his inventory:

For each controlled substance in finished form:

1. The name of the substance.
2. Each finished form of the substance (e.g., 10-milligram tablet or 10-milligram concentration per fluid ounce or milliliter).
3. The number of units or volume of each finished form in each commercial container (e.g., 100-tablet bottle or 3-milliliter vial).
4. The number of commercial containers of each such finished form (e.g., four 100-tablet bottles or six 3-milliliter vials).

For other controlled substances (e.g., damaged, defective, or impure substances awaiting disposal, substances held for quality control purposes, or substances maintained for extemporaneous compoundings):

1. The name of the substance.
2. The total quantity of the substance to the nearest metric unit weight or the total number of units of finished form.
3. The reason for the substance being maintained by the registrant and whether such substance is capable of use in the manufacture of any controlled substance in finished form.

Inventories of Dispensers and Researchers (304.17)

Each person registered or authorized to dispense or conduct research with controlled substances must include in his inventory the same information required of manufacturers. In determining the number of units of each finished form of a controlled substance in a commercial container that has been opened, the dispenser must do as follows:

1. If the substance is listed in Schedule I or II, he shall make an exact count or measure of the contents.
2. If the substance is listed in Schedule III, IV, or V, he must make an estimated count or measure of the contents. If the container holds more than 1000 tablets or capsules, he must make an exact count of the contents.

CONTINUING RECORDS

General Requirements (304.21)

Every registrant is required to maintain on a current basis a complete and accurate record of each such substance manufactured, imported, received, sold, delivered, exported, or otherwise disposed of by him. No registrant, however, is required to maintain a perpetual inventory. Separate records must be maintained for each independent activity as well as for each registered location. In the event controlled substances are in a location that is not registered, the substances shall be included in the records of the registered location at which they are subject to control or at which the person possessing the substance is responsible. In recording dates of receipt, importation, distribution, exportation, or other transfers, the date on which the controlled substances are actually transferred must be used as the date of receipt or distribution of any documents of transfer (e.g., invoices or packing slips).

Records for Dispensers and Researchers (304.24)

Each person registered or authorized to dispense or conduct research with controlled substances must maintain records with the following information for each controlled substance:

1. The name of the substance.
2. Each finished form (e.g., 10-milligram tablet or 10-milligram concentration per fluid ounce or milliliter) and the number of units or volume of finished form in each commercial container (e.g., 100-tablet bottle or 3-milliliter vial).
3. The number of commercial containers of each finished form received from other persons, including the date of and number of containers in each receipt and the name, address, and registration number of the person from whom the containers were received.
4. The number of units or volume of the finished form dispensed, including the name and address of the person to whom it was dispensed, the date of dispensing, the number of units or volume dispensed, and the written or typewritten name or initials of the individual who dispensed or administered the substance on behalf of the dispenser.
5. The number of units or volume of the finished forms and/or commercial containers disposed of in any other manner by the registrant, including the date and manner of disposal and the quantity of the substance in finished form disposed.

ORDER FORMS

Distributions Requiring Order Forms (305.03)

An order form (DEA Form 222c) is required for the purchase of a controlled substance listed in Schedule I or II, except for the following:

1. The exportation of controlled substances from the United States in conformity with the Act.
2. The delivery of controlled substances to or by a common or contract carrier for carriage in the lawful and usual course of its business. The delivery to or by a warehouseman for storage in the lawful and usual course of its business (but excluding such carriage or storage by the owner of the substance in connection with distribution to a third person).
3. The procurement of a sample of controlled substances by an exempt law enforcement official provided that the receipt required is used and is preserved in the manner prescribed for order forms.
4. The procurement of controlled substances by a civil defense or disaster relief organization provided that the Civil Defense Emergency Order Form required is used and is preserved with other records of the registrant.
5. The purchase of controlled substances by the master of a vessel provided that the special order form provided by the United States Public Health Service is used and preserved in the manner prescribed on this order form.
6. The delivery of controlled substances to a registered analytical laboratory, from an anonymous source for the analysis of the drug sample, provided the laboratory has obtained a written waiver of the order form requirement from the Regional DEA Director of the region in which the laboratory is located.

Persons Entitled to Obtain and Execute Order Forms (305.04)

Order forms may be obtained only by persons who are registered to handle controlled substances listed in Schedules I and II, and by persons who are registered to export such substances. Persons not registered are not entitled to obtain order forms. An order form may be executed only on behalf of the registrant and only if his registration as to the substances being purchased has not expired or been revoked or suspended.

Procedure for Obtaining Order Forms (305.05)

Order forms are issued in books of six forms, each form containing an original, duplicate, and triplicate copy (respectively, Copy 1, Copy 2, and Copy 3). A limit of three books of forms will be furnished on any requisition, unless additional books are specifically requested and a reasonable need for such additional books is shown. Any person applying for a registration that would entitle him to obtain order forms may requisition such forms by so indicating on the application form. In this case, order forms will be supplied upon the registration of the applicant. Any person holding a registration entitling him to obtain order forms may requisition such forms for the first time on DEA Form 222d, which may be obtained from the Registration Branch of the DEA. Any person already holding order forms may requisition additional forms only on DEA Form 222b, which is contained in each book of order forms. All requisitions must be submitted to the Registration Branch of the DEA, Washington, D.C.

Each requisition must show the name, address, and registration number of the registrant and the number of books of order forms desired. Each requisition must be signed and dated by the same person who signed the most recent application for registration or for reregistration, or by any person authorized to obtain and execute order forms by a power of attorney. Order forms will be serially numbered and issued with the name, address, and registration number of the registrant and the authorized activity and schedules of the registrant. This information cannot be altered or changed by the registrant. Any errors must be submitted for correction by the Registration Branch of the DEA by returning the forms with notification of the error.

Procedure for Executing Order Forms (305.06)

Order forms may be prepared and executed by the purchaser simultaneously in triplicate by means of the interleaved carbon sheets that are part of DEA Form 222c. Only one item can be entered on each numbered line. There are five lines on each order form. If one order form is not sufficient to include all items in an order, additional forms must be used. Order forms for etorphine hydrochloride and cyprenorphine must contain only these substances. The total number of items ordered must be noted on that form in the space provided.

An item consists of one or more commercial or bulk containers of the same finished or bulk form and quantity of the same substance. A separate item must be made for each commercial or bulk container of different finished or bulk form, quantity, or substance. For each item, the form must show the name of the article ordered, the finished or bulk form of the article (e.g., 10-milligram tablet, 10-milligram concentration per fluid ounce or milliliter, or U.S.P.), the number of units or volume in each commercial or bulk container (e.g., 100-tablet bottle or 3-milliliter vial) or the quantity or volume of each bulk container (e.g., 10 kilograms), the number of commercial or bulk containers ordered, and the name and quantity per unit of the controlled substance or substances contained in the article if not in pure form. The catalogue number of the article may be included at the discretion of the purchaser. The name and address of the supplier from whom the controlled substances are being ordered must be entered on the form. Only one supplier may be listed on any one form. Each order form must be signed and dated by a person authorized to sign a requisition for order forms on behalf of the purchaser. The name of the purchaser, if different from the individual signing the order form, must also be inserted in the signature space. Unexecuted order forms may be kept and executed at a location different from the registered location printed on the form, provided that all unexecuted forms are delivered promptly to the registered location on an inspection of that location.

Power of Attorney (305.07)

Any purchaser may authorize one or more individuals, whether or not located at the registered location of the purchaser, to obtain and execute order forms on his behalf by executing a power of attorney for each such individual. The power of attorney must be signed by the same person who signed the application for registration or reregistration and by the individual being authorized to obtain and execute order forms. The power of attorney must be filed with the executed order forms of the purchaser, and retained for the same period as any order form bearing the signature of the attorney. The power of attorney must be available for inspection together with other order form records. The power of attorney may be revoked at any time by executing a notice of revocation. This notice must be signed by the person who signed the power of attorney or by a successor, whoever signed the most recent application for registration or reregistration. The revocation must be filed with the power of attorney being revoked. Sample forms for the power of attorney and notice of revocation are shown on the following page.

Persons Entitled to Fill Order Forms (305.08)

An order form may be filled only by a person registered as a manufacturer or distributor of controlled substances listed in Schedules I and II or as an

Power of Attorney

_____
(Name of registrant)

_____
(Address of registrant)

_____
(DEA registration number)

I, _____, the undersigned, who is authorized to sign the
(Name of person granting power)
current application for registration of the above-named registrant under the
Controlled Substances Act or the Controlled Substances Import and Export
Act, have made, constituted, and appointed, and by these presents, do make,
constitute, and appoint _____, my true and lawful attorney for
(Name of attorney-in-fact)
me in my name, place, and stead, to execute applications for books of official
order forms and to sign such order forms in requisition for Schedule I and II
controlled substances, in accordance with section 308 of the Controlled
Substances Act (21 U.S.C. 828) and Part 305 of Title 21 of the Code of
Federal Regulations. I hereby ratify and confirm all that said attorney shall
lawfully do or cause to be done by virtue hereof.

_____
(Signature of person granting power)

I, _____, hereby affirm that I am the person named herein as
(Name of attorney-in-fact)
attorney-in-fact and that the signature affixed hereto is my signature.

_____
(Signature of attorney-in-fact)

Witnesses:
1. _____
2. _____

Signed and dated on the _____ day of _____,
19____, at _____.

Notice of Revocation

The foregoing power of attorney is hereby revoked by the undersigned, who
is authorized to sign the current application for registration of the above-
named registrant under the Controlled Substances Act or the Controlled
Substances Import and Export Act. Written notice of this revocation has
been given to the attorney-in-fact, _____,
this same day.

_____
(Signature of person revoking power)

I, _____, hereby affirm that I am in receipt of this notice and
(Name of attorney-in-fact)
that the signature affixed hereto is my signature.

_____
(Signature of attorney-in-fact)

Witnesses:
1. _____
2. _____

Signed and dated on the _____ day of _____,
19____, at _____.

importer of such substances. However, under certain circumstances, other persons may be allowed to fill order forms. For example, a person registered to dispense or export controlled substances may dispose of Schedule I or II substances if he is discontinuing business or if his registration is expiring without reregistration. He must, however, submit in person or by registered or certified mail, return receipt requested, to the Regional Director of the DEA in his region, at least 14 days in advance of the date of the proposed transfer (unless the Regional Director waives this time limitation in individual instances), the following information:

1. The name, address, registration number, and authorized business activity of the registrant discontinuing the business (registrant–transferor).
2. The name, address, registration number, and authorized business activity of the person acquiring the business (registrant–transferee).
3. Whether the business activities will be continued at the location registered by the person discontinuing business, or moved to another location (if the latter, the address of the new location should be listed).
4. Whether the registrant–transferor has a quota to manufacture or procure any controlled substance listed in Schedule I or II (if so, the basic class or class of the substance should be indicated).
5. The date on which the transfer of controlled substances will occur.

The transfer may not take place unless the registrant–transferor is informed by the Regional Director before the date on which the transfer was stated to occur.

On the date of transfer of the controlled substances, a complete inventory of all controlled substances being transferred shall be taken.

This inventory will serve as the final inventory of the registrant–transferor and the initial inventory of the registrant–transferee. A copy of the inventory must be included in the records of each person. It is not necessary to file a copy of the inventory with the DEA unless requested by the Regional Director. Transfers of any substances listed in Schedule I or II require the use of order forms. On the date of transfer of the controlled substances, all records required to be kept by the registrant–transferor with reference to the controlled substances being transferred must be transferred to the registrant–transferee. Responsibility for the accuracy of records prior to the date of transfer remains with the transferor, but responsibility for custody and maintenance rests on the transferee.

A person who has obtained any controlled substance in Schedule I or II by order form may return the substance to the person from whom he obtained it providing he has an order form from that person.

A person registered to dispense such substances may distribute such substances to another dispenser provided that the practitioner to whom the controlled substance is to be distributed is registered under the Act to dispense that controlled substance. The distribution must be recorded by the distributing practitioner and by the receiving practitioner. If the substance is listed in Schedule I or II, an order form is used.

The additional total number of dosage units of all controlled substances distributed by the receiving practitioner during the twelve-month period in which the practitioner is registered to dispense must not exceed 5 percent of the total number of dosage units of all controlled substances distributed and dispensed by the practitioner during that twelve-month period.

If, at any time during the twelve-month period, the practitioner has reason to believe that the additional total number of dosage units of all controlled substances that will be distributed by him will exceed 5 percent, the practitioner must obtain an additional registration to distribute controlled substances.

Procedure for Filling Order Forms (305.09)

The purchaser must submit Copy 1 and Copy 2 of the order form to the supplier, and retain Copy 3 in his own files. The supplier will then fill the order and record on Copies 1 and 2 the number of commercial or bulk containers furnished on each item and the date on which the containers are shipped to the purchaser. If any order cannot be filled in its entirety, it may be filled in part and the balance supplied by additional shipments within 60 days following the date of the order form. No order form is valid more than 60 days after its execution by the purchaser. The controlled substances will be shipped only to the purchaser and only to the location noted on the order form. The supplier retains Copy 1 of the order form for his own files and forwards Copy 2 to the Regional Director of the DEA in the region in which the supplier is located. Copy 2 may be forwarded at the close of the month during which the order is filled. If an order is filled by partial shipments, Copy 2 may be forwarded at the close of the month during which the final shipment is made or during which the 61-day validity period expires. The purchaser must record on Copy 3 of the order form the number of commercial or bulk containers furnished on each item and the dates on which such containers are received by the purchaser.

An order form made out to any supplier who cannot fill all or a part of the order within the time limitation may be endorsed to another supplier for filling. The endorsement must be made only by the supplier to whom the order form was first made. It must state the name and address of the second supplier, and be signed by a person authorized to obtain and execute order forms on behalf of the first supplier. The first supplier may not fill any part of an order on an endorsed form. The second supplier must fill the order if possible and ship the substances directly to the purchaser.

Distributions made on endorsed order forms are reported by the second supplier in the same manner as all other distributions except that where the name of the supplier is requested on the reporting form, the second supplier records the name, address, and registration number of the first supplier.

Unaccepted and Defective Order Forms (305.11)

No order form may be filled if it is not complete, legible, or properly prepared, executed, or endorsed. In addition, it may not be filled if it shows any alteration, erasure, or change of any description.

If an order form cannot be filled for any reason, the supplier must return Copies 1 and 2 to the purchaser with a statement as to the reason (e.g., illegible or altered). A supplier may for any reason refuse to accept any order.

When received by the purchaser, Copies 1 and 2 or the order form and the statement are attached to Copy 3 and retained in the files of the purchaser. A defective order form is not to be corrected. It must be replaced by a new order form for the order to be filled.

Lost and Stolen Order Forms (305.12)

If a purchaser ascertains that an unfilled order form has been lost, he must execute another in triplicate. A statement containing the serial number and date of the lost form, and stating that the goods covered by the first order form were not received through loss of that order form must accompany the second order form. Copy 3 of the second form and a copy of the statement are retained with Copy 3 of the order form first executed. A copy of the statement must be attached to Copies 1 and 2 of the second order form sent to the supplier. If the first order form is subsequently received by the supplier to whom it was directed, the supplier must mark on the face thereof "Not accepted" and return Copies 1 and 2 to the purchaser, who then attaches them to Copy 3 and the statement.

Whenever any used or unused order forms are stolen from or lost (other than in the course of transmission) by any purchaser or supplier, he must immediately report it to the Registration Branch of the DEA, Washington, D.C., stating the serial number of each form stolen or lost. If the theft or loss includes any original order forms received from purchasers and the supplier is unable to state the serial numbers of such order forms, he must report the date or approximate date of receipt and the names and addresses of the purchasers. If an entire book of order forms is lost or stolen, and the purchaser is unable to state the serial numbers of the order forms contained therein, he must report, in lieu of the numbers of the forms contained in such book, the date or approximate date of issuance thereof. If any unused order form reported stolen or lost is subsequently recovered or found, the Registration Branch of the DEA must immediately be notified.

Preservation of Order Forms (305.13)

The purchaser must retain Copy 3 of each order form that has been filled. He must also retain in his files all copies of each unaccepted or defective order form and each statement attached thereto. The supplier must retain Copy 1 of each order form that he has filled.

Order forms must be maintained separately from all other records of the registrant. Order forms are required to be kept available for inspection for a period of two years. If a purchaser has several registered locations, he must retain Copy 3 of the executed order forms and any attached statements or other related documents (not including unexecuted order forms, which may be kept elsewhere) at the registered location printed on the order form.

The supplier of etorphine hydrochloride and cyprenorphine must maintain order forms for these substances separately from all other order forms and records required to be maintained by the registrant.

Return of Unused Order Forms (305.14)

If the registration of any purchaser terminates (because the purchaser dies, ceases legal existence, discontinues business or professional practice, or changes his name or address as shown on the registration) or is suspended or revoked as to all controlled substances listed in Schedules I and II for which he is registered, all unused order forms for such substances, must be returned to the nearest office of the DEA.

Cancellation and Voiding of Order Forms (305.15)

A purchaser may cancel part or all of an order on an order form by notifying the supplier in writing of such cancellation. The supplier must indicate the cancellation on Copies 1 and 2 of the order form by drawing a line through the canceled items and printing "canceled" in the space provided for number of items shipped. A supplier may void part or all of an order on an order form by notifying the purchaser in writing. The supplier may indicate the voiding in the same manner prescribed for cancellation. No cancellation or voiding will affect in any way contract rights of either the purchaser or the supplier.

PRESCRIPTIONS

Persons Entitled to Issue Prescriptions (306.03)

A prescription for a controlled substance may be issued only by an individual practitioner who is authorized to prescribe controlled substances by the jurisdiction in which he is licensed to practice his profession and is either registered or exempted from registration.

A prescription issued by an individual practitioner may be communicated to a pharmacist by an employee or agent of the individual practitioner.

Purpose of Issue of Prescription (306.04)

A prescription for a controlled substance, to be effective, must be issued for a legitimate medical purpose by an individual practitioner acting in the usual course of his professional practice. The responsibility for the proper prescribing and dispensing of controlled substances is on the prescribing practitioner, but a corresponding responsibility rests with the pharmacist who fills the prescription. An order purporting to be a prescription issued not in the usual course of professional treatment or in legitimate and authorized research is not a prescription within the meaning and intent of the law. The person knowingly filling such a purported prescription, as well as the person issuing it, shall be subject to the penalties provided for violations of the provisions of law relating to controlled substances.

A prescription may not be issued by an individual practitioner to obtain controlled substances for the purpose of general dispensing to patients.

A prescription may not be issued for the dispensing of narcotic drugs listed in any schedule to a narcotic-drug-dependent person for the purpose of continuing his dependence on such drugs, in the course of conducting an authorized clinical investigation in the development of a narcotic addict rehabilitation program.

Manner of Issuance of Prescriptions (306.05)

All prescriptions for controlled substances must be dated as of, and signed on, the day when issued and bear the full name and address of the patient, and the name, address, and registration number of the practitioner. A practitioner may sign a prescription in the same manner as he would sign a check or legal document (e.g., J. H. Smith or John H. Smith). Where an oral order is not permitted, prescriptions must be written with ink or indelible pencil or typewriter and manually signed by the practitioner. The prescriptions may be prepared by a secretary or agent for the signature of a practitioner, but the prescribing practitioner is responsible in case the prescription does not conform in all essential respects to the law and regulations. A corresponding liability rests on the pharmacist who fills a prescription not prepared in the form prescribed by these regulations.

An intern, resident, or foreign-trained physician, or physician on the staff of a Veterans Administration facility, exempted from registration must include on all prescriptions issued by him the registration number of the hospital or other institution and the special internal code number assigned to him by the hospital or other institution. This number is in lieu of the registration number of the practitioner. Each written prescription must have the name of the physician stamped, typed, or hand-printed on it, as well as the signature of the physician.

An official exempted from registration must include on all prescriptions issued by him his branch of service or agency (e.g., "U.S. Army" or "Public Health Service") and his service identification number, in lieu of the registration number. Each prescription must have the name of the officer stamped, typed, or hand-printed on it, as well as the signature of the officer.

Persons Entitled to Fill Prescriptions (306.06)

A prescription for controlled substances may be filled only by a pharmacist acting in the usual course of his professional practice and either registered individually or employed in a registered pharmacy or registered institutional practitioner.

Dispensing of Narcotic Drugs for Maintenance Purposes (306.07)

The administering or dispensing directly (but not prescribing) of narcotic drugs listed in any schedule to a narcotic-drug-dependent person for the purpose of continuing his dependence on such drugs in the course of conducting an authorized clinical investigation in the development of a narcotic addict rehabilitation program is within the meaning of the term "in the course of his professional practice or research." This is indeed true provided that approval is obtained prior to the initiation of such a program by submission of a Notice of Claimed Investigational Exemption for a New Drug to the FDA. It will be reviewed concurrently by the FDA for scientific merit and by the DEA for drug-control requirements.

CONTROLLED SUBSTANCES LISTED IN SCHEDULE II

Requirement of Prescription (306.11)

A pharmacist may dispense directly a controlled substance listed in Schedule II that is a prescription drug as determined under the Federal Food, Drug, and Cosmetic Act only pursuant to a written prescription signed by the prescribing individual practitioner, except in cases of emergency. An individual practitioner may administer or dispense directly a controlled substance listed in Schedule II in the course of his professional practice without a prescription.

An institutional practitioner may administer or dispense directly (but not prescribe) a controlled substance listed in Schedule II only pursuant to a written prescription signed by the prescribing individual practitioner or to an order for medication made by an individual practitioner that is dispensed for immediate administration to the ultimate user.

In the case of an emergency situation, a pharmacist may dispense a controlled substance listed in Schedule II on receiving oral authorization of a prescribing individual practitioner, provided that:

1. The quantity prescribed and dispensed is limited to the amount adequate to treat the patient during the emergency period (dispensing beyond the emergency period must be pursuant to a written prescription signed by the prescribing individual practitioner).
2. The prescription is immediately reduced to writing by the pharmacist and contains all information required except for the signature of the prescribing individual practitioner.
3. If the prescribing individual practitioner is not known to the pharmacist, he must make a reasonable effort to determine that the oral authorization came from a registered individual practitioner, which may include a callback to the prescribing individual practitioner using his phone number as listed in the telephone directory and/or other good-faith efforts to ensure his identity.

4. Within 72 hours after authorizing an emergency oral prescription, the prescribing individual practitioner must provide a written prescription for the emergency quantity prescribed to be delivered to the dispensing pharmacist. The prescription must have written on its face "Authorization for Emergency Dispensing," and the date of the oral order. The written prescription may be delivered to the pharmacist in person or by mail, but if delivered by mail it must be postmarked within the 72-hour period. On receipt of the prescription, the dispensing pharmacist must attach it to the oral emergency prescription that had earlier been reduced to writing. The pharmacist must notify the nearest office of the DEA if the prescribing individual practitioner fails to deliver a written prescription to him.

Refilling of Prescriptions (306.12)

The refilling of a prescription for a controlled substance listed in Schedule II is prohibited.

Partial Filling of Prescriptions (306.13)

The partial filling of a prescription for a controlled substance listed in Schedule II is permissible, if the pharmacist is unable to supply the full quantity called for in a written or emergency oral prescription and he makes a notation of the quantity supplied on the face of the written prescription (or written record of the emergency oral prescription). The remaining portion of the prescription may be filled within 72 hours of the first partial filling; however, if the remaining portion is not or cannot be filled within the 72-hour period, the pharmacist must notify the prescribing individual practitioner. No further quantity may be supplied beyond 72 hours without a new prescription.

Labeling of Substances (306.14)

The pharmacist filling a written or emergency oral prescription for a controlled substance listed in Schedule II shall affix to the package a label showing date of filling, the pharmacy name and address, the serial number of the prescription, the name of the patient, the name of the prescribing practitioner, and directions for use and cautionary statements, if any, contained in such prescription or required by law. These requirements do not apply when a controlled substance listed in Schedule II is prescribed for administration to an ultimate user who is institutionalized, provided that:

1. Not more than a 7-day supply of the controlled substance listed in Schedule II is dispensed at one time.
2. The controlled substance listed in Schedule II is not in the possession of the ultimate user prior to the administration.
3. The institution maintains appropriate safeguards and records regarding the proper administration, control, dispensing, and storage of the controlled substance listed in Schedule II.
4. The system employed by the pharmacist in filling a prescription is adequate to identify the supplier, the product, and the patient, and to set forth the directions for use and cautionary statements, if any, contained in the prescription or required by law.

CONTROLLED SUBSTANCES LISTED IN SCHEDULES III AND IV

Requirement of Prescription (306.21)

A pharmacist may dispense directly a controlled substance listed in Schedule III or IV that is a prescription drug as determined under the Federal Food, Drug, and Cosmetic Act. This is accomplished by either a written prescription signed by or an oral prescription made by a prescribing individual practitioner. The latter must be promptly reduced to writing by the pharmacist and contain all required information except for the signature of the prescribing individual practitioner.

An individual practitioner may administer or dispense directly a controlled substance listed in Schedule III or IV in the course of his professional practice without a prescription if such is an authorized clinical investigation. This must be within the meaning of the term "in the course of his professional practice or research."

An institutional practitioner may administer or dispense directly (but not prescribe) a controlled substance listed in Schedule III or IV pursuant to a written prescription signed by, or pursuant to an oral prescription made by, a prescribing individual practitioner and promptly reduced to writing by the pharmacist. In addition, this may be conducted pursuant to an order for medication made by an individual practitioner that is dispensed for immediate administration to the patient.

Refilling of Prescriptions (306.22)

No prescription for a controlled substance listed in Schedule III or IV shall be filled or refilled more than six months after the date on which such prescription was issued. No such prescription authorized to be refilled may be refilled more than five times. Each refilling of a prescription shall be entered on the back of the prescription, or on another appropriate uniformly maintained, readily retrievable record, such as a medication record, that indicates by the number of the prescription the following information:

1. The name and dosage form of the controlled substance.
2. The date of each refilling.
3. The quantity dispensed.
4. The identity or initials of the dispensing pharmacist in each refilling.
5. The total number of refills for that prescription, initialed and dated by the pharmacist as of the date of dispensing, and the amount dispensed.

If the pharmacist merely initials and dates the back of the prescription, he shall be deemed to have dispensed a refill for the full face amount of the prescription. Additional quantities of controlled substances listed in Schedule III or IV may be authorized only by a prescribing practitioner through issuance of a new prescription.

Partial Filling of Prescriptions (306.23)

The partial filling of a prescription for a controlled substance listed in Schedule III, IV, or V is permissible, provided that:

1. Each partial filling is recorded in the same manner as a refilling.
2. The total quantity dispensed in all partial fillings does not exceed the total quantity prescribed.
3. No dispensing occurs after six months after the date on which the prescription was issued.

Labeling of Substances (306.24)

The pharmacist filling a prescription for a controlled substance listed in Schedule III or IV must place a label on the package showing the pharmacy name and address, the serial number and date of initial filling, the name of the patient, the name of the practitioner issuing the prescription, and directions for use and cautionary statements, if any, contained in such prescription as required by law.

These requirements do not apply if the controlled substance is prescribed for an institutionalized patient. However, in the latter case, the following requirements must be met:

1. Not more than a 34-day supply or 100 dosage units, whichever is less, of the controlled substance listed in Schedule II or IV is dispensed at one time.
2. The controlled substance listed in Schedule III or IV is not in the possession of the patient prior to administration.
3. The institution maintains appropriate safeguards and records the proper administration, control, dispensing, and storage of the controlled substance listed in Schedule III or IV.
4. The system employed by the pharmacist in filling a prescription is adequate to identify the supplier, the product, and the patient, and to set forth the directions for use and cautionary statements, if any, contained in the prescription or required by law.

CONTROLLED SUBSTANCES LISTED IN SCHEDULE V

Requirement of Prescription (306.31)

A pharmacist may dispense a controlled substance listed in Schedule V pursuant to a prescription as required for controlled substances listed in Schedules III and IV. A prescription for a controlled substance listed in Schedule V may be refilled only as expressly authorized by the prescribing individual practitioner on the prescription. If no such authorization is given, the prescription may not be refilled. A pharmacist dispensing such substance pursuant to a prescription must label the substance and file the prescription as described for Schedule III and IV substances.

An individual practitioner may administer or dispense directly a controlled substance listed in Schedule V in the course of his professional practice without a prescription if such is an authorized clinical investigation. This must be within the meaning of the term "in the course of his professional practice or research."

An institutional practitioner may administer or dispense directly (but not prescribe) a controlled substance listed in Schedule V only pursuant to a written prescription signed by, or an oral prescription made by, a prescribing individual practitioner and promptly reduced to writing by the pharmacist. In addition, this may be conducted pursuant to an order for medication made by an individual practitioner that is dispensed for immediate administration to the patient.

Dispensing without Prescription (306.32)

A controlled substance listed in Schedule V, and a controlled substance listed in Schedule II, III, or IV that is not a prescription drug as determined under the Federal Food, Drug, and Cosmetic Act, may be dispensed by a pharmacist without a prescription to a purchaser at retail. Such dispensing must be done only by a pharmacist. However, if the pharmacist has fulfilled his professional and legal responsibilities, the actual cash or credit transaction or delivery may be completed by a nonpharmacist.

The following limitations apply to the amounts of Schedule V controlled substances that may be dispensed at retail to the same purchaser in any given 48-hour period:

1. Not more than 240 cc (8 ounces) or 48 dosage units of any controlled substance containing opium
2. Not more than 120 cc (4 ounces) or 24 dosage units of any other controlled substance

The purchaser must be at least 18 years of age and must furnish suitable identification.

A bound record book for dispensing of Schedule V controlled substances must be maintained by the pharmacist. The book must contain the name and address of the purchaser, the name and quantity of controlled substance purchased, the date of each purchase, and the name or initials of the pharmacist who dispensed the substance to the purchaser.

A prescription is not required for distribution or dispensing of the substance pursuant to any other Federal, state, or local law.

Schedule V drugs consist of certain narcotic drugs containing a non-narcotic active medicinal ingredient. Specifically they are any compound, mixture, or preparation containing:

1. Not more than 200 milligrams of codeine per 100 milliliters or per 100 grams
2. Not more than 100 milligrams of dihydrocodeine per 100 milliliters or per 100 grams
3. Not more than 100 milligrams of ethylmorphine per 100 milliliters or per 100 grams
4. Not more than 2.5 milligrams of diphenoxylate and not less than 25 micrograms of atropine sulfate per dosage unit
5. Not more than 100 milligrams of opium per 100 milliliters or per 100 grams

These amounts are limited to weight quantities of the narcotic drug as the free base or a salt derivative. The one or more nonnarcotic active medicinal ingredients must be in sufficient proportion to contribute valuable medicinal qualities other than those possessed by the narcotic drug alone. All the ingredients named above may be designated by any official name, common or usual name, chemical name, or brand name.

5

Excluded Substances

EXCLUSION FROM A SCHEDULE

A nonnarcotic substance is excluded from any schedule if the substance may lawfully be sold over the counter without a prescription as described under the Federal Food, Drug and Cosmetic Act.

EXCLUDED SUBSTANCES

Amodrine[R] (Searle)—Tablet containing 8 mg phenobarbital, 100 mg aminophylline and 25 mg racephedrine

Amodrine[R] E C (Searle)—Enteric coated tablet containing 8 mg phenobarbital, 100 mg aminophylline, and 25 mg racephedrine

Anodyne[R] (Zemmer)—Ointment containing 0.69 g per 30 g chloral hydrate

Anti-Asthma[R] (Ormont Drug & Chem.)—Tablet containing 8 mg phenobarbital, 130 mg theophylline, and 25 mg ephedrine hydrochloride

Antiasthmatic[R] (Zenith)—Tablet containing 8.10 mg phenobarbital, 24 mg ephedrine hydrochloride, and 130 mg theophylline

Asma-Ese[R] (Parmed Pharm.)—Tablet containing 8.10 mg phenobarbital, 129.6 mg theophylline, and 24.30 mg ephedrine hydrochloride

Asma-Lief[R] (Columbia Medical Co.)—Tablet containing 8.10 mg phenobarbital, 24.30 mg ephedrine hydrochloride, and 129.60 mg theophylline

Asma-Lief[R] Pediatric (Columbia)—Suspension containing 4 mg per 5 ml phenobarbital, 12 mg per 5 ml ephedrine hydrochloride, and 65 mg per 5 ml theophylline

Asma Tuss[R] (Halsey)—Syrup containing 4 mg per 5 ml phenobarbital, 50 mg per 5 ml glyceryl guaiacolate, 1 mg per 5 ml chlorpheniramine maleate, 12 mg per 5 ml ephedrine sulfate, and 15 mg per 5 ml theophylline

Azma-Aid^R (Rondex)—Tablet containing 8 mg phenobarbital, 129.6 mg theophylline, and 24.3 mg ephedrine hydrochloride

Azmadrine^R (U.S. Ethicals)—Tablet containing 8 mg phenobarbital, 24 mg ephedrine hydrochloride, and 130 mg theophylline

Bet-U-Lol^R (Huxley Pharm.)—Liquid containing 0.54 g per 30 ml chloral hydrate, 30.1 g per 30 ml methyl salicylate, and 0.69 g per 30 ml menthol

Bronkolixir^R (Breon)—Elixir (5 cc) containing 4 mg phenobarbital, 12 mg ephedrine, 50 mg glyceryl guaiacolate, 15 mg theophylline, and 1 mg chlorpheniramine

Bronkotabs^R (Breon)—Tablet containing 8 mg phenobarbital, 24 mg ephedrine, 100 mg glyceryl guaiacolate, and 100 mg theophylline

Bronkotabs^R-Hafs (Breon)—Tablet containing 4 mg phenobarbital, 50 mg glyceryl guaiacolate, 50 mg theophylline, and 12 mg ephedrine sulfate

Ceepa^R (Geneva Drugs)—Tablet containing 8 mg phenobarbital, 130 mg theophylline, and 24 mg ephedrine hydrochloride

Chlorasal^R (Wisconsin Pharmacal.)—Ointment containing 648 mg per 30 g chloral hydrate, 972 mg per 30 g menthol, and 4.277 g per 30 g methyl salicylate

Choate's Leg Freeze^R (Bickmore, Inc.)—Liquid containing 7.4 g per 30 ml chloral hydrate, 10.3 ml per 30 ml ether, 6.3 g per 30 ml menthol, and 8.7 g per 30 ml camphor

Chlorosalicylate^R (Kremers-Urban Co.)—Ointment containing 648 mg per 30 g chloral hydrate, 6.66 g per 30 g methyl salicyclate, and 1.13 g per 30 g menthol

Menthalgesic^R (Blue Line Chem.)—Ointment containing 0.45 g per 30 g chloral hydrate, 0.45 g per 30 g menthol, 3.6 g per 30 g methyl salicylate, and 0.45 g per 30 g camphor

Neoasma^R (Termac)—Tablet containing 10 mg phenobarbital, 130 mg theophylline, and 24 mg ephedrine hydrochloride

P.E.C.T.^R (Halsom)—Tablet containing 8.1 mg phenobarbital, 2 mg chlorpheniramine maleate, 24.3 mg ephedrine sulfate, and 129.6 mg theophylline

Rynal^R (Blaine)—Spray containing 0.11 g per 50 ml *dl*-methamphetamine hydrochloride, 0.14 g per 50 ml antipyrine, 0.005 g per 50 ml pyrilamine maleate, and 0.01 g per 50 ml hyamine 2389

S-K Asthma^R (S-K Research)—Tablet containing 8 mg phenobarbital, 24.3 mg ephedrine hydrochloride, and 129.6 mg theophylline

Tedral^R (Warner-Chilcott)—Tablet containing 8 mg phenobarbital, 130 mg theophylline, and 24 mg ephedrine hydrochloride

Tedral^R Anti H (Warner-Chilcott)—Tablet containing 8 mg phenobarbital, 2 mg chlorpheniramine maleate, 130 mg theophylline, and 24 mg ephedrine hydrochloride

Tedral[R] Antiasthmatic (Parke-Davis)—Tablet containing 8 mg phenobarbital, 130 mg theophylline, and 24 mg ephedrine hydrochloride

Tedral[R] Elixir (Warner-Chilcott)—Elixir containing 2 mg per 5 ml phenobarbital, 6 mg per 5 ml ephedrine hydrochloride, and 32.5 mg per 5 ml theophylline

Tedral[R] One-Half Strength (Warner-Chilcott)—Tablet containing 4 mg phenobarbital, 65 mg theophylline, and 12 mg ephedrine

Tedral[R] Pediatric (Warner-Chilcott)—Suspension (5 cc) containing 4 mg phenobarbital, 12 mg ephedrine, and 65 mg theophylline

Tedral[R] Suppositories Double Strength (Warner-Chilcott)—Suppository containing 16 mg phenobarbital, 130 mg theophylline, and 48 mg ephedrine

Tedral[R] Suppositories Regular Strength (Warner-Chilcott)—Suppository containing 8 mg phenobarbital, 130 mg theophylline, and 24 mg ephedrine

Teephen[R] (Robinson)—Tablet containing 8 mg phenobarbital, 24 mg ephedrine hydrochloride, and 130 mg theophylline

Teephen[R] Pediatric (Robinson)—Suspension containing 4 mg per 5 ml phenobarbital, 12 mg per 5 ml ephedrine hydrochloride, and 65 mg per 5 ml theophylline anhydrous

T.E.P.[R] Compound (Stanlabs)—Tablet containing 8.1 mg phenobarbital, 129.6 mg theophylline, and 24.3 mg ephedrine hydrochloride

Thedrizem[R] (Zemmer)—Tablet containing 8 mg phenobarbital, 25 mg ephedrine hydrochloride, and 100 mg theophylline

Theobal[R] (Halsey)—Tablet containing 8 mg phenobarbital, 24 mg ephedrine hydrochloride, and 130 mg theophylline

Val-Tep[R] (Vale)—Tablet containing 8 mg phenobarbital, 24 mg ephedrine hydrochloride, and 130 mg theophylline

Verequad[R] (Knoll)—Suspension (5 cc) containing 4 mg phenobarbital, 12 mg ephedrine hydrochloride, 65 mg theophylline calcium salicylate, and 50 mg glyceryl guaiacolate

Verequad[R] (Knoll)—Tablet containing 8 mg phenobarbital, 24 mg ephedrine hydrochloride, 100 mg glyceryl guaiacolate, and 130 mg theophylline calcium salicylate

Vicks[R] Inhaler (Vick)—Inhaler containing 113 mg L-desoxyephedrine

6

Excepted Substances

REQUIREMENTS FOR EXCEPTION

The Federal Controlled Substances Act specifically defines and lists pharmaceutical preparations that are excepted from the application of all or any part of the Act. This list, published annually in the Code of Federal Regulations-T21, is an administrative action, as specific criteria have not been established for exact definitions. For a preparation to be excepted from application of all or any part of the Act, an application must be made giving detailed information about the preparation. As set forth by Federal regulations, each application will contain the following information:

1. The complete quantitation composition of the dosage form
2. Description of the unit dosage form together with complete labeling
3. A summary of the pharmacology of the product, including animal investigations and clinical evaluations and studies, with emphasis on the psychic or physiological (or both) dependence liability (this must be done for each of the active ingredients separately and for the combination product)
4. Details of synergisms and antagonisms among ingredients
5. Deterrent effects of the noncontrolled ingredients
6. Complete copies of all literature in support of claims
7. Reported instances of abuse
8. Reported and anticipated adverse effects
9. Number of dosage units produced for the past two years

An exception may be revoked at any time pursuant to Section 202(d) of the Act [21 U.S.C. 812(d)] (Lowry and Barklow, 1976).

The following groups of drugs list the approved pharmaceutical preparations classified as excepted preparations. Although these preparations are excepted from the Controlled Substances Act, each bears the legend "Caution:

Federal law prohibits dispensing without prescription." Thus, in this text, they are classified as "dangerous drugs." It should be noted, however, that if any dosage form of any excepted preparation has been altered, such as the possibility in a criminal matter, then the trade name would no longer be valid, resulting in the automatic removal of the exception.

Most states have incorporated the exception clause into their drug laws. Since pharmaceutical companies do not apply to the states for exception of drug preparations, but only to the Federal government, many regulatory problems may develop—especially in criminal matters (Lowry and Barklow, 1976).

EXCEPTED SUBSTANCES

Allobarbital Preparations

Diatraegus[R] (Buffington)—Tablet containing $\frac{1}{4}$ gr allobarbital, $\frac{1}{250}$ gr nitroglycerine, 1 gr sodium nitrite, and tincture of crataegus

Dis-Tropine[R] (Buffington)—Tablet containing $\frac{1}{4}$ gr allobarbital, $\frac{1}{300}$ gr atropine sulfate, $2\frac{1}{2}$ gr magnesium carbonate, and 1 gr bismuth subcarbonate

Phedorine[R] (Buffington)—Tablet containing 16 mg allobarbital, 8 mg stramonium extract (alkaloids 0.0015 gr), 8 mg ephedrine, and 100 mg theophylline

Vasorutin[R] (Buffington)—Tablet containing $\frac{1}{4}$ gr allobarbital, $\frac{1}{250}$ gr nitroglycerin, 1 gr sodium nitrite, 20 mg rutin, and tincture of crataegus

Amobarbital Preparations

A.E.A.[R] (Haack)—Tablet containing 25 mg amobarbital, 120 mg aminophylline, and 25 mg ephedrine

Amesec[R] (Lilly)—Amesec contains a mixture of 130 mg aminophylline, 25 mg ephedrine, and 25 mg amobarbital
   Tablets—round, unscored, red, coated, labeled "Lilly," and coded A27
   Pulvules—capsules, orange with dark blue cap, labeled "Lilly," and coded F47

Aminophylline[R] and Amytal (Lilly)—Capsule containing 32 mg amobarbital and 0.1 g aminophylline

Amobarbital[R] and PETN (Meyer)—Capsule containing 50 mg amobarbital and 30 mg pentaerythritol

Barbeloid[R] (Vale)—Tablet containing 20 mg sodium amobarbital, 0.125 mg hyoscyamine, 0.007 mg hyoscine, and 0.5 mg homatropine

Belap[R] Ty-Med (Haack)—Tablet containing 50 mg amobarbital and 7.5 mg homatropine methylbromide

Buffadyne^R A-S (Lemmon)—Tablet containing 15 mg amobarbital, 300 mg asprin, 150 mg phenacetin, 30 mg caffeine, 2.5 mg homatropine methylbromide, 75 mg aluminum hydroxide gel, and 45 mg magnesium hydroxide

Buffadyne^R w/barbiturate (Lemmon)—Tablet containing 8 mg sodium secobarbital, 8 mg amobarbital, 300 mg aspirin, 150 mg phenacetin, and 30 mg caffeine

Co-Elorine^R 25 (Lilly)—Capsule containing 8 mg amobarbital and 100 mg tricyclamol chloride

Co-Elorine^R 100 (Lilly)—Capsule containing 16 mg amobarbital and 100 mg tricyclamol chloride

Hydrochol^R Plus (Elder)—Tablet containing 15 mg amobarbital, 200 mg denydrocholic acid, 0.8 mg scopolamine methylnitrate, and 50 mg desiccated ox bile

Sed-Tens^R (Lemmon)—Tablet containing 50 mg amobarbital and 7.5 mg homatropine methylbromide

Amphetamine Preparations

Bamadex^R (Lederle)—Sustained release capsules, two-toned orange, labeled "Lederle," containing 15 mg amphetamine sulfate and 300 mg meprobamate

Aprobarbital Preparations: None excepted.*

Barbital Preparations

Tetralute^R I (Miles)—Buffer compound containing 4.15 g sodium barbital and 0.75 g barbital f.a. and other drugs and components

Butabarbital Preparations

Algoson^R (McNeil)—Tablet containing 7.5 mg butabarbital and 300 mg acetaminophen

Aludrox^R S.A. (Wyeth)—Suspension, each teaspoon (5 ml) containing 3 mg butabarbital and 2.5 mg ambutonium bromide

Ampyrox^R (Elder)—Tablet containing 15 mg butabarbital and 2 mg scopolamine methylnitrate; elixir containing 10 mg butabarbital and 1 mg scopolamine methylnitrate

* Here and hereafter, the notation "None excepted" indicates that there is no pharmaceutical preparation containing the substance that has been approved pursuant to Federal regulations to be classified as an "excepted substance."

Asmabar^R (Blue Line)—Tablet containing 20 mg butabarbital, 25 mg ephedrine sulfate, and 130 mg theophylline hydroxide

Asmacol^R (Vale)—Tablet containing 15 mg butabarbital, 180 mg aminophylline, 25 mg phenylpropanolamine hydrochloride, 2 mg chlorpheniramine maleate, 60 mg aluminum hydroxide, and 60 mg magnesium trisilicate

Bellatol^R (Zemmer)—Elixir containing 20 mg butabarbital and 83 ml tincture belladonna

Binitrin^R (Vale)—Tablet containing 15 mg butabarbital, 0.3 mg nitroglycerin, and 10 mg pentaerythritol tetranitrate

Bunesia^R (McNeil)—Tablet containing 10 mg butabarbital, 2.5 mg homatropine methylbromide, and 300 mg magnesium hydroxide

Buren^R (Ascher)—Tablet containing 15 mg butabarbital, 150 mg phenazopyridine hydrochloride, 6.5 μg scopolamine hydrobromide, 19.4 μg atropine, and 103.7 μg hyoscyamine

Burrizem^R (Zemmer)—Tablet containing 10 mg butabarbital, 0.1 mg reserpine, 20 mg rutin, and 30 mg mannitol hexanitrate

Butabarbital^R and Hyoscyamine Sulfate (McNeil)—Tablet or elixir containing 15 mg butabarbital and 0.125 mg hyoscyamine; capsule containing 45 mg butabarbital and 0.375 mg hyoscyamine

Butibel^R (McNeil)—Tablet or elixir containing 15 mg butabarbital and 15 mg belladonna extract

Butibel^R R-A (McNeil)—Tablet containing 30 mg butabarbital and 30 mg belladonna extract

Butibel^R-Gel (McNeil)—Suspension containing 7.5 mg butabarbital, 7.5 mg belladonna extract, 1.5 mg activated attapulgite, and 75 mg pectin; tablet containing 7.5 mg butabarbital, 7.5 mg belladonna extract (t. alkaloids, 0.0935 mg)

Butibel^R-Zyme (McNeil)—Tablet containing 15 mg butabarbital, 15 mg belladonna extract, and a combination of proteolytic, amylolytic, cellulolytic, and lipolytic enzymes

Butigetic^R (McNeil)—Tablet containing 15 mg butabarbital, 200 mg acetaminophen, 150 mg phenacetin, and 30 mg caffeine

Covadil^R (Blue Line)—Tablet containing 20 mg butabarbital and 15 mg pentaerythritol tetranitrate

Dolonil^R (Warner-Chilcott)—Tablet containing 15 mg butabarbital, 150 mg phenazopyridine, and 0.3 mg hyoscyamine

Metamine^R w/butabarbital (Pfizer)—Tablet: One containing 16 mg butabarbital and 2 mg trolnitrate; one containing 48 mg butabarbital and 10 mg trolnitrate

Nactisol^R (McNeil)—Tablet containing 15 mg butabarbital and 4 mg poldine

Pentraline^R (McNeil)—Tablet containing 10 mg butabarbital, 0.05 mg reserpine, and 10 mg pentaerythritol tetranitrate

Perbuzem^R (Zemmer)—Tablet containing 15 mg butabarbital and 10 mg pentaerythritol tetranitrate

Sibena^R (Plough)—Tablet containing 16 mg butabarbital, 25 mg simethicone, and 16 mg belladonna extract

Tedral-25^R (Warner-Chilcott)—Tablet containing 25 mg butabarbital, 130 mg theophylline, and 24 mg ephedrine

Zem-Dab^R (Zemmer)—Tablet containing 10 mg butabarbital, 60 mg dehydro-chloric acid, 120 mg desiccated ox bile, and 2.5 mg homatropine

Rx No. 4184 (Zemmer)—Capsule containing 15 mg butabarbital and 15 mg belladonna extract

Butalbital Preparations

Buff-A-Comp^R (Mayland)—Tablet, labeled "M/R," containing 48.6 mg butalbital, 648 mg aspirin, 130 mg phenacetin, and 43.2 mg caffeine

Kengesin^R (Kenwood)—Tablet containing 30 mg butalbital, 60 mg caffeine, and 450 mg aspirin

Butallylonal Preparations: None excepted.

Buthalital Preparations: None excepted.

Butobarbital Preparations: None excepted.

Chloral Betaine Preparations: None excepted.

Chlordiazepoxide Preparations

Librax^R (Roche)—Capsule containing 5 mg chlordiazepoxide and 2.5 mg clidinium bromide

Menrium^R (Roche)—Tablets: One tablet containing 5 mg chlordiazepoxide and 0.2 mg water-soluble esterified estrogens; one tablet containing 5 mg chlordiazepoxide and 0.4 mg water-soluble esterified estrogens; one tablet containing 10 mg chlordiazepoxide and 0.4 mg water-soluble esterified estrogens

Clonazepam Preparations: None excepted.

Clorazepate Preparations: None excepted.

Cyclobarbital Preparations: None excepted.

Cyclopentylallylbarbituric Acid Preparations

Zantrate^R (Upjohn)—Tablet containing $\frac{1}{2}$ gr cyclopentylallylbarbituric acid, $\frac{3}{8}$ gr ephedrine sulfate, and 2 gr theophylline

Diazepam Preparations: None excepted.

Ethchlorvynol Preparations: None excepted.

Ethinamate Preparations: None excepted.

Flurazepam Preparations: None excepted.

Glutethimide Preparations: None excepted.

Heptobarbital Preparations: None excepted.

Hexobarbital Preparations: None excepted.

Ibomal Preparations: None excepted.

Lysergic Acid Preparations: None excepted.

Lysergic Acid Amide Preparations: None excepted.

Mebutamate Preparations: None excepted.

Meprobamate Preparations

Bamadex^R (Lederle)—Sustained-release capsules, two-toned orange, labeled "Lederle," containing 15 mg amphetamine sulfate and 300 mg meprobamate

Milpath^R (Wallace)—Tablets: Yellow, scored, labeled "Wallace 37-5001," containing 400 mg meprobamate and 25 mg tridihexethyl chloride; yellow, coated, labeled "Wallace 37-5101," containing 200 mg meprobamate and 25 mg tridihexethyl chloride

Milprem[R] (Wallace)—Tablets: Dark pink, coated, containing 400 mg meprobamate and 0.45 mg conjugated estrogens; light pink, coated, containing 200 mg meprobamate and 0.45 mg conjugated estrogens

Miltrate[R] (Wallace)—Tablets: White, labeled "Wallace 37-5201," containing 200 mg meprobamate and 10 mg pentaerythritol tetranitrate; orange, labeled "Wallace 37-5301," containing 200 mg meprobamate and 20 mg pentaerythritol tetranitrate

PMB[R] (Ayerst)—Tablets: Green, elongated, coated, labeled "AYERST 880," containing 200 mg meprobamate and 0.45 mg conjugated estrogens; pink, elongated, coated, labeled "AYERST 881," containing 400 mg meprobamate and 0.45 mg conjugated estrogens

Pathibamate[R] (Lederle)—Tablets: Yellow, coated, labeled "Lederle," containing 200 mg meprobamate and 25 mg tridihexethyl chloride; yellow, scored, labeled "Lederle," containing 400 mg meprobamate and 25 mg tridihexethyl chloride

Methamphetamine Preparations: None excepted.

Methaqualone Preparations: None excepted.

Metharbital Preparations: None excepted.

Methohexital Preparations: None excepted.

Methylphenidate Preparations: None excepted.

Mephobarbital Preparations

Ethrava-trate[R] (North American)—Tablet containing 10 mg methylphenobarbital, 20 mg pentaerythritol tetranitrate, and 30 mg ethaverine hydrochloride

Hocalm[R] (Warren-Teed)—Tablet containing 30 mg methylphenobarbital, 2.5 mg methscopolamine nitrate, and 25 mg calcium pantothenate

Monomeb[R] (Winthrop)—Tablet containing 32 mg methylphenobarbital and 5 mg penthienate bromide

Methyprylon Preparations: None excepted.

Narcobarbital Preparations: None excepted.

Nealbarbital Preparations: None excepted.

Oxazepam Preparations: None excepted.

Paraldehyde Preparations: None excepted.

Pentobarbital Preparations

Aminophylline[R] w/pentobarbital (Searle)—Suppository containing 100 mg pentobarbital sodium and 500 mg aminophylline

Aqualin-plus[R] (Webster)—Suppositories: one containing $\frac{3}{8}$ gr pentobarbital sodium and $1\frac{7}{8}$ gr theophylline; one containing $\frac{3}{4}$ gr pentobarbital sodium and $3\frac{3}{4}$ gr theophylline; one containing $1\frac{1}{2}$ gr pentobarbital sodium and $7\frac{1}{2}$ gr theophylline; and one containing $\frac{3}{4}$ gr pentobarbital sodium and $7\frac{1}{2}$ gr theophylline

Cafergot[R] P-B (Sandoz)—Suppository containing 60 mg pentobarbital, 2 mg ergotamine tartrate, 100 mg caffeine, and 0.25 mg alkaloids of belladonna

Cholarace[R] (Warner-Chilcott)—Tablet containing 27.5 mg pentobarbital, 200 mg oxtriphylline, and 20 mg racephedrine

Dainite[R] (Mallinckrodt)—Tablet containing $\frac{1}{4}$ gr pentobarbital sodium, 3 gr aminophylline, $\frac{1}{4}$ gr ephedrine hydrochloride, and $\frac{1}{4}$ gr benzocaine

Dainite[R] Night (Mallinckrodt)—Tablet containing $\frac{1}{2}$ gr pentobarbital sodium, $\frac{3}{8}$ gr phenobarbital, 4 gr aminophylline, $2\frac{1}{2}$ gr aluminum hydroxide gel, dried, and $\frac{1}{4}$ gr benzocaine

Homechol[R] (Lemmon)—Tablet containing 8.0 mg pentobarbital sodium, 2.5 mg homatropine methylbromide, 60 mg dehydrocholic acid, and 150 mg ox bile extract

Homopent[R] (Lemmon)—Tablet containing 15 mg pentobarbital sodium, 2.5 mg homatropine methylbromide, and 300 mg magnesium trisilicate

Kanumodic[R] (Dorsey)—Tablet containing 8 mg pentobarbital, 2 mg methscopolamine nitrate, 9 mg cellulose, 500 mg pancrestin, 200 mg glutamic acid hydrochloride, 100 mg ox bile extract, and 150 mg pepsin

Matropinal[R] (Comatic)—Suppository containing 15 mg pentobarbital, 10 mg homatropine methylbromide, and 8 mg pyrilamine maleate

Matropinal Forte[R] (Comatic)—Suppository containing 90 mg pentobarbital, 10 mg homatropine methylbromide, and 8 mg pyrilamine maleate; tablet containing 10 mg homatropine methylbromide, 12.5 mg methapyrilene fumarate, and 90 mg pentobarbital

Symirin[R] (Wm. P. Poythress)—Tablet containing 8 mg pentobarbital and 324 mg aspirin

Rx No. 36^R (Stayner)—Tablet containing $\frac{3}{4}$ gr pentobarbital sodium, $\frac{3}{8}$ gr ephedrine sulfate, and 3 gr aminophylline

Rx No. 4126^R (Zemmer)—Capsule containing 15 mg pentobarbital sodium and 10 mg belladonna extract

Petrichloral Preparations: None excepted.

Phencyclidine Preparations: None excepted.

Phenmetrazine Preparations: None excepted.

Phenobarbital Preparations

Alased^R (Norgine)—Tablet containing 16.2 mg phenobarbital, 3.6 mg homatropine methylbromide, $7\frac{1}{2}$ gr aluminum hydroxide, and $2\frac{1}{3}$ gr magnesium trisilicate

Alcitex^R (Elder)—Tablet containing $\frac{1}{8}$ gr phenobarbital, $\frac{1}{5000}$ gr atropine sulfate, $3\frac{1}{2}$ gr calcium carbonate, $2\frac{1}{4}$ gr magnesium carbonate, and $\frac{1}{2}$ gr cerium oxalate

Alhydrox^R (Physicians Supply)—Tablet containing $\frac{1}{8}$ gr phenobarbital, 5 gr aluminum hydroxide, and $\frac{1}{325}$ gr atropine sulfate

Alkasans^R (Noyes)—Tablet containing 8.0 mg phenobarbital, 0.06 mg atropine sulfate, and 500 mg kaolin-alumina gel

Alsical^R (Dorsey)—Powder (60 gr) containing $\frac{1}{4}$ gr phenobarbital, $\frac{1}{4}$ gr belladonna extract, 24 gr calcium carbonate, 15 gr magnesium trisilicate, 10 gr magnesium oxide, and 10 gr aluminum hydroxide gel, dried

Alubelap^R (Haack)—Tablet containing 8 mg phenobarbital, 2300 mg aluminum hydroxide gel, dried, and 4 mg belladonna extract

Alu-Mag^R (Norsal)—Tablet containing $\frac{1}{8}$ gr phenobarbital, $2\frac{1}{2}$ gr aluminum hydroxide gel, dried, $2\frac{1}{2}$ gr magnesium trisilicate, and $\frac{1}{8}$ gr belladonna leaf extract

Alumazen^R (Zemmer)—Tablet containing 8 mg phenobarbital, 0.06 mg atropine sulfate, 500 mg magnesium trisilicate, 250 mg aluminum hydroxide gel, dried, and 0.12 mg saccharin sodium

Aluminum hydroxide, magnesium trisilicate, and kaolin with phenobarbital and atropine sulfate^R (Buffalo)—Tablet containing $\frac{1}{8}$ gr phenobarbital, 2 gr aluminum hydroxide, 4 gr magnesium trisilicate, 2 gr kaolin colloidal, and $\frac{1}{300}$ gr atropine sulfate

Aminodrox^R w/phenobarbital (Massengill)—Tablet containing 15 mg phenobarbital, 0.1 g aminophylline, and 0.12 g aluminum hydroxide gel, dried

Aminodrox^R-forte w/phenobarbital (Massengill)—Tablet containing 15 mg phenobarbital, 200 mg aminophylline, and 250 mg aluminum hydroxide gel, dried

Aminophylline^R and phenobarbital (Zemmer)—Tablet containing 15 mg phenobarbital and 100 mg aminophylline

Aminophylline^R and phenobarbital (Blue Line)—Tablet containing $\frac{1}{4}$ gr phenobarbital and 100 mg aminophylline

Aminophylline w/phenobarbital^R (Dubin)—Tablet containing 16 mg phenobarbital and 100 mg aminophylline

Aminophylline w/phenobarbital^R (Searle)—Tablet containing 15 mg phenobarbital and 100 mg aminophylline; tablet containing 15 mg phenobarbital and 200 mg aminophylline; tablet containing 30 mg phenobarbital and 200 mg aminophylline

Amsed^R (NAP-37) (North American)—Tablet containing $\frac{1}{4}$ gr phenobarbital, 0.0072 mg hyoscine hydrobromide, 0.024 mg atropine sulfate, and 0.128 mg hyoscyamine hydrobromide

Amsodyne^R (Elder)—Tablet containing $\frac{1}{4}$ gr phenobarbital, $\frac{1}{8}$ gr extract belladonna leaves, 5 gr aspirin and $\frac{1}{4}$ gr caffeine

Anaspaz^R PB (Ascher)—Tablet containing 0.125 mg hyoscyamine sulfate and 15 mg phenobarbital; liquid, each teaspoonful (5 ml) containing 0.125 mg hyoscyamine sulfate and 15 mg phenobarbital

Antacia^R No. 3 w/phenobarbital and atropine (Meyers)—Tablet containing $\frac{1}{8}$ gr phenobarbital, $\frac{1}{300}$ gr atropine sulfate, 5 gr calcium carbonate, and 5 gr magnesium hydroxide

Antispasmodic^R (Hydrex)—Tablet (purple) containing 16.2 mg phenobarbital, 0.1037 mg hyoscyamine sulfate, 0.567 mg homatropine methylbromide, and 0.0065 mg hyoscine hydrobromide

Antispasmodic-enzyme^R (Hydrex)—Tablet containing 8.1 mg phenobarbital, 0.0519 mg hyoscyamine sulfate, 0.2885 mg homatropine methylbromide, 0.0033 mg hyoscine hydrobromide, 100 mg pancreatin, and 150 mg pepsin

Antrocol^R (Poythress)—Tablet or capsule containing 16 mg phenobarbital, 0.324 mg atropine sulfate, and 22 mg colloidal sulfur

Arco-Lase Plus^R (Arco)—Tablet containing 8.1 mg phenobarbital, 0.02 mg atropine sulfate, 0.10 mg hyoscyamine sulfate, 25 mg lipase, and 38 mg trizyme

Asminyl^R (Cole)—Tablet containing 5 mg phenobarbital, 32 mg ephedrine sulfate, and 130 mg theophylline

Asperease^R, modified with phenobarbital (Noyes)—Tablet containing 0.008 g phenobarbital and 0.5 g acetylsalicylic acid

Atropal^R (Mallinckrodt)—Tablet containing $\frac{1}{8}$ gr phenobarbital, $\frac{1}{300}$ gr atropine sulfate, $2\frac{1}{2}$ gr magnesium trisilicate, and $2\frac{1}{2}$ gr aluminum hydroxide gel, dried

Atrosilital[R] (Zemmer)—Tablet containing 15 mg phenobarbital, 0.12 mg atropine sulfate, 0.5 g magnesium trisilicate, and 0.12 mg saccharin sodium

Banthinine[R] w/phenobarbital (Searle)—Tablet containing 15 mg phenobarbital and 50 mg methantheline bromide

Barbatro[R] No. 1 (Massengill)—Tablet containing 15 mg phenobarbital and 0.12 mg atropine sulfate

Barbatro[R] No. 2 (Massengill)—Tablet containing 15 mg phenobarbital and 0.25 mg atropine sulfate

Barbidonna[R] elixir (Mallinckrodt)—Elixir (5 cc) containing 16 mg phenobarbital, 0.1286 mg hyoscyamine sulfate, 0.0250 mg atropine sulfate, and 0.0074 mg scopolamine hydrobromide

Barbidonna[R] tablets (Mallinckrodt)—Tablet containing 16 mg phenobarbital, 0.1286 mg hyoscyamine sulfate, 0.0250 mg atropine sulfate, and 0.0074 mg scopolamine hydrobromide

Barboma[R] elixir (Blue Line)—Elixir (100 cc) containing 0.4 g phenobarbital and 33.8 mg homatropine methylbromide

Barboma[R] tablets (Blue Line)—Tablet containing 16.2 mg phenobarbital and 1.35 mg homatropine methylbromide

Bardase[R] (Parke-Davis)—Tablet or elixir (4 cc) containing 16.2 mg phenobarbital, 0.1 mg hyoscyamine, 0.007 mg hyoscine hydrobromide, 0.020 mg atropine, and 162.0 mg Taka-Diastase

Bar-Don[R] elixir (Warren-Teed)—Elixir (30 cc) containing 100 mg phenobarbital, 0.60 mg hyoscyamine hydrobromide, 0.042 mg hyoscine hydrobromide, and 0.12 mg atropine sulfate

Bar-Don[R] tablets (Warren-Teed)—Tablet containing 16.670 mg phenobarbital, 0.10 mg hyoscyamine hydrobromide, 0.007 mg hyoscine hydrobromide, and 0.020 mg atropine sulfate

Bar-Tropin[R] (Fellows)—Tablet containing 16.2 mg phenobarbital and 0.3 mg atropine

Belap[R] No. 0 (Lemmon)—Tablet containing 8 mg phenobarbital and 8 mg belladonna extract

Belap[R] No. 1 (Lemmon)—Tablet containing 15 mg phenobarbital and 8 mg belladonna extract

Belap[R] elixir (Lemmon)—Elixir containing 15 mg phenobarbital and 0.033 ml belladonna extract (equivalent to Belap No. 1)

Belladenal[R] (Sandoz)—Tablet containing 50 mg phenobarbital and 0.25 mg bellafoline; elixir (15 cc) containing 15.6 mg phenobarbital and 0.078 mg bellafoline

Bellergal[R] (Sandoz)—Tablet containing 20 mg phenobarbital, 0.3 mg ergotamine tartrate, and 0.1 mg levorotatory alkaloids of belladonna; tablet containing 40 mg phenobarbital, 0.6 mg ergotamine tartrate, and 0.2 mg levorotatory alkaloids of belladonna

Bentyl^R (Merrell-National)—Capsule, blue and white, containing 15 mg phenobarbital and 10 mg dicyclomine hydrochloride; tablet containing 15 mg phenobarbital and 20 mg dicyclomine; syrup, amber, each teaspoon (5 ml) containing 15 mg phenobarbital and 10 mg dicyclomine

Beplete^R w/belladonna elixir (Wyeth)—Elixir (4 cc) containing 15 mg phenobarbital, 1.5 mg vitamin B_1, 1 mg vitamin B_3, 0.33 mg vitamin B_6, 1.66 mg vitamin B_{12}, 10 mg niacinamide, 0.2 mg pantothenol, and 0.2 mg belladonna alkaloids

Bexadonna^R (Bexar)—Tablet containing 16 mg phenobarbital, 10 mg homatropine methylbromide, 0.0065 mg hyoscine hydrobromide, and 0.1 mg hyoscyamine sulfate

Bilamide^R (Norgine)—Tablet containing $\frac{1}{8}$ gr phenobarbital, 2 gr dried ox bile, 2 gr dehydrocholic acid, and $\frac{1}{48}$ gr homatropine methylbromide

Bioxatphen^R (Zemmer)—Tablet containing 8 mg phenobarbital, 0.06 mg atropine sulfate, 120 mg bismuth subnitrite, and 120 mg cerium oxalate

Bismuth^R, belladonna and phenobarbital (Bernard)—Capsule containing $\frac{1}{4}$ gr phenobarbital, 5 gr bismuth subgallate, and $\frac{1}{8}$ gr extract belladonna leaf

Cafergot^R P-P (Sandoz)—Tablet containing 30 mg phenobarbital sodium, 1 mg ergotamine tartrate, 100 mg caffeine, and 0.125 mg levorotatory alkaloids of belladonna

Cal-Ma-Phen^R (Physicians Supply)—Tablet containing $\frac{1}{4}$ gr phenobarbital, 5 gr calcium-carbonate, 5 gr magnesium hydroxide, and $\frac{1}{300}$ gr atropine sulfate

Cantil^R w/phenobarbital (Lakeside)—Tablet containing 16 mg phenobarbital and 25 mg mepenzolate bromide

Carbonates^R No. 3 w/phenobarbital and atropine (Noyes)—Tablet containing 8 mg phenobarbital, 0.11 mg atropine sulfate, 224 mg calcium carbonate, 160 mg magnexium carbonate, and 32 mg bismuth subcarbonate

Cardalin-Phen^R (Mallinckrodt)—Tablet containing $\frac{1}{4}$ gr phenobarbital, 5 gr aminophylline, $2\frac{1}{2}$ gr aluminum hydroxide gel, dried, and $\frac{1}{2}$ gr benzocaine

Cardilate^R-P (Burroughs-Wellcome)—Tablet containing 15 mg phenobarbital and 10 mg erythrityl tetranitrate

Cholan^R HMB (Pennwalt)—Tablet, pink, containing 8 mg phenobarbital, 250 mg dehydrocholic acid, and 2.5 mg bromatropine methylbromide

Cold Preparation^R, special (Knight)—Tablet containing 8.1 mg phenobarbital, 2 mg chlorpheniramine maleate, 60 mg pseudoephedrine hydrochloride, and 300 mg salicylamide, powder

Dactil^R w/phenobarbital (Lakeside)—Tablet containing 16 mg phenobarbital and 50 mg piperidolate hydrochloride

Dainite-KI^R (Mallinckrodt)—Tablet containing $\frac{1}{4}$ gr phenobarbital, 3 gr aminophylline, $\frac{1}{4}$ gr ephedrine hydrochloride, 5 gr potassium iodide, $2\frac{1}{2}$ gr aluminum hydroxide gel, dried, and $\frac{1}{4}$ gr benzocaine

Dainite[R] Night (Mallinckrodt)—Tablet containing $\frac{3}{8}$ gr phenobarbital, $\frac{1}{2}$ gr pentobarbital sodium, 4 gr aminophylline, $2\frac{1}{2}$ gr aluminum hydroxide gel, dried, and $\frac{1}{4}$ gr benzocaine

Daricon[R] PB (Pfizer)—Tablet containing 15 mg phenobarbital and 6 mg oxyphencyclimine hydrochloride

Dilantin[R] w/phenobarbital (Parke-Davis)—Capsule containing $\frac{1}{4}$ gr phenobarbital and 0.1 g diphenylhydantoin sodium

Donabarb[R] (Elder)—Tablet containing $\frac{1}{4}$ gr phenobarbital and $\frac{1}{8}$ gr powder extract belladonna

Donaphen[R] new special donaphen (Krone)—Tablet containing 15 mg phenobarbital, 0.024 mg atropine sulfate, 0.0072 mg scopolamine hydrobromide, and 0.128 mg hyoscyamine hydrobromide

Donna-Sed[R] elixir (North America)—Elixir (5 cc) containing 16.2 mg phenobarbital, 0.1038 mg hyoscyamine hydrobromide, 0.0194 mg atropine sulfate, and 0.0065 mg hyoscine hydrobromide

Donnasep[R] (Robins)—Tablet containing 8.1 mg phenobarbital, 50.0 mg phenazopyridine hydrochloride, 500 mg methenamine mandelate, 0.0519 hyoscyamine sulfate, 0.0097 mg atropine sulfate, and 0.0033 mg hyoscine hydrobromide

Donnatal[R] (Robins)—Tablet, white, containing 16.2 mg phenobarbital, 0.1037 mg hyoscyamine sulfate, 0.0194 mg atropine sulfate, and 0.0065 mg hyoscine hydrobromide; elixir, green, each teaspoon (5 ml) containing same as tablets; tablet, green, containing 32.4 mg phenobarbital and belladonna alkaloids as in white tablets

Donnatal[R] Plus (Robins)—Tablet, green, containing 16.2 mg phenobarbital, belladonna alkaloids as in Donnatal[R], and vitamins; elixir, honey-colored, each teaspoon (5 ml) containing equivalent of one tablet

Donphen[R] (Lemmon)—Tablet containing 15 mg phenobarbital, 0.1 mg hyoscyamine sulfate, 0.02 mg atropine sulfate, and 8 μg scopolamine hydrobromide

Dormital-HM[R] (Buffington's)—Tablet containing $\frac{1}{4}$ gr phenobarbital, $\frac{1}{84}$ gr homatropine methylbromide, and 1 gr strontium bromide

Drostrate[R] (Marion)—Capsule, black and light green, containing 45 mg phenobarbital and 30 mg pentaerythritol tetranitrate; capsule, black and light orange, containing 48.8 mg phenobarbital and 45 mg pentaerythritol tetranitrate

Dynapin[R] w/phenobarbital (Key)—Tablet containing 15 mg phenobarbital, 0.5 mg nitroglycerin, and 15 mg pentaerythritol tetranitrate

Elmaloin[R] w/phenobarbital (Elder)—Capsule containing 15 mg phenobarbital and $1\frac{1}{2}$ gr diphenylhydantoin

Ephedrine[R] and sodium phenobarbital (Vale)—Tablet containing $\frac{1}{4}$ gr sodium phenobarbital and $\frac{3}{8}$ gr ephedrine sulfate

Ephedrine^R sulfate and phenobarbital (Zemmer)—Tablet containing 15 mg phenobarbital and 25 mg ephedrine sulfate

Ephedrine^R w/phenobarbital (Noyes)—Tablet containing $\frac{1}{4}$ gr phenobarbital and $\frac{3}{8}$ gr ephedrine sulfate

Ercafital^R (Blue Line)—Tablet containing 7.5 mg phenobarbital, 0.5 mg ergotamine tartrate, and 60 mg caffeine

Eu-Phed-Amin^R (Warren-Teed)—Tablet containing 30 mg phenobarbital, 0.1 g aminophylline, 30 mg ephedrine sulfate, and 0.1 g extract euphorbia

Eu-Phed-Ital^R (Warren-Teed)—Tablet containing 30 mg phenobarbital sodium, 30 mg ephedrine sulfate, and 0.12 g extract euphorbia

Fensobel^R (U.S. Vitamin & Pharmaceutical)—Tablet containing 8.1 mg phenobarbital, 2.95 mg belladonna extract, 63 mg aluminum hydrochloride gel, dried, 63 mg magnesium trisilicate, 32.5 mg bismuth subcarbonate, 252 mg magnesium carbonate, 203.5 mg precipitated calcium carbonate, 12.5 mg malt diastase, and 3 mg peppermint oil

Franol^R (Winthrop)—Tablet containing 8 mg phenobarbital, 130 mg theophylline, and 32 mg benzylephedrine hydrochloride

Gaysal^R (Geriatric)—Tablet containing 4 mg phenobarbital, 8 mg secobarbital, 300 mg sodium salicylate, 180 mg acetaminophen, and 60 mg aluminum hydroxide

Gustase-Plus^R (Geriatric)—Tablet containing 8.1 mg phenobarbital, 2.5 mg bromatropine methylbromide, 30 mg gerilase, 6 mg geriprotase, and 2 mg gericellulase

Homapin^R (Mission)—Tablets: Orange, containing 16 mg phenobarbital and 5 mg homatropine methylbromide; tablets, pink, containing 16 mg phenobarbital and 10 mg homatropine methylbromide; wafer (liquitab), pink, containing 8 mg phenobarbital and 3 mg homatropine methylbromide

H-P-A^R (modified) (Paine)—Tablet containing $\frac{1}{4}$ gr phenobarbital, 5 gr aspirin, and $\frac{1}{8}$ gr extract hyoscyamus

Hybephen^R (Massengill)—Tablet containing 15 mg phenobarbital, 0.1277 mg hyoscyamine sulfate, 0.0233 mg atropine sulfate, and 0.0094 mg hyoscine hydrobromide; elixir (5 cc) containing 15 mg phenobarbital, 0.1277 mg hyoscyamine sulfate, 0.0233 mg atropine sulfate, and 0.0094 mg hyoscine hydrobromide

Hytrona^R (Pitman-Moore)—Elixir (5 cc) containing 16 mg phenobarbital and 0.2 mg belladonna alkaloids; tablet containing 16 mg phenobarbital and 0.2 mg belladonna alkaloids

Iso-Asminyl^R (Cole)—Tablet containing 8 mg phenobarbital, 10 mg isoproterenol hydrochloride, 32 mg ephedrine sulfate, and 130 mg theophylline

Isordil^R w/phenobarbital (Ives)—Tablet containing 15 mg phenobarbital and 10 mg isosorbide dinitrate

Isufranol[R] (Winthrop)—Tablet containing 8 mg phenobarbital, 130 mg theophylline, 32 mg benzylephedrine, and 10 mg isoproterenol hydrochloride; tablet containing 8 mg phenobarbital, 130 mg theophylline, 32 mg benzylephedrine, and 5 mg isoproterenol hydrochloride

Isuprel[R] compound elixir (Winthrop)—Elixir (15 cc) containing 6 mg phenobarbital, 2.5 mg isoproterenol hydrochloride, 12 mg ephedrine sulfate, 45 mg theophylline, and 150 mg potassium iodide

Kaphebel[R] (Elder)—Tablet containing $\frac{1}{8}$ gr phenobarbital, $\frac{1}{4}$ gr belladonna root, and $7\frac{1}{2}$ gr kaolin colloidal

Kavatrate[R] (Key)—Tablet containing $\frac{1}{4}$ gr phenobarbital sodium, $\frac{1}{4}$ gr veratrum veride, $\frac{1}{2}$ gr mistletoe, 30 minims hawthorn tincture, and 1 gr sodium nitrite

Kie[R] w/phenobarbital (Laser)—Tablet containing 16 mg phenobarbital, 400 mg potassium iodide, and 24 mg ephedrine sulfate

Kinesed[R] (Stuart)—Tablet, orange, oval, fruit flavored, containing 16 mg phenobarbital, 0.1 mg hyoscyamine sulfate, 0.02 mg atropine sulfate, 0.007 mg scopolamine hydrobromide, and 40 mg simethicone

Kiophyllin[R] (Searle)—Tablet containing 15 mg phenobarbital, 150 mg aminophyllin, and 125 mg potassium iodide

Leosin[R] (Kremers-Urban)—Tablets: pink, scored, containing 15 mg phenobarbital and 0.125 mg hyoscyamine sulfate; elixir: red, raspberry flavored, each teaspoon (5 ml) containing 15 mg phenobarbital and 0.125 mg hyoscyamine sulfate; ampules, each 1 ml containing 15 mg phenobarbital and 0.25 mg hyoscyamine sulfate; capsule: pink and clear, containing 45 mg phenobarbital and 0.375 mg hyoscyamine sulfate

Levsin[R] w/phenobarbital (Kremers-Urban)—Tablet containing 0.125 mg hyoscyamine sulfate and 15 mg phenobarbital; elixir, each teaspoon (5 ml) containing 0.125 mg hyoscyamine sulfate and 15 mg phenobarbital; drops, 15 ml, cherry flavored, red, containing 0.125 mg hyoscyamine sulfate and 15 mg phenobarbital; injection, each 1 ml containing 0.25 mg hyoscyamine and 15 mg phenobarbital

Levsinex[R] w/phenobarbital (Kremers-Urban)—Capsule, brown and clear, containing 0.375 mg hyoscyamine sulfate and 45 mg phenobarbital

Luftodil[R] suspension (Mallinckrodt)—Suspension (5 cc) containing 8 mg phenobarbital, 50 mg theophylline, 12 mg ephedrine hydrochloride, and 100 mg glyceryl guaiacolate; tablet containing 16 mg phenobarbital, 100 mg theophylline, 24 mg ephedrine hydrochloride, and 200 mg glyceryl guaiacolate

Lufyllin-EP[R] (Mallinckrodt)—Tablet containing 16 mg phenobarbital, 100 mg glyphylline (dyphylline), and 16 mg ephedrine hydrochloride

Magnesium hydroxide-phenobarbital compound[R] (McNeil)—Tablet containing 15 mg phenobarbital sodium, 300 mg magnesium hydroxide, and 0.12 mg atropine sulfate with aromatics

Malglyn[R] compound (Brayten)—Tablet or suspension (5 cc) containing 16.2 mg phenobarbital, 0.162 mg belladonna alkaloids, and 0.5 g dihydroxy aluminum aminoacetate

Manniphen[R] (Vale)—Tablet containing 16 mg phenobarbital and 32 mg mannitol hexanitrate; tablet containing 16 mg phenobarbital, 32 mg mannitol hexanitrate, and 20 mg rutin

Mannitol[R] hexanitrate w/phenobarbital (Blue Line)—Tablet containing $\frac{1}{4}$ gr phenobarbital and $\frac{1}{2}$ gr mannitol hexanitrate

Mannitol[R] hexanitrate w/phenobarbital (Noyes)—Tablet containing $\frac{1}{4}$ gr phenobarbital and $\frac{1}{2}$ gr mannitol hexanitrate

Matropinal[R] (Comatic)—Elixir, pink, each teaspoon (5 ml) containing 9 mg phenobarbital, 10 mg homatropine methylbromide, and 0.5 mg chlorpheniramine maleate; tablet containing 8 mg phenobarbital, 10 mg homatropine methylbromide, and 12 mg pyrilamine maleate

Maxitol[R] (Burt Krone)—Tablet containing 15 mg phenobarbital, 15 mg mannitol hexanitrate, 15 mg rutin, and 15 mg ascorbic acid

Meprane[R] phenobarbital (Reed & Carnrick)—Tablet containing 16 mg phenobarbital and 1 mg promethestrol dipropionate

Mesopin[R] PB (Endo)—Tablet or elixir (5 cc) containing 15 mg phenobarbital and 5 mg homatropine methylbromide

Mexal[R] (Massengill)—Tablet containing 16 mg phenobarbital and 32 mg mannitol hexanitrate

Mudrane[R] (Poythress)—Tablet containing 21 mg phenobarbital, 195 mg potassium iodide, 130 mg aminophylline, and 16 mg ephedrine hydrochloride; elixir (5 cc) containing 5.4 mg phenobarbital, 20 mg theophylline, 4 mg ephedrine hydrochloride, and 26 mg glyceryl guaiacolate

Natrona[R] compound (Zemmer)—Tablet containing 15 mg phenobarbital, 30 mg extract hawthorn berries, 15 mg extract mistletoe, 60 mg sodium nitrite, and 0.2 g sodium bicarbonate

Neocholan[R] (Pitman-Moore)—Tablet containing 8 mg phenobarbital, 250 mg dehydrocholic acid, 15 mg bile extract, and 1.2 mg homatropine methylbromide

Nergestic[R] (Massengill)—Tablet containing 8 mg phenobarbital, 0.10 mg atropine sulfate, and 0.5 g magnesium trisilicate

Nophesan[R] (Noyes)—Tablet containing 8 mg phenobarbital and 300 mg acetylsalicylic acid

Novalene[R] (Lemmon)—Tablet containing 16 mg phenobarbital, 24 mg ephedrine sulfate, 162 mg potassium iodide, and 162 mg calcium lactate

Oxsorbil-PB[R] (Ives)—Capsule containing 7.5 mg phenobarbital, 7.5 mg belladonna extract, 32 mg dehydrochloric acid, 32 mg desoxycholic acid, or 65 mg bile extract, 160 mg sorbitan monooleate, and 180 mg oleic acid

Paminal[R] (Upjohn)—Elixir (5 cc) containing 8 mg phenobarbital and 1.25 mg methscopolamine bromide

Pamine[R] PB (Upjohn)—Elixir (5 cc) containing 8 mg phenobarbital and 1.25 mg methscopolamine bromide

Pamine[R] PB, half strength (Upjohn)—Tablet containing 8 mg phenobarbital and 1.25 methscopolamine bromide

Pediatric Piptal[R] antipyretic (Lakeside)—Solution (0.6 cc) containing 3 mg phenobarbital, 5 mg pipenzolate bromide, and 60 mg acetaminophen

Pediatric Piptal[R] w/phenobarbital (Lakeside)—Solution (0.5 cc) containing 3 mg phenobarbital and 2 mg pipenzolate bromide

Pencetylon[R] (Elder)—Tablet containing $\frac{1}{4}$ gr phenobarbital and 5 gr acetylsalicylic acid

Pentaerythritol tetranitrate[R] w/phenobarbital (Noyes)—Tablet containing 16 mg phenobarbital and 10 mg pentaerythritol tetranitrate; tablet containing 16 mg phenobarbital and 20 mg pentaerythritol tetranitrate

Pentratrol[R] w/phenobarbital (North American)—Tablet containing 15 mg phenobarbital and 10 mg pentaerythritol tetranitrate

Peribar[R] L-A No. 1 (Whittier)—Tablet containing 48.6 mg phenobarbital and 30 mg pentaerythritol tetranitrate

Peritrate[R] w/phenobarbital (Warner-Chilcott)—Tablet containing 15 mg phenobarbital and 10 mg pentaerythritol tetranitrate; tablet containing 15 mg phenobarbital and 20 mg pentaerythritol tetranitrate; tablet containing 45 mg phenobarbital and 80 mg pentaerythritol tetranitrate

Phenaphen[R] plus (Robins)—Tablet containing 16.2 mg phenobarbital, 194 mg phenacetin, 162 mg aspirin, 0.031 mg hyoscyamine sulfate, 12.5 mg pheniramine maleate, and 10 mg phenylephrine hydrochloride

Phenobarbital[R] and atropine (Blue Line)—Tablet containing $\frac{1}{4}$ gr phenobarbital and $\frac{1}{500}$ gr atropine sulfate

Phenobarbital[R] and atropine (Meyers)—Tablet containing $\frac{1}{4}$ gr phenobarbital and $\frac{1}{500}$ gr atropine sulfate

Phenobarbital[R] and atropine (Paine)—Tablet containing $\frac{1}{4}$ gr phenobarbital and $\frac{1}{500}$ gr atropine sulfate

Phenobarbital[R] and atropine (Vale)—Tablet containing $\frac{1}{4}$ gr phenobarbital and $\frac{1}{250}$ gr atropine sulfate

Phenobarbital[R] and atropine No. 1 (Pitman-Moore)—Tablet containing 16 mg phenobarbital and 0.13 mg atropine sulfate

Phenobarbital[R] and atropine No. 2 (Pitman-Moore)—Tablet containing 8 mg phenobarbital and 0.65 mg atropine sulfate

Phenobarbital[R] w/atropine sulfate (Zemmer)—Tablet containing 8 mg phenobarbital and 0.06 mg atropine sulfate

Phenobarbital^R w/atropine sulfate (Zemmer)—Tablet containing 15 mg phenobarbital and 0.12 mg atropine sulfate

Phenobarbital^R and atropine sulfate (Buffington)—Tablet containing $\frac{1}{4}$ gr phenobarbital and $\frac{1}{200}$ gr atropine sulfate

Phenobarbital^R and atropine tablets (Noyes)—Tablet containing 8 mg phenobarbital and $\frac{1}{1000}$ gr atropine sulfate; tablet containing 16 mg phenobarbital and $\frac{1}{500}$ gr atropine sulfate

Phenobarbital^R and atropine tablets No. 2 (Noyes)—Tablet containing $\frac{1}{4}$ gr phenobarbital and $\frac{1}{200}$ gr atropine sulfate

Phenobarbital^R and atropine tablets No. 3 (Noyes)—Tablet containing $\frac{1}{2}$ gr phenobarbital and $\frac{1}{300}$ gr atropine sulfate

Phenobarbital^R and belladonna (Vale)—Tablet containing $\frac{1}{4}$ gr phenobarbital and $\frac{1}{2}$ gr belladonna leaves (total alkaloids 0.0015 gr)

Phenobarbital^R and belladonna (Lilly)—Tablet containing 16 mg phenobarbital and 8 mg belladonna extract

Phenobarbital^R and belladonna (Paine)—Tablet containing $\frac{1}{4}$ gr phenobarbital and $\frac{1}{8}$ gr belladonna extract

Phenobarbital^R and belladonna No. 2 (Upjohn)—Tablet containing $\frac{1}{4}$ gr phenobarbital and $\frac{1}{8}$ gr belladonna extract (alkaloids 0.00156 gr)

Phenobarbital^R w/mannitol hexanitrate (Elder)—Tablet containing 7.5 mg phenobarbital, 15 mg mannitol hexanitrate, 25 mg ascorbic acid powder, and 25 mg rutin

Phenobarbital^R and mannitol hexanitrate (Meyer)—Tablet containing $\frac{1}{4}$ gr phenobarbital and $\frac{1}{2}$ gr mannitol hexanitrate

Phenobarbital^R sodium atropine No. 1 (McNeil)—Tablet containing 8 mg phenobarbital sodium and 60 μg atropine sulfate

Phenobarbital^R sodium atropine No. 2 (McNeil)—Tablet containing 15 mg phenobarbital sodium and 120 μg atropine sulfate

Phenobarbital^R sodium atropine No. 3 (McNeil)—Tablet containing 20 mg phenobarbital sodium and 200 μg atropine sulfate

Phenobarbital^R and sodium nitrite (Noyes)—Tablet containing $\frac{1}{4}$ gr phenobarbital and 1 gr sodium nitrite

Phenobarbital^R theocalcin (Knoll)—Tablet containing 15 mg phenobarbital and 0.5 g theobromide calcium salicylate

Phenodonna^R tablets (Flint)—Tablet containing $\frac{1}{4}$ gr phenobarbital and 6 minims tincture belladonna

Phenodrox^R (North American)—Tablet containing $\frac{1}{4}$ gr phenobarbital, $\frac{1}{500}$ gr atropine sulfate, 4 gr magnesium trisilicate, and 4 gr aluminum hydroxide gel, dried

Phyldrox^R (Lemmon)—Tablet containing 15 mg phenobarbital, 100 mg neothylline, and 25 mg ephedrine sulfate

Piptal[R] PHB (Lakeside)—Elixir (5 cc) containing 16 mg phenobarbital and 5 mg pipenzolate bromide

Prantal[R] w/phenobarbital (Schering)—Tablet containing 16 mg phenobarbital and 100 mg diphemanil methylsulfate

Premarin[R] w/phenobarbital (Ayerst)—Tablet containing 32 mg phenobarbital and 6.626 mg conjugated estrogense-equin

Probanthine[R] w/phenobarbital (Searle)—Tablet containing 15 mg phenobarbital and 15 mg probanthine

Probital[R] (Searle)—Tablet containing 15 mg phenobarbital and 7.5 mg probanthine

Propenite[R] (Zemmer)—Tablet containing 12 mg phenobarbital sodium, 60 mg sodium nitrite, 120 mg hawthorn berries extract, and 60 mg mistletoe extract

Prydonnal[R] spansule (Smith & French)—Capsule containing 65 mg phenobarbital, 0.4 mg belladonna alkaloids, 0.305 mg hyoscyamine sulfate, 0.06 mg atropine sulfate, and 0.035 mg scopolamine hydrobromide

Quadrinal[R] (Knoll)—Tablet containing 24 mg phenobarbital, 24 mg ephedrine hydrochloride, 130 mg theophylline calcium salicylate, and 300 mg potassium iodide; suspension (5 cc) containing 12 mg phenobarbital, 12 mg ephedrine hydrochloride, 65 mg theophylline calcium salicylate, and 160 mg potassium iodide

Quintrate[R] w/nitroglycerin and phenobarbital (Elder)—Tablet containing 15 mg phenobarbital and 20 mg pentaerythritol tetranitrate and 0.4 mg nitroglycerin

Quintrate[R] w/phenobarbital (Elder)—Tablet containing 15 mg phenobarbital and 10 mg pentaerythritol tetranitrate; tablet containing 15 mg phenobarbital and 20 mg pentaerythritol tetranitrate

Robinul-PH[R] (Robins)—Tablet containing 16.2 mg phenobarbital and 1.0 mg glycopyrrolate

Robinul-PH[R] forte (Robins)—Tablet containing 16.2 mg phenobarbital and 2.0 mg glycopyrrolate

Ruhexatal[R] (Lemmon)—Tablet containing 15 mg phenobarbital, 30 mg mannitol hexanitrate, 10 mg ascorbic acid, and 20 mg rutin

Rutol[R] (Pitman-Moore)—Tablet containing 8 mg phenobarbital, 16 mg mannitol hexanitrate, and 10 mg rutin

Salisil[R] w/phenobarbital (Elder)—Tablet containing $\frac{1}{4}$ gr phenobarbital, 5 gr acetylsalicyclic acid, and 2 gr magnesium trisilicate

Selbella[R] (Wyeth)—Tablet containing $\frac{1}{8}$ gr phenobarbital, 5 gr aluminum hydroxide, and $\frac{1}{8}$ gr belladonna extract

Sodium nitrite[R] w/phenobarbital (Buffalo)—Tablet containing $\frac{1}{2}$ gr phenobarbital and 1 gr sodium nitrite

Sodium nitrite[R] w/phenobarbital (Paine)—Tablet containing $\frac{1}{8}$ gr phenobarbital, 1 gr sodium nitrite, 2 gr sodium bicarbonate, and $\frac{1}{4}$ minim hawthorn berries, fluid extract

Spasticol[R] PB (Key)—Tablet containing 15 mg phenobarbital and 2.5 mg homatropine methylbromide

Spastosed[R] (North American)—Tablet containing 8 mg phenobarbital, 0.13 mg atropine sulfate, 227 mg calcium carbonate, and 162 mg magnesium hydroxide

TCS[R] (Poythress)—Tablet containing 16 mg phenobarbital, 0.4 g theobromine salicylate, and 0.06 g calcium salicylate

Tedral[R] SA (Warner-Chilcott)—Tablet containing 25 mg phenobarbital, 180 mg theophylline, and 48 mg ephedrine hydrochloride

Tensodin[R] (Knoll)—Tablet containing 15 mg phenobarbital, 30 mg ethaverine hydrochloride, and 200 mg theophylline calcium salicylate

Tensophen[R] (Noyes)—Tablet containing 16 mg phenobarbital, 0.26 mg nitroglycerin, 32 mg sodium nitrite, 1 mg podophyllin, and 16 mg extract beef bile

Thedrizem[R] (Zemmer)—Tablet containing 8 mg phenobarbital, 100 mg theophylline, and 25 mg ephedrine hydrochloride

Theobarb[R] (Mallinckrodt)—Tablet containing 32 mg phenobarbital and 325 mg theobromine

Theobarb[R]-R (Mallinckrodt)—Tablet containing 10 mg phenobarbital, 0.1 mg reserpine, and 324 mg theobromine

Theobarb[R] Special (Mallinckrodt)—Tablet containing 16 mg phenobarbital and 325 mg theobromine

Theobromine[R] and phenobarbital (Noyes)—Tablet containing 16 mg phenobarbital and 0.3 gm theobromine

Theobromine-phenobarbital[R] (Massengill)—Tablet containing 32 mg phenobarbital and 0.3 gm theobromine

Theobromine-phenobarbital[R] (Upjohn)—Tablet containing 32 mg phenobarbital and 324 mg theobromine

Theobromine-phenobarbital[R] compound (Upjohn)—Tablet containing $\frac{1}{4}$ gr phenobarbital, $2\frac{1}{2}$ gr theobromine, $2\frac{1}{2}$ gr potassium iodide, and 2 gr potassium bicarbonate

Theobromine[R] w/phenobarbital No. 1 (Buffington)—Tablet containing 15 mg phenobarbital and 324 mg theobromine

Theobromine[R] and sodium acetate w/phenobarbital (Elder)—Tablet containing $\frac{1}{4}$ gr phenobarbital and 3 gr theobromine and sodium acetate

Theobromine[R] sodium salicylate w/phenobarbital (Zemmer)—Tablet containing 15 mg phenobarbital and 300 mg theobromine sodium salicylate

Theocardone[R] No. 1 (Haack)—Tablet containing 15 mg phenobarbital and 300 mg theobromine

Theocardone^R No. 2 (Haack)—Tablet containing 30 mg phenobarbital and 300 mg theobromine

Theodide^R (Vale)—Tablet containing $\frac{1}{4}$ gr phenobarbital, $2\frac{1}{2}$ gr potassium iodide, and $2\frac{1}{2}$ gr theobromine sodium salicylate

Theoglycinate^R w/phenobarbital (Brayten)—Tablet containing 16 mg phenobarbital and 324 mg theophylline-sodium glycinate

Theoglycinate^R w/racephedrine and phenobarbital (Brayten)—Tablet containing 324 mg theophylline-sodium glycinate and 24 mg racephedrine hydrochloride

Theominal^R (Winthrop)—Tablet containing 32 mg phenobarbital and 320 mg theobromine

Theominal^R M (Winthrop)—Tablet containing 16 mg phenobarbital and 320 mg theobromine

Theominal^R RS (Winthrop)—Tablet containing 10 mg phenobarbital, 320 mg theobromine, and 1.5 mg alseroxylon

Theophen^R (Vale)—Tablet containing $\frac{1}{4}$ gr phenobarbital, 5 gr theobromine sodium salicylate, and $2\frac{1}{2}$ gr calcium carbonate

Theoplaphen^R (Massengill)—Tablet containing 15 mg phenobarbital, 0.2 g theobromine sodium salicylate, and 0.1 mg calcium lactate

Theorate^R (Whittier)—Tablet containing 16.2 mg phenobarbital and 324 mg theobromine

Thymodyne^R (Noyes)—Tablet containing 32 mg phenobarbital, 130 mg theophylline anhydrous, and 24 mg ephedrine sulfate

Tral^R w/phenobarbital (Abbott)—Tablets: "Filmtab," lavender, containing 25 mg hexocyclium methylsulfate and 15 mg phenobarbital; "gradumet," blue, containing 50 mg hexocyclium methylsulfate and 30 mg phenobarbital

Trasentine^R w/phenobarbital (Ciba)—Tablet, yellow, sugar-coated, containing 50 mg adiphenine hydrochloride and 20 mg phenobarbital

Tricoloid^R (Burroughs Wellcome)—Tablet containing 16 mg phenobarbital and 50 mg tricyclamol chloride

Triophen^R (Vale)—Tablet containing $\frac{1}{8}$ gr phenobarbital, $\frac{1}{500}$ gr atropine sulfate, and 7 gr magnesium trisilicate

Trocinate^R w/phenobarbital (Poythress)—Tablet containing 16 mg phenobarbital and 100 mg thiphenamil hydrochloride

Valpin-PB^R (Endo)—Tablet or elixir (5 cc) containing 8 mg phenobarbital and 10 mg anisotropine methylbromide

Veralzem^R (Zemmer)—Tablet containing 15 mg phenobarbital, 50 mg veratrum viride, and 60 mg sodium nitrite

Veratrite^R (Neisler)—Tablet containing $\frac{1}{4}$ gr phenobarbital, 40 CSR (carotid sinus reflex) units cryptenamine, and 1 gr sodium nitrite

Veritag^R (Tutag)—Tablet containing 16 mg phenobarbital, 40 mg veratrum viride, and 65 mg sodium nitrite

Vertegus^R (Krone)—Tablet containing $\frac{1}{4}$ gr phenobarbital, $\frac{3}{4}$ gr veratrum viride, 1 gr sodium nitrite, $\frac{1}{2}$ gr mistletoe, and $\frac{1}{2}$ gr hawthorn berries

Veruphen^R (Zemmer)—Tablet containing 15 mg phenobarbital, 20 mg rutin, 15 mg veratrum viride, and 60 mg sodium nitrite

Viritin^R (Lemmon)—Tablet containing 15 mg phenobarbital, 30 mg mannitol hexanitrate, 1.5 mg veratrum viride alkaloids, and 20 mg rutin

Wesmatic^R (Wesley)—Tablet, green and white, layered, containing 8 mg phenobarbital, 2 mg ephedrine sulfate, and 16 mg chlorpheniramine maleate; tablet (Forte), capsule-shaped, containing 8 mg phenobarbital, 2 mg ephedrine sulfate, 16 mg chlorpheniramine maleate, and 100 mg glyceryl guaiacolate

W-T^R (Warren-Teed)—Powder (4 g) containing 15 mg phenobarbital, 10 mg belladonna extract (0.12 mg belladonna alkaloids), 15 mg benzocaine, 1.55 g calcium carbonate, 0.5 g magnesium oxide, and 60 mg aluminum hydroxide gel, dried; tablet containing $\frac{1}{16}$ gr phenobarbital, $\frac{1}{24}$ gr belladonna extract, $\frac{1}{16}$ gr benzocaine, 6 gr calcium carbonate, $3\frac{3}{4}$ gr magnesium trisilicate, $2\frac{1}{2}$ gr aluminum hydroxide gel, dried, and 1% chlorophyll extract

Xaniophen^R (Pitman-Moore)—Tablet containing 16.2 mg phenobarbital, 162 mg theobromine, and 32.4 mg ethylenediamine dihydriodide

Zallogen^R compound (Massengill)—Tablet containing 8 mg phenobarbital, 75 mg tocamphyl, and 2.5 mg homatropine methylbromide

No. 23 (Stayner)—Tablet containing $\frac{1}{2}$ gr phenobarbital and 3 gr aminophylline

No. 35 (Stayner)—Tablet containing $\frac{1}{8}$ gr phenobarbital, 1.5 gr aminophylline, and $\frac{3}{8}$ gr ephedrine sulfate

No. 65 (Stayner)—Tablet containing $\frac{1}{4}$ gr phenobarbital and $\frac{1}{4}$ gr extract belladonna

No. 66 (Stayner)—Tablet containing $\frac{1}{4}$ gr phenobarbital and $\frac{1}{4}$ gr extract belladonna

No. 75 (Bariatric)—Tablet containing $\frac{1}{4}$ gr phenobarbital and $\frac{1}{8}$ gr belladonna

No. 88 (Stayner)—Tablet containing $\frac{1}{4}$ gr phenobarbital and 1.5 gr aminophylline

No. 89 (Stayner)—Tablet containing $\frac{1}{2}$ gr phenobarbital and 1.5 gr aminophylline

No. 111 (Stayner)—Tablet containing $\frac{1}{2}$ gr phenobarbital and $\frac{3}{8}$ gr ephedrine sulfate

No. 136 (Stayner)—Tablet containing 20 mg phenobarbital and 5 mg homatropine methylbromide

No. 643 (Stayner)—Tablet containing $\frac{1}{8}$ gr phenobarbital, 2 gr theophylline, and $\frac{3}{8}$ gr ephedrine hydrochloride

Rx No. 4104 (Zemmer)—Tablet containing $\frac{1}{4}$ gr phenobarbital, $7\frac{1}{2}$ gr calcium carbonate, 4 gr magnesium oxide, and $\frac{1}{300}$ gr atropine sulfate

Rx No. 4105 (Zemmer)—Tablet containing $\frac{1}{4}$ gr phenobarbital, 10 gr calcium carbonate, and $\frac{1}{300}$ gr atropine sulfate

Rx No. 4108 (Zemmer)—Capsule containing $\frac{1}{4}$ gr phenobarbital, $\frac{1}{300}$ gr atropine sulfate, $6\frac{1}{2}$ gr calcium carbonate, and 2 gr magnesium oxide, heavy

Rx No. 4123 (Zemmer)—Capsule containing $\frac{1}{4}$ gr phenobarbital, 5 gr bismuth subgallate, and $\frac{1}{8}$ gr extract belladonna

Rx No. 4134 (Zemmer)—Capsule containing $\frac{1}{4}$ gr phenobarbital, 1.5 gr aminophylline, and 1 gr potassium iodide

Rx No. 4152 (Zemmer)—Tablet containing $\frac{1}{4}$ gr phenobarbital and $\frac{1}{200}$ gr atropine sulfate

Rx No. 4155 (Zemmer)—Tablet containing $\frac{1}{8}$ gr phenobarbital, $\frac{1}{1000}$ gr atropine sulfate, $3\frac{3}{4}$ gr aluminum hydroxide, and $3\frac{3}{4}$ gr kaolin

Rx No. 4170 (Zemmer)—Tablet containing $\frac{1}{2}$ gr phenobarbital, $\frac{1}{200}$ gr atropine sulfate, and 10 gr calcium carbonate

Probarbital Preparations: None excepted.

Secobarbital Preparations

Buffadyne[R] w/barbiturates (Lemmon)—Tablet containing 8 mg secobarbital, 8 mg amobarbital, 300 mg aspirin, 150 mg phenacetin, 30 mg caffeine, 75 mg aluminum hydroxide, and 45 mg magnesium hydroxide

Carovas[R] Tymcaps (Amfre-Grant)—Capsule, orange and red, containing 50 mg secobarbital and 30 mg pentaerythritol tetranitrate

Gaysal[R] (Geriatric)—Tablet containing 8 mg secobarbital, 4 mg phenobarbital, 300 mg sodium salicylate, 180 mg acetaminophen, and 60 mg aluminum hydroxide

Nitrased[R] (Lemmon)—Tablet containing 15 mg secobarbital, 0.4 mg nitroglycerin, and 15 mg pentaerythritol tetranitrate

Sulfodiethylmethane Preparations: None excepted.

Sulfonethylmethane Preparations: None excepted.

Sulfonmethane Preparations: None excepted.

Thialbarbital Preparations: None excepted.

Thiamylal Preparations: None excepted.

Thiopental Preparations: None excepted.

Vinbarbital Preparations: None excepted.

7
Drug Isomers and Derivatives

SCHEDULE I (308.11)

Under Schedule I [308.11 (b)], the preface to the drug listings states that unless specifically excepted or unless listed in another schedule, any of the opiates listed in Schedule I include the isomers, esters, ethers, salts, and salts of the isomers, esters, and ethers of the opiates. Included in this listing are:

Acetylmethadol	Etoxeridine
Allylprodine	Furethidine
Alphacetylmethadol	Hydroxypethidine
Alphamethadol	Ketobemidone
Benzethidine	Levomoramide
Betacetylmethadol	Levophenacylmorphan
Betameprodine	Morpheridine
Betamethadol	Noracymethadol
Clonitazene	Norlevorphanol
Dextromoramide	Normethadone
Dextrorphan	Norpipanone
Diampromide	Phenadoxone
Diethylthiambutene	Phenampromide
Dimenoxadol	Phenomorphan
Dimepheptanol	Phenoperidine
Dimethylthiambutene	Piritramide
Dioxaphetylbutyrate	Proheptazine
Dipipanone	Properidine
Ethylmethylthiambutene	Racemoramide
Etonitazene	Trimeperidine

It should be noted that the term "opiate" is used to classify these drugs. This term is chemically incorrect, as the drugs listed above are synthetically produced and are not necessarily opiate derivatives. "Narcotic" would be a more appropriate term.

Following the opiates under Schedule I are the opium derivatives [308.11 (c)]. These include any of the opium derivatives listed below, and their salts, isomers, and salts of isomers, unless they are specifically excepted or listed in another schedule. Unlike the opiates, the opium derivatives exclude the esters, ethers, and salts of the esters and ethers.

Acetorphine	Hydromorphinol
Acetyldihydrocodeine	Methyldesorphine
Benzylmorphine	Methyldihydromorphine
Codeine methylbromide	Morphine methylbromide
Codeine-N-oxide	Morphine methylsulfonate
Cyprenorphine	Morphine-N-oxide
Desomorphine	Myrophine
Dihydromorphine	Nicocodeine
Drotebanol	Nicomorphine
Etorphine (except hydrochloride salt)	Normorphine
	Pholcodine
Heroin	Thebacon

The hallucinogenic substances [308.11 (d)] include any material, compound, mixture, or preparation that contains any quantity of the substances listed below, or any of their salts, isomers, and salts of their isomers, unless the substance is specifically excepted or listed in another schedule. For hallucinogenic substances only, the term "isomer" includes the optical, positional, and geometrical isomers. This designation implies a restriction on types of isomers included in other sections. It is unknown to these authors, however, what isomers would be excluded from the other sections.

4-Bromo-2,5-dimethoxyamphetamine
    (Some trade or other names: 4-bromo-2,5-dimethoxy-α-methyl-phenethylamine; 4-bromo-2,5-DMA)
2,5-Dimethoxyamphetamine
    (Some other names including 2,5-dimethoxy-α-methylphenethyl-amine; 2,5-DMA)
4-Methoxyamphetamine
    (Some other names including 4-methoxy-α-methylphenethyl-amine; paramethoxyamphetamine; PMA)
5-Methoxy-3,4-methylenedioxyamphetamine
4-Methyl-2,5-dimethoxyamphetamine
    (Some other names including 4-methyl-2,5-dimethoxy-α-methyl-phenethylamine; "DOM"; "STP")
3,4-Methylenedioxy amphetamine

3,4,5-Trimethoxy amphetamine
Bufotenine
  [Some other names including 3-(2-di-methylaminoethyl)-5-hydroxyindole; 3-(2-dimethylaminoethyl)-5-indolol; *N,N*-dimethylserotonin; 5-hydroxy-*N,N*-dimethyltryptamine; mappine]
Diethyltryptamine
  (Some other names including *N,N*-diethyltryptamine; DET)
Dimethyltryptamine
  (Some other names including DMT)
Ibogaine
  [Some other names including 7-ethyl-6,6,7,8,9,10,12,13-octa-hydro-2-methoxy-6,9-methano-5H-pyrido(1′,2′:1,2)azepino(5,4-b)indole; *Tabernanthe iboga*]
Lysergic acid diethylamide
Marijuana
Mescaline
Peyote
  (Meaning all parts of the plant presently classified botanically as *Lophophora williamsii* Lemaire, whether growing or not; the seeds thereof; any extract from any part of such plant; and every compound, manufacture, salt, derivative, mixture, or preparation of such plant, its seeds or extracts)
N-Ethyl-3-piperidyl benzilate
N-Methyl-3-piperidyl benzilate
Psilocybin
Psilocyn
Tetrahydrocannabinols
  (Synthetic equivalents of the substances contained in the plant, or in the resinous extractives of *Cannabis* sp. and/or synthetic substances, derivatives, and their isomers with similar chemical structure and pharmacological activity such as the following: 1 *cis* or *trans* tetrahydrocannabinol, and optical isomers; 6 *cis* or *trans* tetrahydrocannabinol, and their optical isomers; 3,4 *cis* or *trans* tetrahydrocannabinol, and its optical isomers)
    (Since nomenclature of these substances is not internationally standardized, compounds of these structures, regardless of numerical designation of atomic positions covered)
Thiophene analogue of phencyclidine
  [Some other names including 1-(1-(2-thienyl) cylohexyl) piperidine; 2-thienyl analog of phencyclidine; TPCP]

The depressants [308.11 (e)] include any material, compound, mixture, or preparation that contains any quantity of mecloqualone, its salts, isomers, and salts of its isomers, unless specifically excepted or listed in another schedule.

SCHEDULE II (308.12)

Under the substances from vegetable origin or chemical synthesis [308.12 (b)] is listed coca leaves. This includes any salt, compound, derivative, or preparation of coca leaves, and any salt, compound, derivative, or preparation thereof that is chemically equivalent to or identical with any of these substances. This does not include decocainized coca leaves or coca leaf extracts that do not contain cocaine or ecgonine. This implies that the naturally occurring isomer of cocaine is controlled only (see Cocaine in Chapter 9). Cocaine is specifically listed under "Basic Class" definition [301.02 (xiv)].

The opiates [308.12 (c)], as under Schedule I, include the isomers, esters, ethers, salts, and salts of isomers, esters, and ethers of the substances listed below, unless they are specifically excepted or listed in another schedule.

Alphaprodine
Anileridine
Benzitramide
Dihydrocodeine
Diphenoxylate
Fentanyl
Isomethadone
Levomethorphan
Levorphanol
Metazocine
Methadone
Methadone-intermediate,
    4-cyano-2-dimethylamino-
    4,4-diphenyl butane
Moramide-intermediate,
    2-methyl-3-morpholino-1,1-
    diphenylpropane-carboxylic
    acid

Pethidine
Pethidine-intermediate-A,
    4-cyano-1-methyl-4-
    phenylpiperidine
Pethidine-intermediate-B,
    ethyl-4-phenylpiperidine-4-
    carboxylate
Pethidine-intermediate-C,
    1-methyl-4-phenylpiperidine-
    4-carboxylic acid
Phenazocine
Piminodine
Racemethorphan
Racemorphan

The stimulants [308.12 (d)] include any material, compound, mixture, or preparation that contains any quantity of the substances listed below, unless they are specifically excepted or listed in another schedule.

Amphetamine, its salts, optical isomers, and salts of its optical isomers
Methamphetamine, its salts, isomers, and salts of its isomers
Phenmetrazine and its salts
Methylphenidate

The depressants [308.12 (e)] include any material, compound, mixture, or preparation that contains any quantity of the substances listed below, their salts, isomers, and salts of isomers, unless they are specifically excepted or listed in another schedule.

Methaqualone
Amobarbital
Secobarbital
Pentobarbital
Phencyclidine

SCHEDULE III (308.13)

The stimulants [308.13] include any material, compound, mixture, or preparation that contains any quantity of the substances listed below, their salts, isomers, and salts of their isomers, unless specifically excepted or listed in another schedule. Under this section, the term "isomer" includes optical, positional, or geometrical.

Benzphetamine
Chlorphentermine
Clortermine
Mazindol
Phendimetrazine

It should be noted here that the depressants [308.13 (c)] listed under Schedule III have no specific isomer designation.

SCHEDULE IV (308.14)

The depressants [308.14 (b)] include any material, compound, mixture, or preparation that contains any quantity of the substances listed below, their salts, isomers, and salts of their isomers. Under this section, the term "isomer" does not have any specific limitation.

Barbital	Mebutamate
Chloral betaine	Meprobamate
Chloral hydrate	Methohexital
Chlordiazepoxide	Methylphenobarbital
Clonazepam	Oxazepam
Clorazepate	Paraldehyde
Diazepam	Petrichloral
Ethchlorvynol	Phenobarbital
Ethinamate	Prazepam
Flurazepam	Propoxyphene

Under Schedule IV [308.14 (c)], fenfluramine is listed designating control of optical, positional, and geometrical isomers and salts of these isomers that may be included within any material, compound, mixture, or preparation in any quantity.

Under Schedule IV [308.14 (d)] are listed other stimulants, including:

> Diethylpropion
> Phentermine
> Pemoline

and the organometallic complexes and chelates of pemoline in any material, compound, mixture, or preparation containing any quantity of these substances unless they are specifically excepted. These include the salts, optical isomers, positional isomers, geometrical isomers, and the salts of these isomers.

SCHEDULE V (308.15)

Under Schedule V [308.15 (b)] are listed certain narcotic drugs containing nonnarcotic active medicinal ingredients. These narcotic drugs have no isomer designation and include any compound, mixture, or preparation containing any of the limited quantities of narcotic drugs listed below, or their salts, along with one or more nonnarcotic active medicinal ingredients in sufficient proportion to confer on the compound, mixture, or preparation valuable medicinal qualities other than those possessed by the narcotic drug alone:

1. Not more than 200 milligrams of codeine per 100 milliliters or per 100 grams
2. Not more than 100 milligrams of dihydrocodeine per 100 milliliters or per 100 grams
3. Not more than 100 milligrams of ethylmorphine per 100 milliliters or per 100 grams

4. Not more than 2.5 milligrams of diphenoxylate and not less than 25 micrograms of atropine sulfate per dosage unit
5. Not more than 100 milligrams of opium per 100 milliliters or per 100 grams

OPTICAL ISOMERS

Stereoisomers are identical compounds with the exception of having different three-dimensional structures that are not interchangeable. These three-dimensional structures are termed "configurational isomers." Stereo-isomerism includes both optical isomerism and geometrical isomerism.

An optically active substance is one that rotates the plane of polarized light. A pure optically active compound is nonsuperimposable on its mirror image. If a molecule is nonsuperimposable on its mirror image, then the two isomers (called "enantiomers") must be different molecules. The difference in structure is only in the left- and right-handedness (called "chirality") of their orientations. Enantiomers have identical chemical and physical properties, with two exceptions: (1) They rotate the plane of polarized light equally but in opposite directions. The isomer that rotates the plane of polarized light to the left is called the *levo* isomer and has a (−) designation. The isomer that rotates the plane of polarized light to the right is called the *dextro* isomer and has a (+) designation. (2) The second property is that the isomers react at different rates with optically active compounds. These rates may be so nearly equal that it is almost impossible to distinguish between them. However, one isomer may react at a reasonable rate while the other may be so slow that for all practical purposes, it may not react at all. It is for this latter reason that many medicinal substances and other biological compounds are physiochemically active while their enantiomers are not.

Thus, enantiomers have identical properties in a symmetric environment but differ if the environment is asymmetric.

Equal mixtures of enantiomers are optically inactive. These equal mixtures are called racemic mixtures and most of the time have different properties than the individual enantiomers.

The amount of rotation (α) observed is variable for a given enantiomer, this variability being dependent on several factors. These factors include the length of the sample vessel, the temperature, the solvent and concentration (for solutions), and the wavelength of light used. However, if the conditions are constant, rotations for the same compound may be determined. This rotation is called "specific rotation" ($[\alpha]$), where the concentration and length of the vessel determine the number of molecules in the path of the beam that is linear with α. Thus, for solutions

$$[\alpha] = \frac{\alpha}{lc}$$

where α is the observed rotation, l is the cell length in decimeters, and c is the concentration in grams per milliliter. Specific rotation is usually noted with the temperature and wavelength under which it was determined (e.g., $[\alpha]_{589}^{25°}$). Basically, there should be no change in $[\alpha]$ with concentration; however, association, dissociations, and solute–solvent interactions may cause nonlinear behavior (March, 1968).

GEOMETRICAL ISOMERS

Geometrical isomers do not rotate the plane of polarized light, unless they also happen to be dissymmetric. The physical and chemical properties of geometrical isomers are different. The two major types of geometrical isomerism are those resulting from double bonds and those resulting from rings (March, 1968).

In an alkene, rotation about the σ bond is restricted by the overlap of p orbital comprising the π bond, resulting in a rigid configuration about the double bond that is planar. In this case, only two isomers can exist, noted as *cis* and *trans*. Each isomer is superimposable on its mirror image unless one group happens to have an asymmetric center.

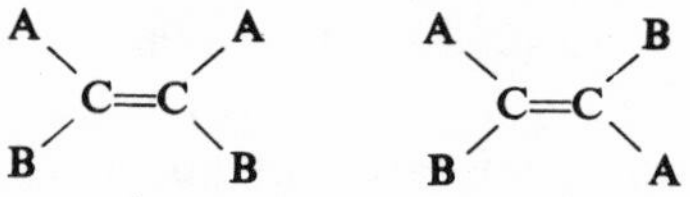

Due to the presence of symmetry, therefore, this type of geometrical isomerism is not usually associated with optical activity.

Another type of geometrical isomerism is found in ring compounds, the ring taking the place of the rigid double bond. For example, *trans*-2-phencyclopropylamine is more stable than the *cis* isomer and is a potent monoamine oxidase inhibitor.

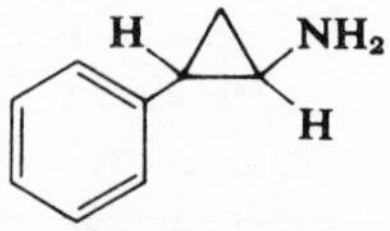

trans-Phenylcyclopropylamine
(Tranylcypromine)

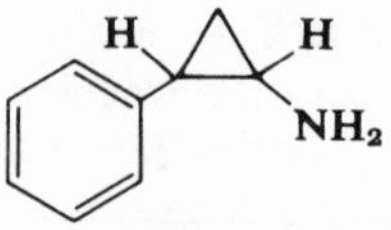

cis-Phenylcyclopropylamine

POSITIONAL ISOMERS

Compounds having the same number and kind of atoms are called isomers. However, the position or location of these atoms within the molecule determine what the compound is and what its properties will be. For example, dimethyl ether and ethyl alcohol are isomers with the general formula C_2H_6O:

$$CH_3—O—CH_3 \qquad CH_3—CH_2—OH$$
Dimethyl ether   Ethyl alcohol

It is well known, though, that each substance is different—separate compounds altogether. Phentermine and methamphetamine are isomers, having the same general formula $C_{10}H_{15}N$:

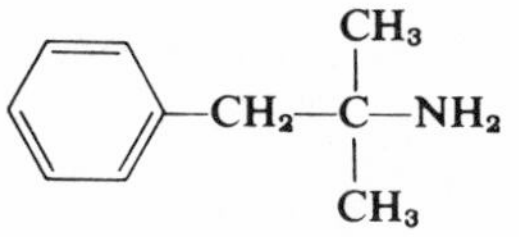

Phentermine 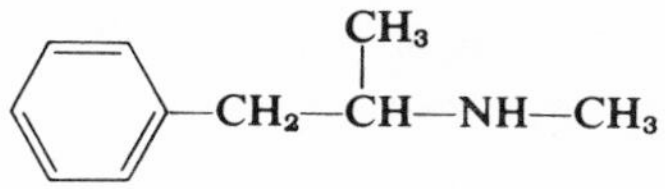   Methamphetamine

Again, although they are isomers, the difference in the position of the methyl group makes these two substances different and distinct compounds. Both are listed separately in the Controlled Substances Act: phentermine, in Schedule IV; methamphetamine, in Schedule II. Theoretically, since Schedule II specifies "unless listed in another schedule..., methamphetamine, including its salts, *isomers*, and salts of isomers," the listing of phentermine under Schedule IV would automatically remove methamphetamine from the Act.

ESTERS

Esters are functional derivatives of alcohols and/or carboxylic acid and have the chemical designation

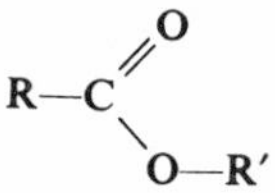

where R may be alkyl or aryl. An example of such a derivative is the esterification of morphine to form heroin:

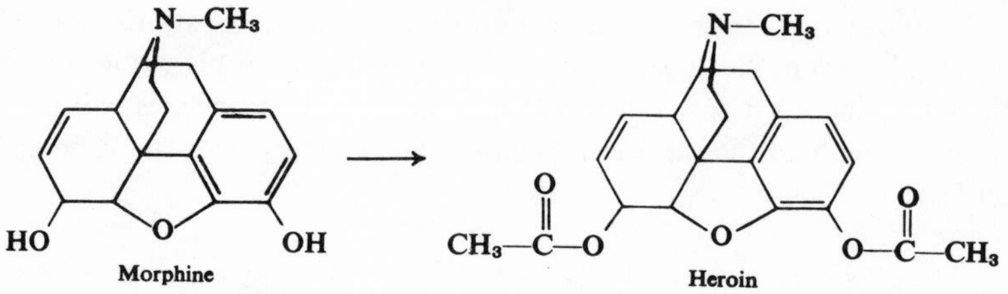

Morphine   Heroin

ETHERS

Ethers are functional derivatives of alcohols and have the chemical designation

$$R—O—R$$

where R may be alkyl or aryl. An example of such a derivative is the etherification of morphine to form codeine:

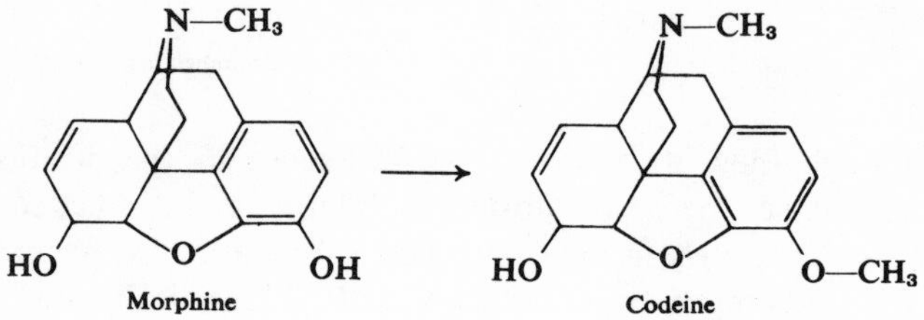

Morphine   Codeine

SALTS

An acid is a proton donor and a base is a proton acceptor. The electron-attracting or electron-repelling properties of other atoms in the molecule determine the bond strength of the proton and base, which in turn determines the extent of ionization at a given pH. The negative logarithm of the acid dissociation constant, termed pKa, reflects this bond strength:

$$\text{acid} \underset{k_2}{\overset{k_1}{\rightleftharpoons}} \text{base} + \text{H}^+$$

At equilibrium

$$k_1 \, (\text{acid}) = k_2 \, (\text{base}) \, (\text{H}^+)$$

$$(\text{H}^+) = \frac{k_1}{k_2} \frac{(\text{acid})}{(\text{base})} = Ka \frac{(\text{acid})}{(\text{base})}$$

and

$$pH = -\log (H^+) = pKa + \log \left(\frac{base}{acid}\right)$$

At 50% ionization, log (base)/(acid) = 0; thus

$$pKa = pH$$

The ionization states of most drugs depend on the pKa values of the substance and the ambient pH, as most drugs have weak acidic and/or weak basic groups.

Nitrogen plays a central role in the ionization of drugs with its property of an unshared pair of electrons. Compounds containing nitrogen in the trivalent state can associate with a hydrogen ion and acquire a positive charge. For example, phentermine contains a primary amino group, methamphetamine contains a secondary amino group, and morphine contains a tertiary amino group. However, all can become cations under acidic conditions.

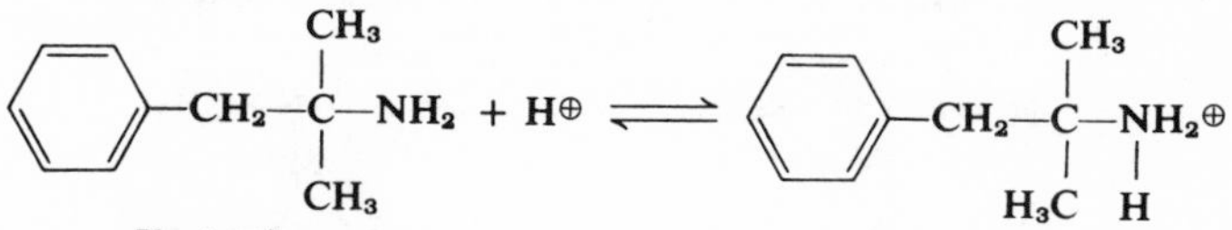

Phentermine

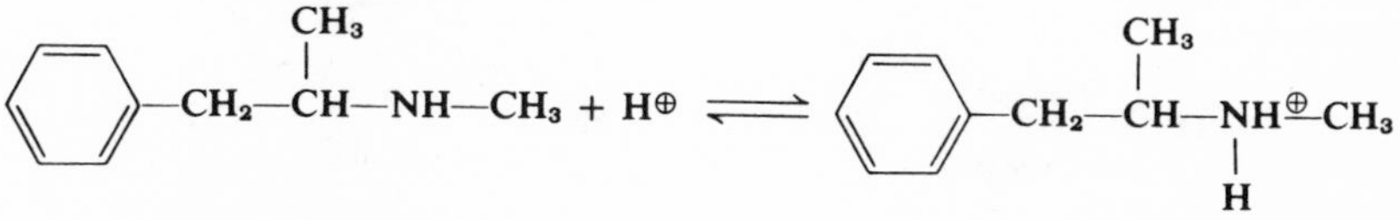

Methamphetamine

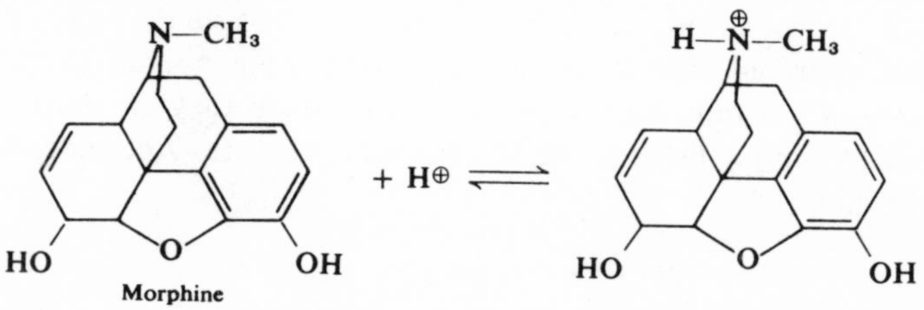

Morphine

Drugs of this type in the free base form tend to be poorly soluble in water. However, if they are treated with acid and form the acid salt, their solubility is greatly enhanced. It should be noted and understood that the resulting salt has no influence on the drug's biological action, with the exception of its rate of absorption.

If a nitrogen donates its unshared electron pair to an atom other than hydrogen, a coordinate covalent bond is formed. When this happens, the nitrogen atom is said to be "quaternized." Drugs of this type, containing a quaternary nitrogen, are not bases, but are permanent organic cations. They cannot lose their positive charge at any pH. The difference between tertiary and quaternary nitrogen compounds has important implications for the passage of drugs across membranes. It is for this reason that morphine methylbromide and morphine methylsulfonate are not accepted medicinal drugs in the United States and are Schedule I drugs, whereas morphine and morphine sulfate (the morphine salt of sulfuric acid, which is essentially the same as morphine free base) are Schedule II drugs.

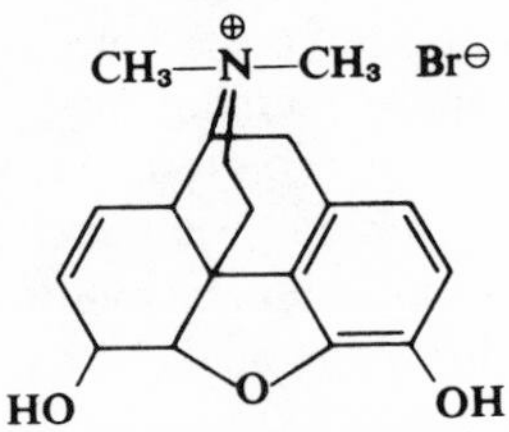

Morphine methylbromide

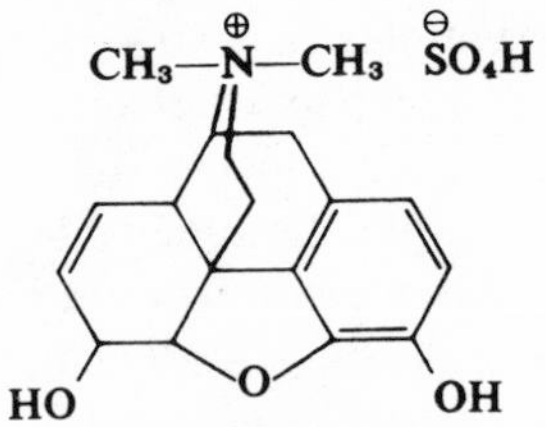

Morphine methylsulfonate

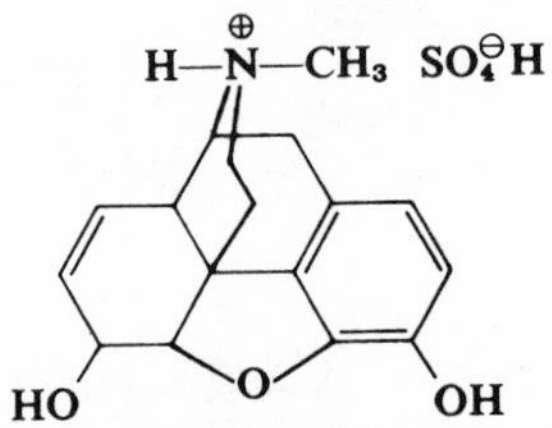

Morphine sulfate

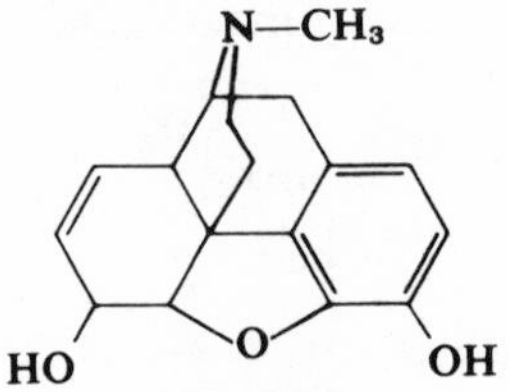

Morphine

Considering this premise, the scheduling of etorphine in Schedule I and etorphine hydrochloride in Schedule II is inconsistent, especially since morphine hydrochloride is not accepted any more by the *United States Pharmacopeia* but morphine sulfate is, even though they are essentially the same and are simply listed in the Controlled Substances Act under Schedule II as morphine.

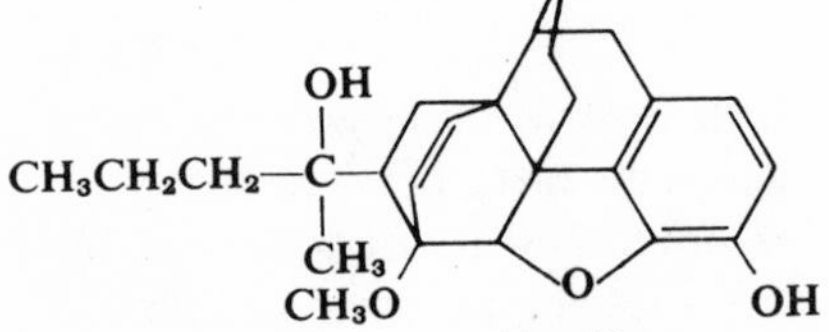

Etorphine

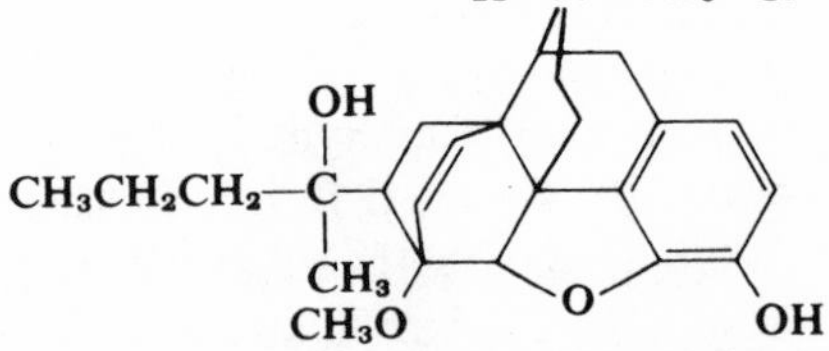

Etorphine hydrochloride

8

Techniques and Instrumentation for Analysis of Drugs

CHROMATOGRAPHY: THIN-LAYER, PAPER, AND COLUMN

Chromatographic techniques are extremely useful in identification and quantitation of many molecular structures, and have been extensively applied to the evaluation of drug substances. Chromatography may be interpreted literally as "writing or display in colors," since the original applications were in separation of mixtures into colored components. Although in thin-layer and paper chromatography, color development of components is a major identification factor, in some forms of chromatography, such as gas–liquid chromatography, color is no longer a feature and the ability to separate mixtures is the common bond among all chromatographic techniques.

Paper chromatography was the first form of chromatography to be applied to identification of drugs and toxins. Various grades of adsorbant paper (even newspaper) can be used for this process. The most commonly used paper is laboratory filter paper of varying thicknesses. The paper serves as the stationary phase, while the developing solvent serves as the mobile phase. A solution of a mixture of substances to be separated and identified is applied as a small spot to the paper by applying droplets a little at a time, drying the spots between applications. The paper with the concentrated spots is then lowered so that it dips into the mobile solvent phase to a depth not touching the spots. The solvent then travels up the paper by diffusion, carrying with it the components of the concentrated spot. When the liquid has reached a specified distance (usually 10–15 cm), the paper is removed and allowed to dry. The process is carried out in a closed chamber, such as a sealed jar, as saturation of the atmosphere with the mobile phase is necessary for optimal separation. Saturation of the atmosphere and increased temperature both shorten the development time. The paper is then allowed to dry, and the components of the originally applied substances, which will have ascended the paper, are usually visualized by spraying the paper with a reagent that reacts with the substances to produce a colored spot. Substances that fluoresce or adsorb ultraviolet light can be located by simply looking at the paper under an ultraviolet lamp.

The distance the spot travels up the paper and the color it develops with the reagent are characteristics used for identification of the substance. Spots of known composition must be applied to the same paper each time this procedure is followed for comparison with the unknown sample.

In thin-layer chromatography, the solid phase consists of a fine, granular adsorbant material, most commonly silica gel, spread in a layer of uniform thickness on a glass plate or a polyester fiber. The principles and applications are the same as described for paper chromatography. Thin-layer chromatography is now much preferred over the paper chromatography, however, because of its greater speed and greater flexibility. Layers of various thicknesses and various types of adsorbant materials are employed to separate various types of molecular structures. The solvent phases are usually organic solvents, most commonly benzene, ethyl acetate, acetone, dioxane, or various mixtures of these. Ammonium hydroxide is often added to the solvent to effect better movement of substances with basic properties. After application, development of the components of the mixture is carried out in glass containers that can be sealed to the atmosphere by sintered glass fittings and lubricant to prevent loss of solvents from evaporation, and to effect a saturated atmosphere.

The spots may be visualized by observing the plate under an ultraviolet light, or by spraying the plate with various types of chemicals that react with the substances in question to form colored components. Some commercially available supports have fluorescent indicators. When these are used, the spots appear as opacities in a green or yellow background when viewed under ultra-violet light. By using gel layers of varying thicknesses, one can also utilize thin-layer chromatography to separate components of mixtures to identify by other means. For example, the mixture may be "streaked" at the bottom of the plate, then the bands of unknown material adsorbed on the gel scraped from the plate. The compound in question can be eluted from the gel with a suitable solvent and separated by centrifugation and the resultant solution scanned in an ultraviolet spectrophotometer or analyzed on a gas chromatograph.

A laboratory using thin-layer chromatography as an analytical procedure will probably have many solvent tanks set up, each with a solvent known to separate and develop a particular group of drugs. Likewise, corresponding color reagents for each group of drugs must be available.

Column chromatography is used only for the purpose of separating components within mixtures. It consists of glass cylinders, with stopcocks at the bottom, that are filled with various types of adsorbant materials (often the same as used for thin-layer chromatography) and with a suitable mobile phase consisting of a liquid in which the drugs or mixtures are at least partially soluble.

The flow of solvent is regulated by adjusting the stopcock, and the separation accomplished by collecting fractions of solvent as it flows through the gel. For ideal separation of mixtures, a slow flow rate is desirable, so that a column may be run for 24 hours or more. Automated fraction collectors are available. The components of the mixture now contained in separate fractions can be identified by application of one or more of the techniques described below.

ULTRAVIOLET AND VISIBLE SPECTROPHOTOMETRY

This instrumental capability was probably one of the earliest of the laboratory instruments applied to drug identification. Spectrophotometry entails passage of light of varying wavelengths in the ultraviolet (200–400 nm) or visible (400–800 nm) range through a solution of the compound in question. Organic molecules absorb this light in varying degrees at various wavelengths depending on their molecular structure. By measuring the amount of light transmitted from the light source through the specimen at various wavelengths by use of a photocell, a spectrophotometric wavelength pattern can be obtained. For many substances, this pattern is a unique characteristic, and identification can be accomplished by this means alone. However, the substance must be pure, as spectrophotometry is not a separational instrument. Separations of mixtures may be achieved by the chromatographic technique mentioned above, by selective solvent extractions of samples (such as blood), and by extraction into acidic or alkaline solution. Spectrophotometric techniques (such as ultraviolet and visible) are of great value for quantitative analysis. The organic molecules absorb light proportionately according to the Beer–Lambert Law, so that the concentration of the unknown substance in the solution can be calculated by relating optical density (absorbed light) to the molecular concentration. Thus,

$$\log \frac{I_o}{I} = \text{optical density}$$

where I_o is the intensity of incident light and I is the intensity of transmitted light, or

$$E_{1cm}^{1\%} = \frac{OD}{C}$$

where E is the optical density of a 1% solution in a cell or path length of 1 centimeter, OD is the optical density of the unknown concentration, and C is the unknown concentration.

INFRARED SPECTROPHOTOMETRY

Infrared spectrophotometry is an extremely useful technique in the identification of drugs, since almost all organic compounds produce characteristic absorption spectra in the infrared range (800 to 1×10^6 nm). For the purpose of drug identification, the most useful portion of the infrared spectrum is around 2500–15,400 nm (the midinfrared region). Infrared spectrophotometry is the study of transmitted v. absorbed infrared light through a medium containing organic material to be studied.

For practical considerations, this procedure is a highly specific qualitative technique. Infrared spectra of typical drugs have many absorption maxima in this range, and the positions of these maxima along with their relative intensity provide a "finger-print" identification feature that can often stand alone.

The infrared spectrophotometer is not a separational instrument; thus, it must have a relatively pure preparation for analysis. Since separation and purification from biological specimens may entail losses of from 50 to 95% of the original quantity, infrared is almost useless, or at least impractical, for routine analysis of drugs or toxins from biological specimens. For solid-sample drug analysis such as pharmaceutical preparations, when the starting quantity is in the milligram range, however, infrared indentification is quite useful. The material in question, e.g., an unknown tablet, may be extracted with chloroform and passed through a small column, and the eluate from the column examined by infrared spectrophotometry. Quantitation would have to be carried out by ultraviolet spectrophotometry or another technique, such as gas chromatography, however.

SPECTROFLUORIMETRY

Certain organic compounds including many drugs have inherent fluorescent properties at specific wavelengths, rather than, or in addition to, absorbant characteristics in ultraviolet light. In addition, some compounds not inherently fluorescent can be measured by fluorescence assay by converting the molecule to fluorescent derivatives. Fluorescence assays offer two advantages over other spectrophotometric methods: they are usually more sensitive, and they tend to be more specific. The spectrofluorimeter consists of (1) an exciting light source, (2) a sample container, (3) a photo-detector connected to a gavanometer, and (4) a means of selecting the exciting and/or emission wavelengths.

Those substances with inherent fluorescence that can practically be assayed by fluorimetry include quinine, quinidine, LSD, imipramine, and salicylates.

The chemical formation of a fluorophor, or product with fluorescent properties, enables one to measure a wide range of substances that are not inherently fluorescent. Practical assays exist for the phenothiazines, morphine, chlordiazepoxide, and others.

Fluorescence assays can be highly sensitive and provide an accurate quantitation of the substance in question. For most substances, however, confirmation of the identity of the compound in question should be obtained by another technique.

In contrast to gas chromatography or other chromatographic techniques, the specificity of spectrofluorimetry is a disadvantage in that spectrofluorimetry does not provide a separational mixture or a "screen" for drug substances. Other techniques employing gas chromatography or ultraviolet spectrophotometry should ordinarily be used first. In some cases, however, one will be analyzing for agents, such as morphine in blood, that cannot be detected by most gas chromatographic methods; quinidine as a therapeutic monitoring technique when the patient is known to be taking the drug; and LSD, which has unique fluorescent properties and cannot be practically measured by other methods. In these cases, often spectrofluorimetric identification alone is sufficient.

GAS CHROMATOGRAPHY

Gas chromatography (or gas–liquid chromatography) is an advanced form of chromatography, similar in principle to column chromatography. A column, consisting of a glass or metal tube, usually 3–6 feet in length and only a few millimeters in diameter, is filled with a liquid phase (an organic compound such as high-molecular-weight alcohols, paraffins, etc.) adsorbed on a fine-mesh granular solid-phase material (such as silica compounds). The columns are contained in an oven with carefully regulated temperature control and attached to the injection port at one end and the detector at the other. Gas is fed in near the injection port from a pressurized gas source and travels through the column at a constant flow rate. This carrier gas is usually an inert gas such as nitrogen or helium. The substance or substances to be analyzed are placed on the column by injecting a solution of the mixture into the injection port. The organic molecules become adsorbed on the column material and are forced along the column by the carrier gas. The time it takes to reach the other end of the column is determined by the size and polarity (active groups) of the molecule, the pressure of the carrier gas, the temperature of the oven, and the properties of the stationary phase in the column. This time factor is known as the retention time, and is the major identification feature for identification of compounds by gas chromatography. To determine accurately when each substance is eluted from the column, it is necessary to have a suitable means for detection. As the material comes off the column, it is fed into a detector. This is, for drugs, most characteristically a flame ionization detector (FID). The eluate from the column is mixed with a supply of hydrogen, and the mixture is burned at a small jet in a flow of air sufficient for combustion. Above the jet is an electrode, which may be a wire or an annular ring. The polarizing voltage is applied between the jet and the electrode. When a component appears in the flame, the ionization causes the current between the electrodes to decrease. This increase is detected by measuring the voltage drop across a very high resistance in the circuit using a very high impedance amplifier. The response of the flame detector is roughly dependent on the number of carbon atoms in the substance. This response is usually recorded on chart paper by a sliding pen recorder, resulting in a "peak" as each substance comes through the column, which size is proportional to the amount of substance coming through.

Other detectors are useful for special purposes in gas chromatography. The electron capture detector is a selective detector with a high sensitivity for electrons. Substances containing halogen atoms, nitro groups, carbonyl groups, acids, and esters are detected with much greater sensitivity than by other types of detectors. The greatest practical utility in drug analysis for this detector is in detection of halogenated compounds (such as chloral hydrate) in low quantities such as are found in blood samples.

Thermal conductivity detectors are also commonly used with gas chromatographs. This detector consists of a metal block of high thermal capacity drilled with channels to carry a sample stream and a reference gas stream. In the channels are electrically heated filaments. When a sample component emerges into the sample stream, the thermal conductivity of the system is changed and the resulting change in temperature of the wire causes a change in resistance. The change in signal can be displayed on a chart recorder, indicating the time and magnitude of response of the substance coming off the column. This type of detector is of most value for gases, or low-boiling alcohols. Its disadvantages are that it is not especially sensitive and requires a larger sample than does detection with other detectors.

Gas chromatography provides the most useful form of identification of organic compounds. Its sensitivity is such that most drug agents can be detected in blood samples, when properly extracted and purified. It can separate and enable identification of many compounds present in a simple mixture simultaneously. When standard materials are compared, it provides a highly accurate identification parameter for most organic molecular structures.

The major limitation of gas chromatography is that it provides only a single parameter for identification purposes. A single retention time that is identical to that of the standard compound cannot be used as an unequivocal identification. To correct for this limitation, most laboratories, especially those doing forensic identifications, utilize at least one other parameter for identification purposes. This can be another column in the gas chromatograph, with different support, and different temperature conditions. Thin-layer chromatography and ultraviolet spectrophotometry can also be used to confirm identification made by gas chromatography. The most highly specific procedure in use and the best suited for interface with gas chromatography is the mass spectrometer.

GAS CHROMATOGRAPHY–MASS SPECTROMETRY (GC-MS)

The mass spectrometer interfaced with a gas chromatograph is today the most accurate tool for identification of organic compounds such as pharmaceuticals. The mass spectrometric identification is accomplished by degrading minute quantities of a compound and recording the fragmentation pattern according to the mass of the fragments. The sample is drawn into the low-pressure system of the mass spectrometer, where it is ionized with sufficient energy to cause fragmentation of the chemical bonds of the original molecule. The resulting positively charged ions are accelerated into a magnetic field that disperses and permits relative abundance measurement of ions of a given mass-to-charge ratio. The resulting record of ion abundance across mass constitutes a fragmentation pattern. This spectrum usually has sufficient specific characteristics to identify the molecules without comparison with a known spectrum. With large or more stable molecules, some molecules escape fragmentation, and a molecular ion is recorded, allowing determination of the molecular weight of the structure.

The gas chromatograph permits separation of mixtures of several compounds and purification of each, so that one can choose the peak in question to be analyzed by the mass spectrometer. Thus, if one encounters a response on the gas chromatograph that is not entirely characteristic, by relative time, of known structure, a mass spectrum may be obtained of that substance and the structure determined. Often impurities, putrefactive products, metabolites, or artifacts appear in gas chromatographic analysis and may be confused with drugs or toxic agents. These occur especially when analyzing for drugs in blood or other biological samples. By obtaining a mass spectrum, one can identify most of these unknown substances. Since the mass spectrometer can analyze substances in very minute quantity (low nanogram range), one can identify trace quantities of substances not heretofore possible to identify. Identification of trace quantities of drugs that may remain on syringes or other drug paraphernalia after use for injection is an example of the utility of this procedure.

LIQUID CHROMATOGRAPHY

The liquid chromatograph (high-pressure liquid chromatograph) has the ability to detect and measure trace quantities of substances in various specimens. Its unique advantage is the separation and detection of substances at low temperatures. This permits a "nondestructive" analysis, in contrast to gas chromatography, for example, in which the sample is burned or otherwise destroyed in the detection process as it comes off the column. For certain substances, this is a highly desirable feature due to their lability under higher temperature conditions. Methods are in use in which therapeutic or lower levels of theophylline, carbamazepine, and many other drugs are measured in small volumes of blood (as little as 50 μl).

The organic extract from a sample may be concentrated, then applied to a column. The solvent used to elute the sample is employed at high pressures. As the sample is eluted, it is detected by measuring its adsorbance in ultraviolet light at a specific wavelength.

Those substances difficult to assay by gas chromatography because of decomposition at high temperature can now be measured accurately. Included in the future may be LSD, tetrahydrocannabinol and metabolites, chlordiazepoxide, methaqualone, and their respective metabolites, and other substances.

RADIOIMMUNOASSAY

Although radioimmunoassay (RIA) has just recently been applied to drug detection and assay in biological specimens, it has found widespread use for several speciality determinations. Substances such as hormones, insulin, and others that have biochemical parameters preventing their detection by other techniques due to separational difficulties lend themselves readily to RIA. Digoxin and digitoxin cannot be detected by any other methods at the therapeutic concentrations found in blood (2 ng/ml). LSD and THC, both widely used substances, are effective in very low biological concentrations (a few ng/ml). They cannot be detected in blood at present by any other laboratory technique, excepting perhaps GC-MS. RIA kits, however, are now available to detect these substances in urine or other biological substances.

RIA enables one to analyze a large number of samples with a minimum of preparation time and with accurate quantitation. Morphine can be measured by several techniques using previously described instrumentation. However, many such techniques are time-consuming and impractical when a large number of samples, such as urine, must be analyzed routinely.

RIA offers the advantage of being an automated analytical capability for which prepared reagents and kits are commercially available. Also, most samples can be assayed directly, without risking the losses entailed with extractions or other separations. Therefore, a minimum of the analyst's time is consumed and high-quality, accurate results can be obtained. All immuno-assay procedures have certain limitations in specificity, however. For example, certain molecules when present in large concentrations and similar in structure to morphine can give a false positive for this drug. Codeine and naloxone are among these. For this reason, it is highly desirable to confirm all positive specimens detected by RIA by another method, especially when results are to be used for medicolegal purposes.

EMIT, HI, AND FRAT

Other immunoassay techniques of current usefulness in toxicology include the EMIT (Enzyme Multiplied Immunoassay Technique), HI (Hemagglutination Inhibition), and FRAT [Free Radical Assay Technique or electron spin resonance (ESR)].

These techniques are utilized to screen large numbers of specimens for certain selected drug substances for which tests have been developed. As with RIA, they offer specific testing for the particular agent or agents for which test kits have been developed by the manufacturers.

Initially, morphine was the target molecule and kits were developed to detect small quantities of morphine in urine or other biological specimens. More recently, other drugs that can serve as antigens for the development of antibodies have been employed for the development of test kits. For example, the EMIT system (available through SYVA Corporation) has kits available to detect morphine, barbiturates, methadone, amphetamine, benzoylecgonine, diphenylhydantoin, and others. A small volume of urine is added to a test tube containing a solution with the antibody specific to the substance being tested. Enzyme-labeled molecules of the substance to be tested along with the substrate are added to the urine. If the unknown molecule is present, the enzyme is released and reacts with the substrate. The resulting reaction can be measured spectrophotometrically. The HI test is performed in the well of a "spot plate." A small volume of urine is incubated with morphine-specific antibody. Red blood cells sensitized with morphine are then added. If morphine is absent, the cells aggregate and stick to the sides of the well. If present, the antibody is neutralized, the agglutination is inhibited, and the cells settle in a disk at the bottom of the well.

The FRAT, also an immunoassay technique, utilizes spin labels. The spin label is a molecule containing a "free radical" or having an unpaired electron. This unpaired electron produces a magnetic movement that can be detected and measured in an ESR spectrometer. The spin-labeled haptene and haptene-specific antibody are reacted with the unknown solution (urine) containing unlabled haptene. If present, the spin-labeled haptene is displaced and can be measured by ESR.

This technique is extremely sensitive, detecting morphine in urine for at least four days after use of heroin. On the other hand, other opiates may cross-react, and confirmation of the positive sample would have to be made using more specific procedures. The considerable expense involved in the instrumentation, plus the cost per test, unless large numbers of samples are being run, are disadvantages of this system.

NUCLEAR MAGNETIC RESONANCE (NMR) SPECTROSCOPY

Spinning nuclei create a magnetic dipole with a magnetic moment, μ, along the axis of the nuclei. The angular momentum of the spinning nucleus is characterized by a spin quantum number (I). If the atomic mass number is odd, I will be $\frac{1}{2}$ or an integral multiple of $\frac{1}{2}$. In contrast, nuclei having an I of 1 or more exhibit a nonspherical nuclear charge distribution that is characterized by a nuclear quadrupole moment and results in demonstrable spectral perturbations.

Nuclei with a spin quantum number, 1, when placed in an external uniform static magnetic field of strength, H_0, will tend to be oriented similarly to a bar magnet in $(2I + 1)$ possible orientations. For nuclei with $I = \frac{1}{2}$, there will be two possible orientations, $+\frac{1}{2}$ or $-\frac{1}{2}$, a lower and an upper energy state. Since two energy states exist, transitions from the lower to the higher state should be possible if the proper amount of energy is introduced. In a static magnetic field, the nuclear magnetic axis will spin or precess (Larmor precession) about the external field axis. The precessional angular velocity, ω_0, is related to the external magnetic field strength through the equation

$$\omega_0 = \gamma H_0$$

in which γ is the magnetogyric ratio, which is a constant for each nucleus. If energy from an oscillating radiofrequency field is introduced, the absorption of radiation will take place according to the relationship

$$\Delta E = h\nu_0 = \mu H_0/I$$

and

$$\nu_0 = \omega_0/2\pi = \gamma H_0/2\pi$$

Thus, when the frequency (ν_0) of the external energy ($E = h\nu$) is the same as the precessional angular velocity, resonance is acheived, and the nucleus attains the upper state.

NMR involves energy absorption by nuclei in the radiofrequency range. The range of study possible is limited only by the natural abundance of the isotope and the relative sensitivity for equal numbers of nuclei at constant magnetic field strength. In practice, NMR measurements are generally useful in studies of nuclei such as ^{1}H, ^{19}F, ^{13}C, ^{31}P, and ^{11}B, since they have odd mass numbers and I values of $\frac{1}{2}$ or integral multiples of $\frac{1}{2}$. Of these, the proton, ^{1}H, is by far most often studied and most frequently used in the identification of drugs.

The magnitude of the separation of the frequency of resonance of a proton from that of some standard (tetramethylsilane or sodium 2,2-dimethyl-2-silapentane-5-sulfonate) is called the "chemical shift," which is proportional to the strength of the applied field. The latter is a composite of the external field and the field caused by the circulation of surrounding electrons about the protons. The conventional NMR spectrum is observed with the magnetic field strength increasing in the direction left to right. Thus, a proton that resonates at a high magnetic field strength (near tetramethylsilane) is said to be more shielded (greater electron density) than a proton that resonates at a lower magnetic field strength and is said to be deshielded (lower electron density).

A particular group may exhibit resonance at different field positions and that signal may be separated or split into a related group or multiplet of peaks. The magnitude of the chemical shift of a particular group varies because of intramolecular effects on the individual group or atomic environment. The splitting of a peak results from the influence of other active nuclei that are generally within three valence bonds of the nucleus in question. This interaction between two nuclei is called "coupling."

The coupling activity between two nuclei may be described in terms of the coupling constant, J, which is the separation (in Hz) between the individual peaks of the multiplet. When two nuclei are interacting and causing reciprocal splitting, the measured coupling constant in the two resulting multiplets is equal. J is independent of magnetic field strength.

The possible complication of the spectrum by the introduction of extra peaks not due to the NMR phenomena must be recognized. In an attempt to negate magnetic field inhomogeneity and increase resolution, the sample tube is caused to spin. If this spinning frequency is too low, the desired field-averaging is not complete, and an absorption signal is accompanied by signals of lower intensity called spinning side bands. These side bands are located symmetrically around the main signal, and the separation is equal to the spinning frequency or some integral multiple of that frequency. Thus, spinning side bands may be identified since their location changes with spinning frequency. Side bands can also rise from uneven spinning.

A useful means of simplifying spectra is by use of double resonance or spin decoupling. This technique removes spin coupling between nuclei or groups of nuclei. This provides a convenient way of establishing coupling relationships.

Another valuable property of the recorded spectrum is the peak area. During a single instrumental scan, the intensity of energy absorption is constant for all protons no matter what their particular nature. Thus, the area of a single peak or a multiplet is directly proportional to the number of protons giving rise to the peak or peaks. As a result, it is possible to determine the relative ratio of different kinds of protons that are found in a molecule. If the sample solution is prepared quantitatively and a reference standard is used, the peak areas, measured by instrumental integration, may be used for quantitative analysis.

The utility of NMR lies in the ability to use the spectrum for a variety of analytical purposes. The various types of protons present will be shown as different resonance signals with regard to their absolute different chemical environment. This permits structural information to be gathered. The general appearance of each individual resonance (e.g., singlet, doublet, triplet) adds more structural information, and the combination of position and appearance enables the determination of (1) the number of the atoms being measured, (2) the chemical environment of each, (3) the structural and/or isomeric relationships, and (4) the presence of impurities. The integration of peak areas is an important step in interpretation, since the ratio of areas will yield the relative ratios of the various kinds of resonant nuclei. In addition, the integration may be extended to quantitative analysis.

The quantitative analysis of a compound by NMR is an example of the use of a very specific property for measurement purposes. Once the position of a definite structural unit is known, the area of its resonance peak(s) can be related to other peaks resulting in ratios of the various atoms represented in the spectrum. By employing multiple integration tracings across the entire spectrum, as well as several independent analyses, the relative accuracy of quantitative NMR analyses can be $\pm 2\%$. If small parts of the scan will yield the quantitative information of interest, then these partial scans can be integrated at higher gain to improve the accuracy. The principal advantages of quantitative NMR are: (1) quantities such as molar absorptivity values (which are present in spectrophotometric techniques) are absent; (2) the intensity of a signal for a given nuclear isotope is proportional to the number of nuclei contributing to the signal, but independent of its chemical nature; (3) a compound being analyzed in a mixture need not be available in pure form for use as a standard; and (4) resonance lines are narrow relative to chemical shift differences (line positions).

9

Controlled and Noncontrolled but Commonly Abused Substances

▶ **ACEPROMAZINE**
Dangerous Drug

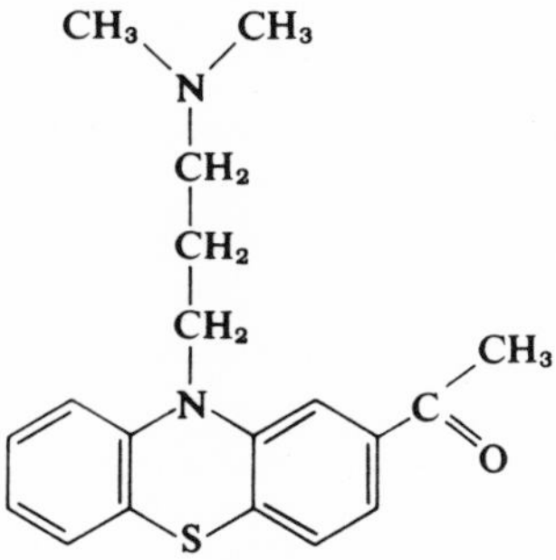

Synonyms: Acetylpromazine, 2-acetyl-10-(3-dimethylaminopropyl) phenothiazine.

Pharmaceutical Preparations: This drug is not found in pharmaceutical preparations sold in the United States. In Europe, acepromazine is produced under the trade name Notensil[R].

General Comment: Acepromazine is classified in this text as a dangerous drug because it is a phenothiazine tranquilizer.

Biochemistry: Janssen et al. (1965) showed that the neuroleptic potency of acepromazine is about three times greater than that of chlorpromazine. This difference is attributed to the different substituents at the 2 position on the phenothiazine ring, $COCH_3$ for acepromazine and Cl for chlorpromazine.

Toxicology–Pharmacology: The usual recommended dose of acepromazine is up to 100 mg per day. It is used in treatment of major psychiatric disturbances. The lethal dose or blood concentrations are not known.

▶ **ACETAMINOPHEN**
Noncontrolled Substance

$$OH$$

$$NH$$
$$C{=}O$$
$$CH_3$$

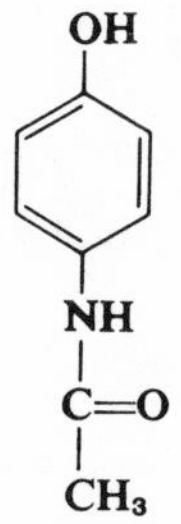

Synonyms: Paracetamol, *p*-hydroxyacetanilide.

General Comments: Acetaminophen, an analgesic and antipyretic, is found in numerous proprietary preparations, including numerous over-the-counter preparations. Therefore, even though it is encountered in many cases of drug abuse mixed with a controlled drug, it is not, itself, controlled by law.

Toxicology–Pharmacology: Plasma levels varied from 0.24 to 0.64 mg% after a dose of 324 mg, i.e., up to 5.0 mg/dl after 2.0 g. Sixty-seven percent of a dose is excreted into the urine as a sulfate or glucuronide conjugate. Toxic hepatitis is often associated with overdose of acetaminophen.

▶ **ACETANILIDE**
Noncontrolled Substance

$$CH_3$$
$$C{=}O$$
$$NH$$

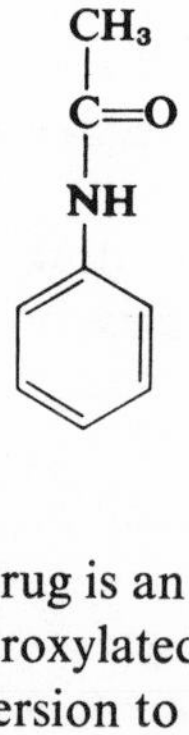

Synonym: *N*-phenylacetamide.

Toxicology–Pharmacology: This drug is an analgesic, comparable in effect to aspirin. Acetanilide is rapidly hydroxylated to acetaminophen, which exerts the therapeutic action. Some conversion to aniline results in methemoglobinemia and consequent cyanosis, and other toxic effects. Consequently, acetanilide has largely been replaced by safer analgesics. Acute lethal dose is between 5 and 20 g.

▶ **ACETOPHENAZINE**
Dangerous Drug

Synonyms: Sch 6673, 2-acetyl-10-(3-[4-(2-hydroxyethyl)piperazinel-y]-propyl) phenothiazine.

Pharmaceutical Preparations: TINDAL^R (Schering)—Tablet: sugar-coated, salmon-colored, containing 20 mg acetophenazine maleate.

General Comments: Acetophenazine is a phenothiazine tranquilizer and thus is classified in this text as a dangerous drug. A registered pharmaceutical preparation containing acetophenazine requires a prescription. Usual dose of acetophenazine is up to 120 mg per day. In extreme cases of psychosis, it may be increased to 600 mg per day.

Biochemistry: From studies of structure–activity relationships, it has been concluded that in the phenothiazine derivatives and analogues, the structural features connected with high antipsychotic potency are: (1) a tricyclic ring system with a six- or seven-membered central ring; (2) a chain of three atoms between the central ring and a terminal amino group; and (3) an electron-attracting atom or group at the 2 position.

Toxicology–Pharmacology: Sudden death has occasionally been reported in patients receiving phenothiazines. In some cases, the death was apparently due to cardiac arrest; in others, the cause appeared to be asphyxia due to failure of the cough reflex. In some patients, the cause could not be determined nor could it be established that the death was due to the phenothiazine.

The central nervous system effects for chronic usage may include pseudo-parkinsonism, akathisia (motor restlessness), and dystonias. Dystonias include spasms of the neck muscles, extensor rigidity of back muscles, carpopedal spasm, eyes rolled back, convulsions, trismus, and swallowing difficulties.

Adverse behavioral effects from chronic use of phenothiazines include abnormal harsh psychotic symptoms, catatonic-like states, paranoid reactions, lethargy, restlessness, hyperactivity, nocturnal confusion, and bizarre dreams.

In case of an overdose, one may observe one of the following symptoms:

1. Extreme somnolence; however, the patient can usually be roused, but if permitted, will fall asleep. The general condition is usually satisfactory. The skin may be pale, warm, and dry. Slight blood pressure, respiratory, and pulse changes may occur, but are not a problem.
2. The patient may have a mild to moderate drop in blood pressure. The patient may or may not be conscious. The skin is markedly gray but warm and dry. The nail beds are pink, and respiration is slow and regular with strong pulse but the rate slightly increased.
3. The patient may have severe hypotension, possibly accompanied by weakness, cyanosis, perspiration, rapid thready pulse, and respiratory depression.

The acute lethal dose is between 1 and 10 g.

▶ **ACETORPHINE**
Schedule I

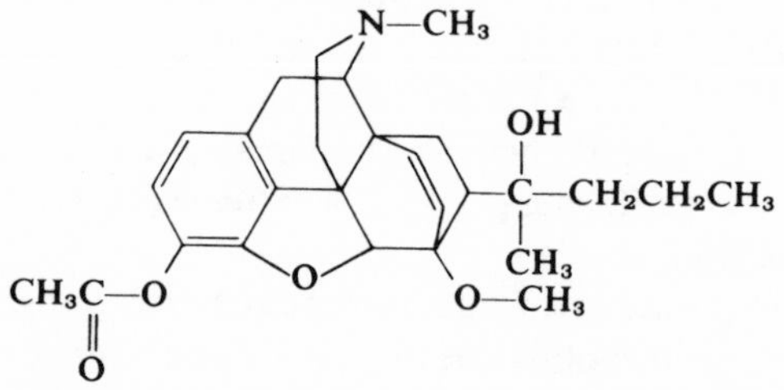

Synonyms: 3-O-Acetyl-19-propylorvinol, M183, 3-O-acetyl-7,8-dihydro-7α-[1(R)-hydroxy-1-methylbutyl]-6-O-methyl-6,14-*endo*-ethenormorphine.

Pharmaceutical Preparations: This drug is not found in pharmaceutical preparations sold in the United States.

General Comments: Acetorphine is a synthetic narcotic analgesic. As a Schedule I substance, it is not legally accepted for medicinal use in the United States.

Biochemistry: Acetorphine has not been studied in depth to describe its metabolism.

Toxicology–Pharmacology: Acetorphine is the O-acetylderivative of ethorphine. Both drugs have been used as immobilizing agents in the capture of wild animals. Acetorphine is capable of leading to a high degree of physical dependence in humans. Acetorphine being pharmacologically classified as a narcotic analgesic, its effects may be antagonized by narcotic antagonists such as cyprenorphine or nalorphine. Since the effective dose for acetorphine is small, it is dangerous to smell or taste this substance.

▶ **ACETYLDIHYDROCODEINE**
Schedule I

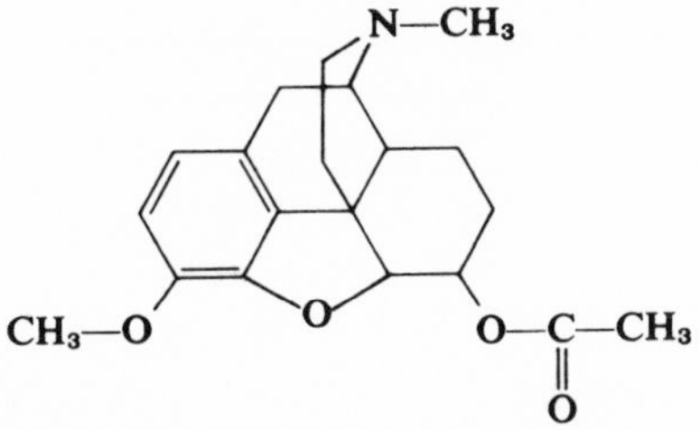

Synonym: 6-Acetoxy-4,5-epoxy-3-methoxy-N-methylmorphinan.
Pharmaceutical Preparations: Acetyldihydrocodeine is not found in any pharmaceutical preparations sold in the United States.
General Comment: Acetyldihydrocodeine is a semisynthetic narcotic analgesic that has no accepted medicinal value in the United States.
Biochemistry: The biochemistry of acetyldihydrocodeine is unknown. However, one would expect general metabolic pathways similar to those of other opiate derivatives.
Toxicology–Pharmacology: Unknown.

▶ **ACETYLMETHADOL**
Schedule I

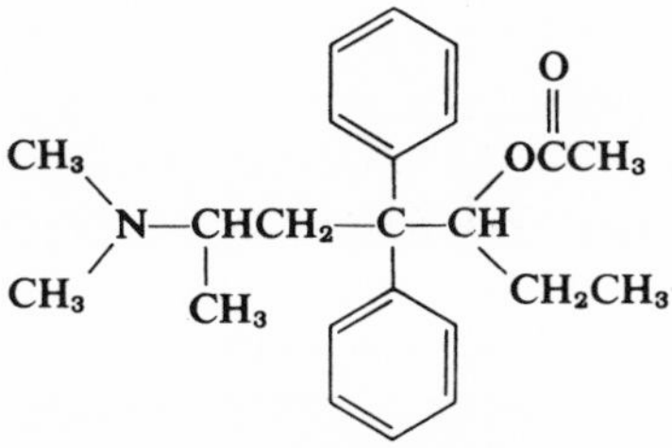

Synonyms: α-Acetylmethadol, β-acetylmethadol, α- or β-acetylmethadone, α- or β-acemethadone, α- or β-amidon acetate, α- or β-methadol acetate, α- or β-dimethylamino-4,4-diphenyl-3-acetoxyheptane.
Pharmaceutical Preparations: Acetylmethadol is not found in any pharmaceutical preparations sold in the United States.
General Comments: Acetylmethadol is the name given to the mixture of α- and β-acetyl esters of the substance methadol. Both the α-acetyl compound, α-acetylmethadol, and the β counterpart, β-acetylmethadol, are known as discrete compounds, and they are both specified in the Federal schedules.

Biochemistry: Two metabolites of α-acetylmethadol have been identified (Booker and Pohland, 1975). These two metabolites were identified as "metabolite I," α-($\pm$)-noracetylmethadol, a *N*-demethylation product, and "metabolite II," α-($\pm$)-6-amino-4,4-diphenyl-3-heptanol acetate, a *N*-demethylation product of metabolite I. The compound noracetylmethadol has been shown to possess potent antinociceptive activity (Smits, 1974). It has been suggested that this biotransformation product of acetylmethadol is responsible for the time–action characteristics of certain of the pharmacological effects of this compound, primarily the relatively long duration of suppression of narcotic withdrawal symptoms following the administration of α-acetylmethadol. In the rat, acetylmethadol is converted to noracetylmethadol about three times as rapidly as noracetylmethadol is metabolized (McMahon *et al.*, 1965). This results in the accumulation of noracetylmethadol in tissues.

Acetylation of methadol establishes the stereospecific dominance of the C-6 center, the 6R-isomers being the most active. α-(−)-Acetylmethadol is far less potent than the *dextro* isomer by intraventricular administration. It has been suggested that the analgetic effects of the *levo* isomer are due to a metabolite and not to the parent drug (Veath *et al.*, 1964).

Toxicology–Pharmacology: L-α-Acetylmethadol (LAAM) and *dl*-acetylmethadol have the same action as methadone, acting as narcotic analgesics. Their much more mildly euphoriant narcotic action allays the desire for heroin in narcotic addicts. The primary use is to treat heroin addicts (at this writing still in experimental programs only).

The long-acting property (72 hours) results in enhanced toxicity, and death from respiratory depression may occur from overdose, or combination with other depressant drugs.

Peak levels are achieved in about 6 hours (as methadone). The half-life in plasma is about 15–17 hours. Eighty percent of the dose is excreted in the feces.

▶ **ALETAMINE**
Noncontrolled Substance

General Comment: Aletamine is not a controlled substance; however, this analgesic has reportedly been abused.

► **ALLOBARBITAL**
Schedule III

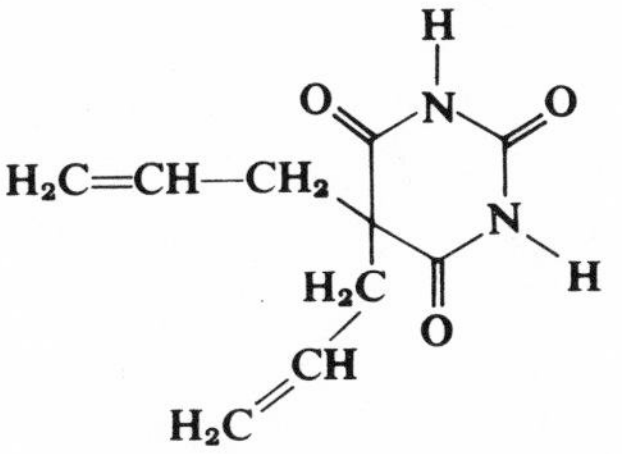

Synonyms: Allobarbitone, diallybarbitone, diallylbarbituric acid, diallyl-malonylurea, 5,5-diallylbarbituric acid.

Pharmaceutical Preparations: Dialog^R (Ciba)—A white, single-scored tablet labeled "CIBA" containing 15 mg allobarbital and 300 mg acetaminophen. Also see Chapter 6.

General Comments: Allobarbital is a Schedule III drug by virtue of its being a "derivative of barbituric acid." It is, however, a long-acting barbiturate similar in duration of action to phenobarbital and should theoretically be listed under Schedule IV.

Biochemistry: The plasma half-life of allobarbital is 2.0 days as compared with 3.4 days for phenobarbital (Lous, 1954; Brilmayer and Loennecken, 1962).

Toxicology–Pharmacology: Blood concentrations of 1.0–4.0 mg/dl are indicative of severe poisoning and overdosage. Overdosage produces symptoms typical of an intermediate-acting barbiturate (central nervous system depression, coma, death from respiratory failure).

► **ALLYLPRODINE**
Schedule I

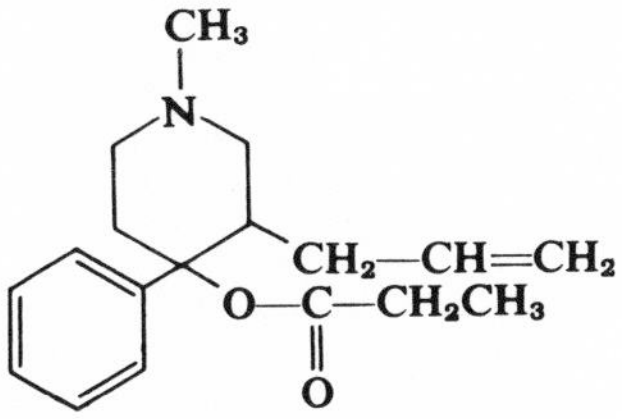

Synonyms: 3-Allyl-1-methyl-4-phenyl-4-propionyloxy-piperidine.

Pharmaceutical Preparations: Allylprodine is not found in pharmaceutical preparations sold in the United States.

General Comments: Allylprodine is a narcotic analgesic chemically related to pethidine (meperidine). Its potency is much greater than that of meperidine, and allylprodine maintains a cross-tolerance to heroin. However, allylprodine has not been accepted for medicinal use in the United States.
Biochemistry: X-ray crystallographic studies have been performed on the two diastereomeric racemates of allylprodine (Portoghese, 1976). This study was conducted to determine the role of conformation in the interaction with analgetic receptor sites. The chiral orientation of the phenyl group in the highly potent isomer, (+)-1, is quantitatively in conformity with the stereo-structure–activity relationship. The data suggest that the very high potency and stereoselectivity that the allylic double bond confers to (+)-1 are due primarily to the interaction of this bond with an accessory site on the receptor.

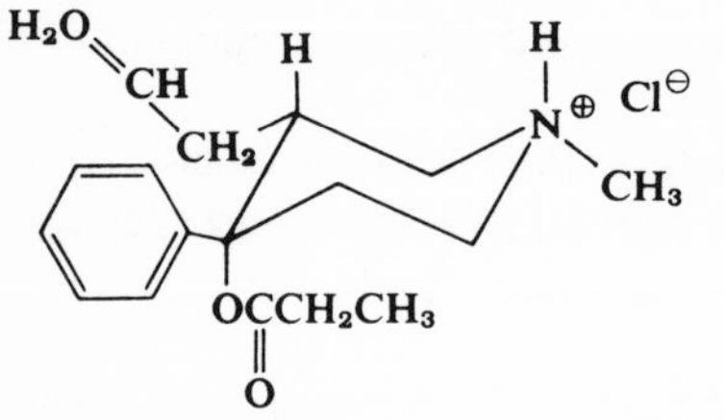

(+)-1

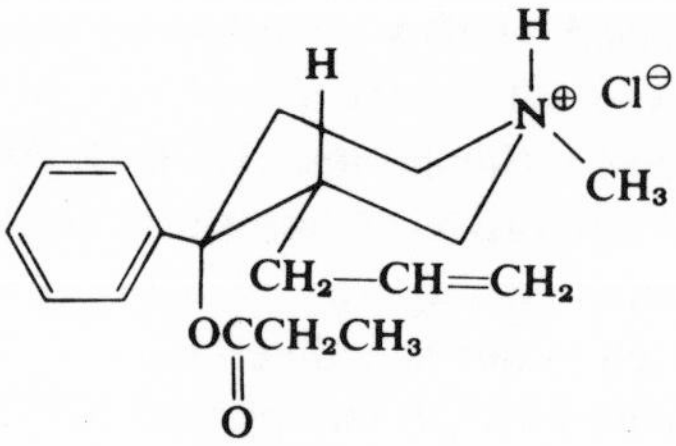

(+)-2

(+)-Allylprodine possesses an analgetic potency 40 times greater than that of morphine with an enantiomeric potency ratio, (+)/(−), of 260. (+)-Allylprodine, (+)-1, is approximately 460 times more potent than its β-diastereomer, (+)-2, which possesses virtually no stereoselectivity.
Toxicology–Pharmacology: See **PETHIDINE.**

▶ **ALPHAACETYLMETHADOL**
Schedule I
See **ACETYLMETHADOL**

▶ **ALPHAMEPRODINE**
Schedule I
See **MEPRODINE**

▶ **ALPHAMETHADOL**
Schedule I
See **METHADOL**

▶ **ALPHAPRODINE**
Schedule II

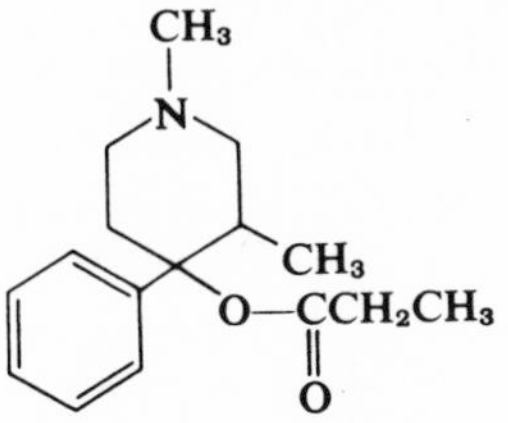

Synonyms: Prisilidene, α-1,3-dimethyl-4-phenyl-4-propionyl-oxypiperidine.
Pharmaceutical Preparations: Nisentil[R] (Roche)—Ampules and vials. Ampules contain 40 mg/ml alphaprodine; vials contain 60 mg/ml alphaprodine.
General Comments: α-Prodine and β-prodine are isomers. Together, they form a racemic mixture of prodine with the same molecular formula. However, α-prodine is an accepted drug for medicinal use whereas β-prodine is not. Therefore, they are listed under Schedules II and I, respectively, of the Controlled Substances Act. The method for distinguishing the two isomers is by optical rotation.

α-Prodine

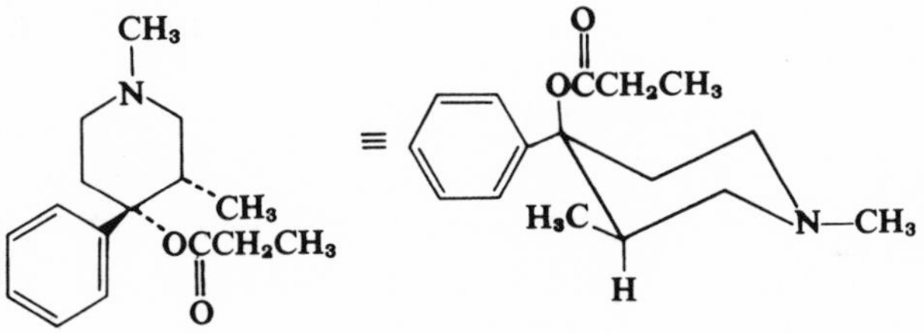

β-Prodine

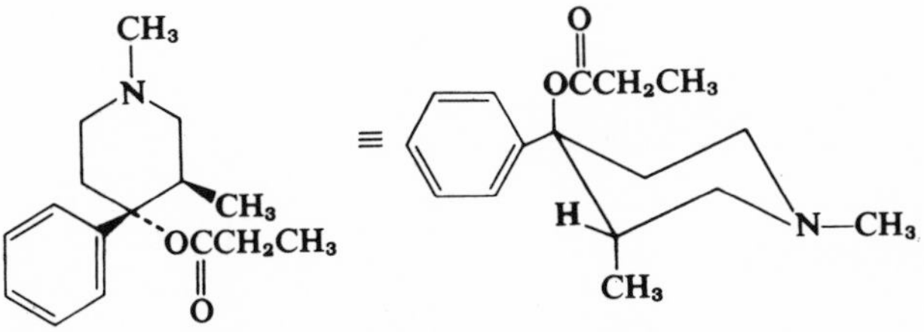

Biochemistry: Extensive quantum chemical calculations have been made of the electronic distribution and confirmation behavior of meperidine (pethidine), (+)-α-prodine, and (+)-β-prodine. These calculations were made using the PCILO semiempirical molecular orbital method (Loew and Jester, 1975). Differences in potency among these compounds were shown to be due solely to receptor interactions and not brain-level concentrations. There are only small structural differences between prodine and meperidine. A difference in potency by a factor of almost 100 is seen in the optical isomers of prodine. For these compounds, the phenyl equitorial confirmation was preferred over the phenyl axial, with the equitorial confirmer most favored and the most potent compound.

α-Prodine is five times as effective as meperidine in animals, and is almost as potent as morphine. β-Prodine is more potent than morphine. α-Prodine has a rapid onset and short duration of action. It may be used for acute pain encountered in childbirth (King, 1956). It is, however, used infrequently because of its strong respiratory-depressant action, dependence liability, and other side effects.

Toxicology–Pharmacology: Usual dose: subcutaneous, 20–40 mg; intravenous, 20 mg. Usual dose range: subcutaneous, 20–60 mg; intravenous, 20–30 mg; oral, 50 mg.

α-Prodine is probably intermediate between morphine and codeine in effectiveness as an analgesic; actions are qualitatively the same as morphine. It is mildly sedative and produces some peripheral vasodilatation; respiratory depression and nausea may be induced. The duration of action is about 1–2 hours. α-Prodine is an addictive drug with withdrawal symptoms similar to those of meperidine. Toxic effects include coma, shallow respiration, cyanosis, hypotension, pinpoint pupils, and early unconsciousness. Specific antidote therapy is administration of nalorphine or levallorphan.

A fatality in a 28-month-old child has been reported after the child was given a total dose of 18 mg α-prodine, 5 mg promethazine, and 5 ml 5% xylocaine in preparation for dental surgery. No α-prodine or promethazine was detected at autopsy (Hine and Pasi, 1972).

▶ **AMBUTONIUM BROMIDE**
Encountered in Excepted Substances

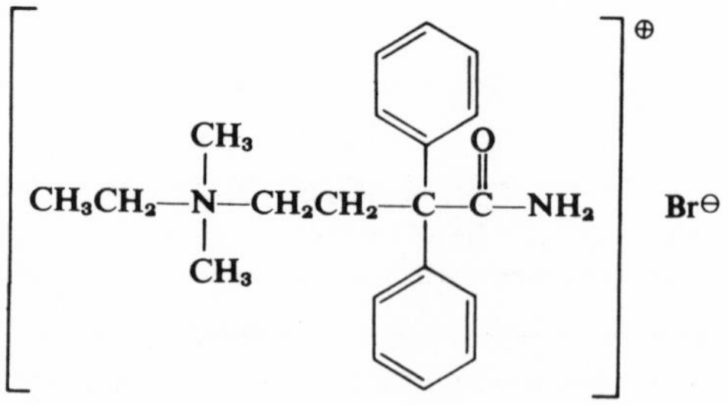

General Comments: Ambutonium bromide, also known as (3-carbamoyl-3,3-diphenyl-propyl) ethyldimethylammonium bromide, is a parasympatholytic drug that has stimulating properties on the central nervous system. It is found in excepted butabarbital preparations with a butabarbital/ambutonium bromide ratio of about 1/0.3.

Pharmacology: Used as an antispasmodic and anticholinergic agent, particularly for gastrointestinal tract ailments (treatment of ulcer).

▶ **AMINOPHYLLINE**
Encountered in Excepted Substances

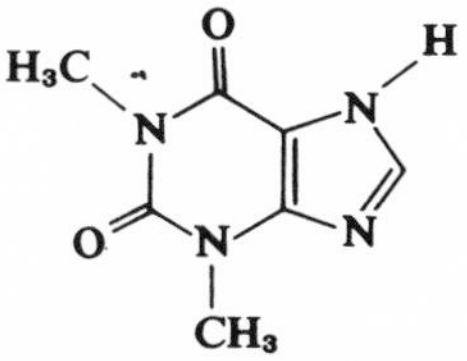

$+ H_2NCH_2CH_2NH_2$

General Comments: Aminophylline is a mixture of theophylline and ethylenediamine, its composition being approximately $(C_7H_8N_4O_2)_2, C_2H_4(NH_2)_2, 2H_2O$. It is encountered in numerous pharmaceutical preparations classified as Excepted Substances. The following table shows the drugs that aminophylline is found with and the drug/aminophylline ratio classifying the preparation as an Excepted Substance.

Drug	Drug/Aminophylline Ratio
Amobarbital	1/3.1
Butabarbital	1/12/0.1 with phenylpropanolamine
Pentobarbital	1/5 (suppository)
Phenobarbital	1/6

Toxicology–Pharmacology: Aminophylline, theophylline, theobromine, and other xanthine compounds are useful as stimulants to the myocardium, or heart muscle. They also have the ability to relax bronchial smooth muscle, and consequently can be used to treat asthma patients. They can be given over prolonged periods of time to reduce the number of asthma attacks. Since aminophylline is essentially a compound of theophylline, the therapeutic comments for theophylline apply here also.

Overdose results in headache, palpitation, dizziness, nausea, and fall in blood pressure. Fatalities can occur in massive overdoses, or rapid intravenous administration, although these have been rare.

▶ **AMITRIPTYLINE**
Dangerous Drug

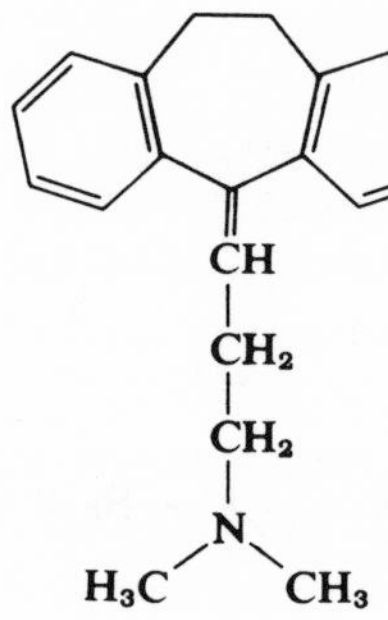

Synonym: 10,11-Dihydro-5-(3-dimethylaminopropylidene)-5*H*-dibenzo-[*a,d*]-cycloheptene.

Pharmaceutical Preparations

Elavil[R] (Merck Sharp & Dohme)—Tablets: blue, round, film-coated, coded MSD23, containing 10 mg amitriptyline; yellow, round, film-coated, coded MSD45, containing 25 mg amitriptyline. Injection: 10 mg/ml amitriptyline.

Etrafon[R] (Schering)—See **PERPHENAZINE**

Triavil[R] (Merck Sharp & Dohme)—See **PERPHENAZINE**

General Comment: Amitriptyline is an antidepressant drug classified in this text as a Dangerous Drug because all pharmaceutical preparations containing amitriptyline require a prescription.

Biochemistry: In the metabolism of amitriptyline, the ethylene bridge adjacent to the aromatic ring is attacked to form the hydroxylated product:

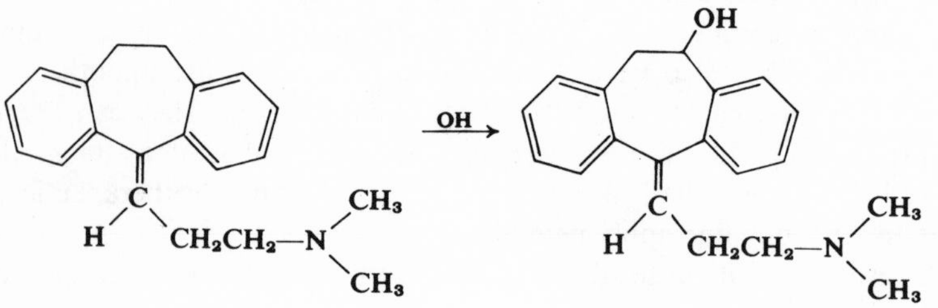

The same hydroxylation occurs with the major metabolite of amitriptyline, nortriptyline (Hucker, 1962; McMahon *et al.*, 1963):

Nortriptyline retains the antidepressant action of the parent drug. The hydroxylated products are excreted in the urine as the glucuronide conjugates.

Stereochemical and conformational considerations appear to be important in determining the kind of psychotropic activity that is elicited by tricyclic compounds. The rigidly planar tricyclic compound, amitriptyline, has no neuroleptic activity but produces distinct clinical antidepressive effects (Poldinger, 1964).

Toxicology–Pharmacology: Amitriptyline is used in the treatment of endogenous depression. In normal individuals, it engenders feelings of fatigue accompanied by atropine-like symptoms (e.g., dryness of the mouth, blurred vision). The mechanism of action in combating depression is not known, but may be due to the anticholinergic effects in the brain. Clinical improvement may not occur prior to several weeks of administration.

Amitriptyline levels in plasma of individuals on therapeutic doses do not usually exceed 0.18 μg/ml (0.018 mg/dl). The major metabolite, nortriptyline, may be found in even larger concentration than the parent compound, and is the major excretion product in the urine. On maintenance therapy of 50 mg amitriptyline administered orally three times a day, blood concentrations of 0.06 mg/dl of amitriptyline and 0.07 mg/dl nortriptyline were found, measured at 2-, 4-, and 6-week intervals (Braithwaite *et al.*, 1972). In urine, several other metabolites are recognized: 5-hydroxy-5-dimethylaminopropyl amitriptyline, didemethylamitriptyline, and amitriptyline *N*-oxide.

Amitriptyline poisoning accounts for a significant number of deaths due to medications each year. Overdose is characterized by predominantly anticholinergic signs, an irritable hyperkinetic state, leading rapidly to coma with respiratory and cardiac arrest being the cause of death. In hospital-treated cases, death may occur up to six days postingestion.

Fatal cases usually have blood levels of greater than 0.20 mg/dl of amitriptyline, with up to five times that concentration of nortriptyline, depending on survival time after ingestion.

▶ **AMOBARBITAL**
Schedule II, Schedule III

Synonyms: Amylobarbitone, pentymalium, 5-ethyl-5-isopentylbarbituric acid.
Pharmaceutical Preparations—Applicable Schedules: The Controlled Substances Act states that unless the substance is listed in another schedule,
Schedule III will apply to any material, compound, mixture, or preparation
that contains any quantity of amobarbital having a potential for abuse associated with a depressant effect on the central nervous system, and that contains, in addition to amobarbital, one or more active medicinal ingredients
that are not scheduled substances. Also, any suppository dosage approved by
the FDA that contains amobarbital falls into Schedule III. Thus, any of the
Schedule III preparations are subject to the excepted substance clause in
Schedule III.
Schedule II Preparations
Amytal^R (Lilly)—Elixirs No. 225, containing 440 mg amobarbital per 100 ml;
   No. 237, containing 880 mg amobarbital per 100 ml. Tablets, capsule-
   shaped and scored: light green, coded T40, containing 15 mg amobarbital; yellow, coded T56, containing 30 mg amobarbital; orange,
   coded T37, containing 50 mg amobarbital; pink, coded T32, containing
   100 mg amobarbital. All tablets are labeled "Lilly."
Amytal^R Sodium Ampoules (Lilly)—Ampules, containing dry powdered
   sodium amobarbital: code No. 361, 65 mg; code No. 362, 125 mg; code
   No. 386, 250 mg; code No. 363, 250 mg; code No. 364, 0.5 g; code No.
   387, 0.5 g.
Amytal^R Sodium Pulvules (Lilly)—Capsules: blue, labeled "Lilly," coded F23
   (containing 65 mg sodium amobarbital), coded F33 (containing 200 mg
   sodium amobarbital)
Dexamyl^R Spansules (Smith Kline & French)—See **AMPHETAMINE**
Dexamyl^R Tablets (Smith Kline & French)—See **AMPHETAMINE**
Dexamyl^R Elixir (Smith Kline & French)—See **AMPHETAMINE**
Tuinal^R (Lilly)—This preparation combines the intermediate-acting sodium
   amobarbital and short-acting sodium secobarbital in equal parts, resulting in an intermediate-acting, rapidly effective hypnotic.

Schedule III Preparations

Ectasule[R] Sr., Jr., and III (Fleming)—Capsules, purple and orange: Sr., containing 30 mg amobarbital and 60 mg ephedrine; Jr., containing 15 mg amobarbital and 30 mg ephedrine; III, containing 8 mg amobarbital and 15 mg ephedrine. The Ectasule[R] should be noted to be different than Ectasule[R] Minus in that Ectasule[R] Minus does not contain amobarbital. Ectasule[R] Minus is found in black and light blue capsules. Also see Chapter 6.

General Comment: From the foregoing information, one can determine the variations in the control status of amobarbital, depending on its formulation. Thus, for scientific–legal purposes, it is necessary to conduct complete laboratory screening for the presence of other medicinal substances for court presentation.

Biochemistry: The major metabolite of amobarbital is the tertiary alcohol 5-ethyl-5-(3'-hydroxy-3'-methylbutyl)barbituric acid (hydroxyamobarbital). Amobarbital is very rapidly metabolized and, in consequence, has only a very short initial hypnotic action of its own. The continued pharmacological activity is due to the metabolite, hydroxyamobarbital, which has weaker but more prolonged hypnotic activity than the parent drug. Two human male subjects who each received a 500-mg dose of ^{15}N-labeled amobarbital excreted a total of 70 and 100% of the dose (51 and 73%, respectively, was ether-extractable) in the urine over 5 days. Both excreted 51% of the dose as hydroxyamobarbital, which accounted for all the ether-soluble material present in the urine of one subject, but only 70% of the ether-soluble material of the second subject (Maynert, 1965).

Amobarbital   Hydroxyamobarbital

Using ^{15}N-labeled amobarbital, it has been shown that the barbiturate ring may undergo scission, and is then metabolized into urea and other products (Maynert and Van Dyke, 1950).

Toxicology–Pharmacology: Amobarbital is a short- to intermediate-acting barbiturate with an approximate duration of effectiveness of 6 hours. Therapeutic dosage may be up to 600 mg per day. It may be used intravenously to control seizures, or orally as a sedative–hypnotic medication.

The usual dosage is 65–200 mg.

Overdosage with amobarbital will cause central nervous system depression. One may see the symptoms of depression of respiration, reflexes, and constriction of the pupils (however, in severe poisoning, the pupils may dilate). Urine formation may decrease, as may the body temperature. The patient may be comatose.

Therapeutic blood levels are usually within the range of 0.2–1.23 mg/dl (Parker *et al.*, 1970). It is excreted in the urine, partly unchanged and partly as the hydroxylated metabolite, 5-ethyl-5(3-hydroxy-3-methylbutyl) barbituric acid.

Toxicity and possible coma begin at a blood level around 3.0 mg/dl, and fatalities usually occur with levels of from 4.0 to 8.0 mg/dl.

▶ **AMPHETAMINE**
Schedule II

$$\text{C}_6\text{H}_5\text{—CH}_2\text{—}\underset{\underset{\text{NH}_2}{|}}{\text{CH}}\text{—CH}_3$$

Synonyms: Isomyn, phenopromine, phenylisopropylamine, racemic deoxynorephedrine, α-methylphenethylamine.

Pharmaceutical Preparations: Amphetamine is found in many pharmaceutical preparations as either the free base, the phosphate salt, or the sulfate salt.

Benzedrine[R] (Smith Kline & French)—Capsule: clear with maroon cap, labeled "SKF," coded A90, containing 15 mg amphetamine. Tablets: orange, triangular, labeled "SKF," coded A92, containing 10 mg amphetamine; coded A91, containing 5 mg amphetamine.

Biphetamine[R] (Pennwalt)—Capsules: white, coded 18-895, containing 3.75 mg amphetamine; black and white, coded 18-878, containing 6.25 mg amphetamine; black, coded 18-875, containing 10 mg amphetamine

Delcobese[R] (Delco)—Tablets or capsules in 5-, 10-, 15-, or 20-mg preparations

Dexamyl[R] (Smith Kline & French)—This preparation contains a mixture of amphetamine and amobarbital. Capsules: clear with green top labeled "SKF" and coded D92, containing 15 mg amphetamine and amobarbital; coded D91, containing 10 mg amphetamine and 65 mg amobarbital. Tablets: light green, triangular, labeled "SKF" and coded D93, containing 5 mg amphetamine and 32 mg amobarbital. Elixir: each 5 ml of the liquid contains 5 mg amphetamine and 32 mg amobarbital.

Obetrol[R] (Obetrol)—Obetrol-10, blue tablet, round, unscored, labeled "OP," containing 5 mg amphetamine and 5 mg methamphetamine; Obetrol-20, orange tablet, round, unscored, labeled "OP," containing 10 mg amphetamine and 10 mg methamphetamine

Also see Chapter 6.

General Comments: Amphetamine is a highly abused drug. The behavior of the amphetamine abuser is characterized by excessive activity. The abuser may be unstable, argumentative, appearing extremely nervous, with difficulty remaining in one position. This drug has a drying effect on the mucous membranes of the mouth and nose, resulting in an unidentifiable odor. As a result of this drying effect, the abuser may constantly lick his lips or rub or scratch his nose.

Because the body develops a tolerance to amphetamine, in time, the abuser must increase the dosage to obtain the psychic effects desired. Tolerance to all the effects does not develop uniformly; thus, the tolerant abuser may develop one or more of the symptoms.

Biochemistry: The major metabolite of amphetamine is *p*-hydroxyamphetamine.

$$HO-\langle\!\!\!\langle\bigcirc\rangle\!\!\!\rangle-CH_2-\overset{\overset{\displaystyle NH_2}{|}}{CH}-CH_3$$

p-Hydroxyamphetamine

This metabolism is a two-step pathway. The formation of *p*-hydroxyamphetamine is the first stage. It is not stereoselective. However, the second stage, β-hydroxylation, is stereoselective and is restricted to the dextro $(+)$ isomer. The metabolite formed is *p*-hydroxyphenylpropanolamine:

$$HO-\langle\!\!\!\langle\bigcirc\rangle\!\!\!\rangle-\overset{\overset{\displaystyle OH}{|}}{CH}-\overset{\overset{\displaystyle NH_2}{|}}{CH}-CH_3$$

p-Hydroxyphenylpropanolamine

The metabolitic selectivity discussed above may account for the more pronounced pharmacological properties of dextro- compared with levo-amphetamine. The dextro isomer is about twice as active as the racemic mixture.

It has been suggested that the central nervous system (CNS) effects of amphetamine are related to its resistance to degradation by monomine oxidase (MAO). However, since amphetamine reduces norepinephrine levels in both peripheral and central tissues, its CNS effects may be related to a lowering of endogenous CNS norepinephrine stores (Stein, 1964).

Toxicology–Pharmacology: Amphetamine has powerful CNS stimulant actions in addition to vasoconstrictive and bronchodilatory actions.

It acts as a respiratory stimulant, cardiac stimulant, and general stimulant. It is used to treat narcolepsy, obesity, fatigue, and parkinsonism. After a usual therapeutic dose of 10–30 mg, the following symptoms are observed: wakefulness, alertness, a decreased sense of fatigue, elevation of mood, increased initiative, confidence, and ability to concentrate, elation and euphoria, and increase in motor and speech activity. Physical performance in athletics is improved.

Prolonged use or large doses are followed by mental depression and fatigue. Tolerance occurs after regular use, resulting in increased dosage to obtain the desired effects. One of its chief uses, in low doses, is suppression of appetite, to encourage weight loss.

Overdose of amphetamine leads to hyperexcitability, paranoia, hyperthermia, headache, hysteria, and final collapse. Death from overdose is extremely rare, and when it occurs is usually the result of intravenous injection. One case of death from oral overdose has been observed, after 150 amphetamine capsules were ingested. A blood level of 1.65 mg/dl of amphetamine was detected at death (DiMaio and Garriott, 1977).

Toxic doses vary widely. However, 5–30 mg is considered to be a therapeutic dose. Maximum therapeutic blood levels of amphetamine are considered to be 0.002–0.010 mg% (Beckett *et al.*, 1969). The minimum toxic blood level of amphetamine is considered to be 0.10 mg%.

▶ **AMYL NITRITE**
Dangerous Drug

$$CH_3\!\!\diagdown\!\!\underset{CH_3\diagup}{CHCH_2CH_2NO_2} + CH_3CH_2\overset{\overset{\displaystyle CH_3}{|}}{CHCH_2NO_2}$$

Pharmaceutical Preparations
Amyl Nitrite[R] (Burroughs-Wellcome)—Vaporole, 5-minute inhaler
Amyl Nitrite[R] (Lilly)—Aspirol, 3-minute inhaler
Amyl Nitrite[R] (Lilly)—Aspirol, 5-minute inhaler
General Comments: Amyl nitrite is classified in this text as a Dangerous Drug because all pharmaceutical preparations require a prescription.

Amyl nitrite consists chiefly of isoamyl nitrite; however, normally one encounters the presence of 2-methylbutyl nitrite also. This coronary vasodilator is abused quite often when the abuser believes it will enhance the sexual orgasm.

The combination of alcohol and amyl nitrite provides a potentially lethal situation.

There are on the market, as "deodorants," substances that produce effects similar to those of amyl nitrite. These "deodorants" (e.g., Bullet, Locker Room, Cat's Meow) contain butyl nitrite, which has an odor similar to dirty socks. On each bottle is the label "Not for Human Consumption." At this time, there is no regulation of butyl nitrite.

Biochemistry: When inhaled, amyl nitrite is rapidly absorbed and its effect is almost immediate. Its action lasts from 2 to 8 minutes, it being metabolized after that time to the nitrite ion and amyl alcohol.

Amyl nitrite will oxidize hemoglobin to methemoglobin. This property enables amyl nitrite to be used in the emergency treatment of cyanide poisoning.

Toxicology–Pharmacology: Amyl nitrite is administered only by inhalation, and is very rapidly absorbed from the lungs. The basic pharmacological property is to relax smooth muscle. The most prominent action and chief therapeutic action is on the vascular smooth muscle, and specifically on the coronary arteries of the heart. By this dilating action, the inhalation of amyl nitrite by a heart attack victim can be life-saving. It is also used for "angina pectoris" or cardiac insufficiency. Side effects are lightheadedness, dizziness, and a temporary fall in blood pressure resulting, in some cases, in syncope. Headache is common.

The nitrite agents are rapidly decomposed in the body, having a therapeutic effect lasting only a few minutes. No deaths or severe toxicity have been reported. No information on blood levels is available.

► **ANHALONIDINE**
Noncontrolled Substance

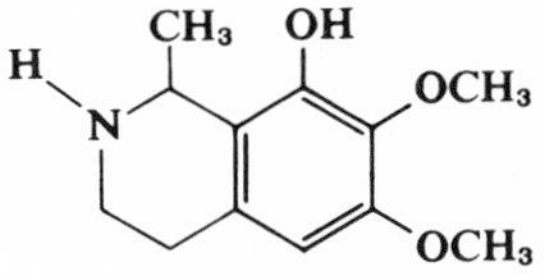

Synonyms: 1,2,3,4-Tetrahydro-6,7-dimethoxy-1-methyl-8-isoquinolinol.
General Comments: This compound is not used medically, and thus is not prepared commercially. It is found in mescal buttons (peyote), the buds of *Lophophora williamsii.*

▶ **ANHALONINE**
Noncontrolled substance

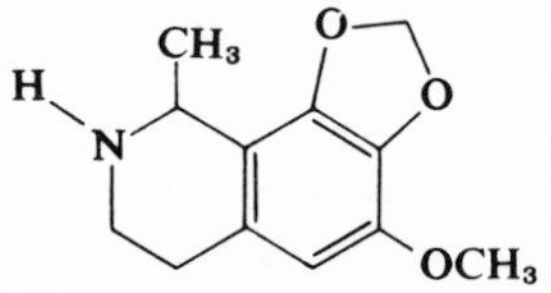

General Comments: This compound is not used medically, and thus is not prepared commercially. It is found in mescal buttons (peyote), the buds of *Lophophora williamsii*. It is not a controlled substance, but is ingested with peyote.

▶ **ANILERIDINE**
Schedule II

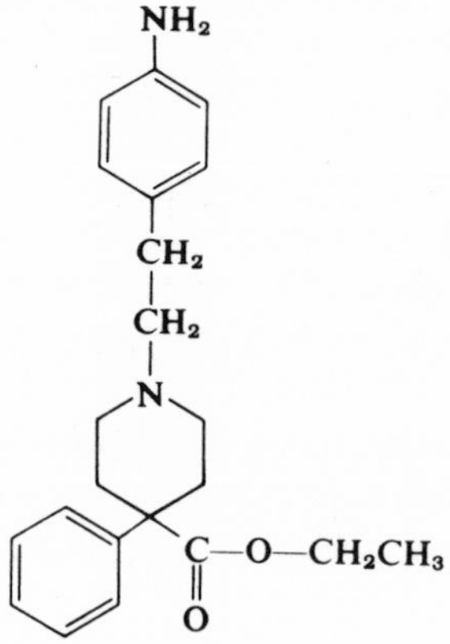

Synonym: Ethyl-1-*p*-aminophenethyl-4-phenylpiperidine-4-carboxylate.
Pharmaceutical Preparations: Leritine^R (Merck Sharp & Dohme)—Tablets and injection
General Comment: Anileridine is a synthetic narcotic analgesic that has been accepted for medicinal use in the United States.
Biochemistry: Anileridine is a piperidine derivative that is $2\frac{1}{2}$ times more active than meperidine. The metabolism of anileridine is also similar to that of meperidine. It undergoes hydrolysis as well as *N*-dealkylation. However, since the structure of anileridine is not rigid like the opiate narcotics, its metabolism becomes more complex.
Toxicology–Pharmacology: Anileridine is a synthetic narcotic analgesic similar in action to meperidine. It has a duration of action of from 2 to 3 hours. The addiction-producing potential is greater than that of meperidine.

Addicts who are tolerant to the depressant effects of anileridine may show the symptoms of tremors, muscle twitches, dilated pupils, hyperactive reflexes, and convulsions. They may be hypersensitive to external stimuli. The person may experience hallucinations.

The recommended oral dose of anileridine is 30–40 mg.

The estimated minimum lethal dose in man is 500 mg. Tolerance to this drug or other narcotic substances enables one to tolerate much larger doses without toxicity. No information on toxic or therapeutic blood levels is available.

▶ ANISOTROPINE
Encountered in Excepted Substances

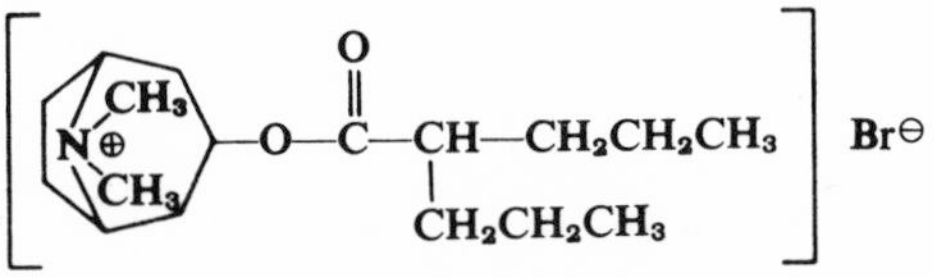

General Comments: Anisotropine is found in pharmaceutical preparations as the methylbromide salt. Anisotropine methylbromide, also known as anisotropine methobromide, octatropine methylbromide, and *N*-methyl-*O*-(2-propyl-pentanoyl)tropinium bromide, is a parasympatholytic drug that, when combined with a depressant drug, decreases the abuse potential of the depressant drug. The preparation may thus be legally classified as an Excepted Substance. The only depressant drug with which anisotropine methylbromide is found in combination that is classified as an Excepted Substance is phenobarbital, in a ratio of 1/1.2 (phenobarbital/anisotropine).

▶ APOMORPHINE
Dangerous Drug

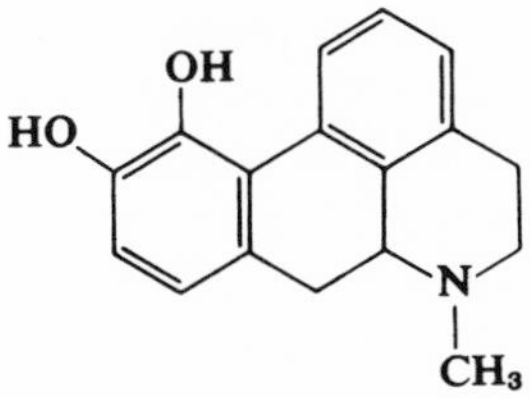

Synonyms: None.
Pharmaceutical Preparations: Apomorphine Hydrochloride[R] (Lilly)—Tablets, containing 6 mg apomorphine hydrochloride

General Comment: Apomorphine was removed from Schedule II of the Controlled Substances Act in September 1976. Since all pharmaceutical preparations containing apomorphine require a prescription, it is classified in this text as a Dangerous Drug.

Toxicology–Pharmacology: Apomorphine is obtained by hydrolyzing morphine with strong mineral acids. It has no analgesic properties, but it can produce a combination of central nervous system excitation and depression. However, apomorphine is not an abused drug, probably because of its primary effects as an emetic. It is used to induce vomiting in cases of poisoning by orally ingested substances. The usual dose is 0.1 mg/kg given subcutaneously.

▶ **APROBARBITAL**
Schedule III

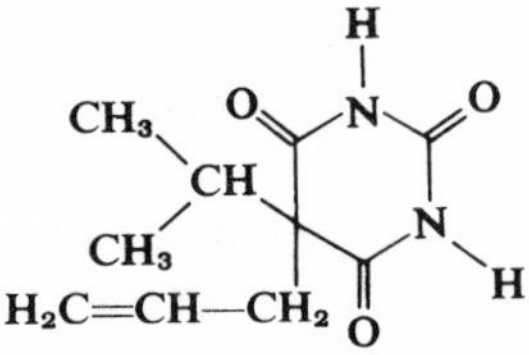

Synonyms: Aprobarbitone, allylisopropylmalonylurea, allypropymal, 5-allyl-5-isopylbarbituric acid.
Pharmaceutical Preparations: Alurate^R (Roche)—Elixir, red. Elixir verdum, green
General Comments: Aprobarbital is an intermediate-acting barbiturate and has toxic actions similar to those of amobarbital. It is listed under Schedule III as a "derivative of barbituric acid."
Biochemistry: See **AMOBARBITAL.**
Toxicology–Pharmacology: Aprobarbital is similar in action to amobarbital, having an onset of action of $\frac{1}{4}$ to $\frac{1}{2}$ hour with a 2–8-hour duration of action. For dosage and toxic data of aprobarbital, see **AMOBARBITAL.**

▶ **ASCORBIC ACID**
Noncontrolled Substance

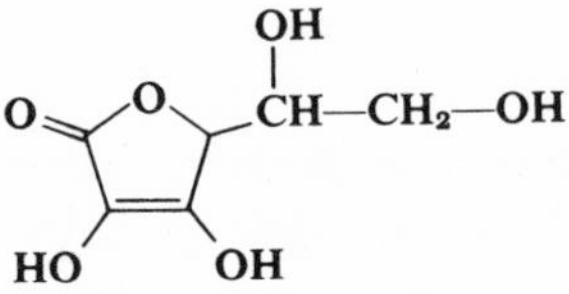

General Comments: Ascorbic acid, also known as vitamin C, cevitamic acid, and 3-oxo-L-gulofuranolacetone (enolicform), is not a Controlled Substance. However, it is frequently mistaken for a controlled drug by law-enforcement officers.

▶ **ATROPINE**
Encountered in Excepted Substances

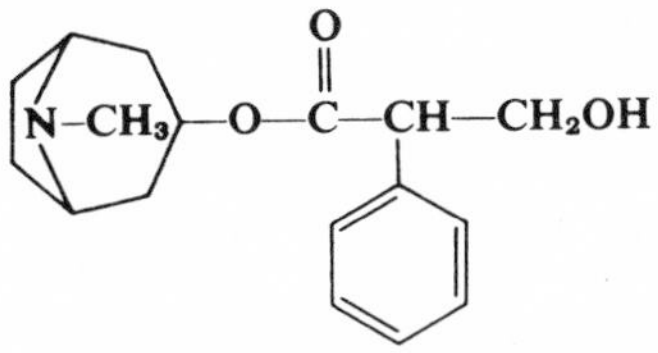

General Comments: Atropine is *dl*-hyoscyamine, which is the racemic form of an alkaloid usually obtained from species of belladonna, hyoscyamus, or stramonium, or prepared synthetically from tropinone.
Pharmaceutical Preparations: It is encountered in numerous pharmaceutical preparations classified as Excepted Substances. The following table shows the drugs with which atropine is found and the drug/atropine ratio classifying the preparation as an Excepted Substance:

Drug	Drug/Atropine Ratio
Allobarbital	1/0.013
Phenobarbital	1/0.0016

Toxicology–Pharmacology: The primary pharmacological action of atropine is to counteract the effects of acetylcholine, the neurotransmitter agent of the parasympathetic nervous system and at the ganglia of the sympathetic nervous system. It is used in the treatment of poisoning from agents that have anticholinesterase activity (e.g., organophosphorous insecticides, "nerve gases"). It also has therapeutic application to suppress motility and secretions of the gastrointestinal tract, as a presurgical medication, and in ulcer therapy, and is used as a mydriatic agent in ophthalmology.

Atropine poisoning may occur from ingestion of belladonna, or from administration of atropine therapeutically to children. Fatalities are rare, but may occur in children. The fatal dose is not known, but up to 200 mg have been used therapeutically, and a 1000-mg dose has been survived. In children, 10 mg may be a lethal dose. Symptoms of atropine intoxication include rapid heart rate, marked dryness of the mouth, dilated pupils, blurring of near vision, flushed, dry, hot skin, ataxia, restlessness, hallucinations, and delirium.

▶ **AZACYCLONOL**
Dangerous Drug

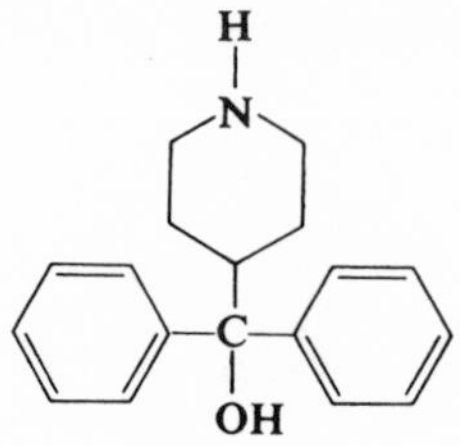

Synonym: α,α-Diphenyl-α-piperid-4-ylmethanol.
Pharmaceutical Preparations: Azacyclonol is not found in any pharmaceutical preparations sold in the United States.
General Comments: Azacyclonol is classified pharmacologically as a tranquilizer. It is therefore classified in this text as a Dangerous Drug. Azacyclonol does not produce any sedative or hypnotic effects.
Biochemistry: Unknown.
Toxicology–Pharmacology: Unknown.

▶ **BARBITAL**
Schedule IV

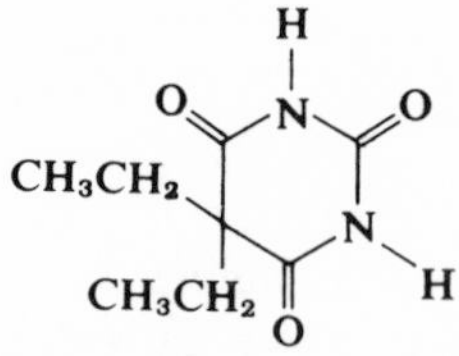

Synonyms: Barbitone, barbiton, diemalum diethylmalonylurea, malonal, malonurea, 5,5-diethylbarbituric acid.
Pharmaceutical Preparations
Plexonal[R] (Sandoz)—Tablet: white, triangular, sugar-coated, labeled "-57," containing 45 mg barbital, 15 mg phenobarbital, 25 mg butalbital, 0.08 mg scopolamine, and 0.16 mg dihydroergotamine. However, because this preparation contains butalbital, Plexonal falls under Schedule III.
Tetralute[R] I (Miles)—See Chapter 6.
General Comments: Barbital is a long-acting barbiturate and as such is less toxic than the short-acting ones. Usually, overdoses of the short- to intermediate-acting barbiturates are the ones requiring hospital treatment.

Biochemistry: Barbital is a long-acting barbiturate. Most of it is excreted almost entirely unchanged in the urine over a period of several days. It has been shown with [^{14}C]barbital that metabolism does occur to a slight extent, and that this results in the hydroxylation, or in the elimination, of one of the ethyl substituent groups:

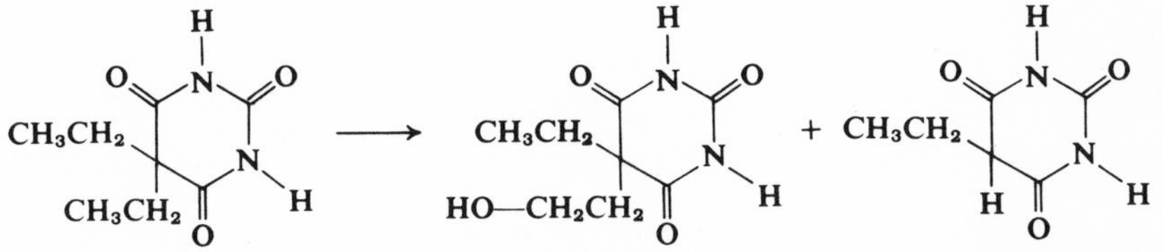

Barbital   Hydroxybarbital   5-Ethylbarbituric acid

Toxicology–Pharmacology: Barbital is a long-acting barbiturate, due to the fact that it is not metabolized to any significant degree in the body, but is eliminated by renal excretion. Its primary use is as a laboratory reagent, and in experimental pharmacology. It is less than half as potent as phenobarbital, and blood levels of greater than 25 mg/dl may be found after overdose.

▶ **BENACTYZINE**
Dangerous Drug

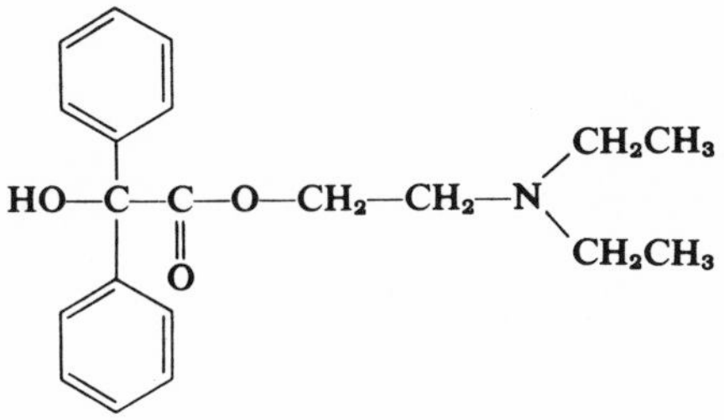

Synonym: 2-Diethylaminoethylbenzilate.
Pharmaceutical Preparations: Benactyzine is found in the pharmaceutical preparation Deprol^R (Wallace). However, because this preparation also contains meprobamate, it is controlled under Schedule IV.
General Comments: Benactyzine is rapidly metabolized and excreted; thus, its action is very short. As a tranquilizer, it is classified in this text as a Dangerous Drug. Benactyzine is referred to as "DMZ" in the drug culture.
Biochemistry: Benactyzine is a tertiary alkylamine. It has a variety of metabolitic pathways including *N*-dealkylation, hydrolysis, and aromatic hydroxylation.

Toxicology–Pharmacology: In addition to being a psychosedative, benactyzine is an anticholinergic drug having antisecretory action about five to six times greater, and antispasmodic action about three to four times greater, than atropine. The effective oral dose in man is indicated to be 3–9 mg.

▶ **BENZETHIDINE**
Schedule I

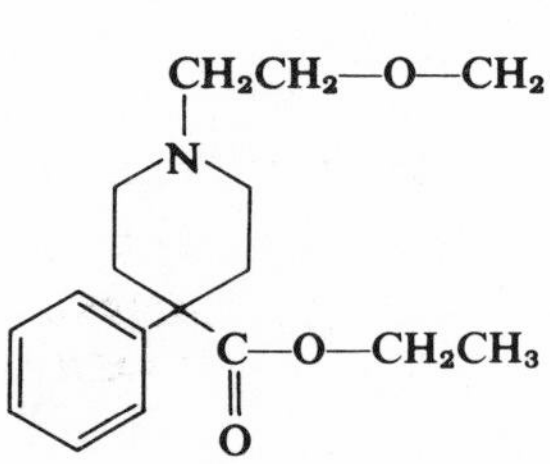

$$CH_2CH_2\!-\!O\!-\!CH_2\!-\!\langle phenyl \rangle$$

(structure: piperidine ring with N bearing $CH_2CH_2\!-\!O\!-\!CH_2\!-$phenyl substituent, and the 4-position bearing a phenyl group and $C(=\!O)\!-\!O\!-\!CH_2CH_3$)

Synonyms: Benzyloxyethylnorpethidine, ethyl-1-(2-benzyloxyethyl)4-phenyl-piperidine-4-carboxylate.
Pharmaceutical Preparations: Benzethidine is not found in any pharmaceutical preparations sold in the United States.
General Comments: Benzethidine is chemically similar to pethidine. It has the properties of a narcotic analgesic, but has not been accepted in the United States for medicinal use.
Biochemistry: Unknown.
Toxicology–Pharmacology: Similar to that of meperidine (pethidine).

▶ **BENZITRAMIDE**
Schedule II
Synonym: 1-(3-Cyano-3,3-diphenylpropyl)-4-(2-oxo-3-propionyl-1-benzimidazolinyl)-piperidine (?).
Pharmaceutical Preparations: Benzitramide is not found in any pharmaceutical preparations sold in the United States.
General Comments: Benzitramide is probably chemically and pharmacologically related to pethidine. Even though this drug is accepted as a medicinal narcotic analgesic, it is not listed in any literature to the knowledge of these authors, much less marketed.
Biochemistry: Unknown.
Toxicology–Pharmacology: Unknown.

▶ **BENZOCAINE**
Noncontrolled Substance

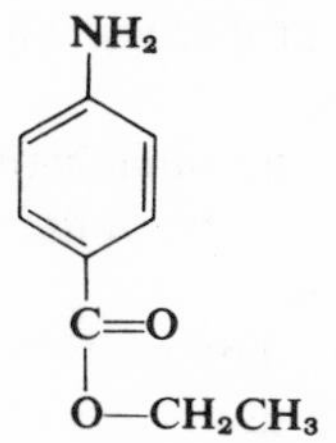

$$NH_2$$

$$C=O$$
$$O-CH_2CH_3$$

General Comments: Benzocaine, also known as ethoforme, ethyl amino-benzoate, noicainam, and ethyl *p*-aminobenzoate, is a local anesthetic. This substance is not controlled by the Controlled Substances Act and is found in over-the-counter (OTC) preparations. It has been found as an adulterant in illicit drug preparations, and as such has been encountered in numerous cases of drug abuse.

Toxicology–Pharmacology: Benzocaine is one of a large number of drugs known as local anesthetics. When these drugs are applied to the skin or mucous membranes, the generation and conduction of nerve impulses is prevented, resulting in loss of sensation or pain. They are absorbed well and may be detected in blood within a short time after application. They are used in minor surgical procedures, or in proprietary preparations to alleviate minor pain or itching. Benzocaine is one of the least soluble of the group. It may be incorporated in oily solutions, ointments, and suppositories. It is probably not very toxic due to low solubility.

▶ **BENZPHETAMINE**
Schedule III

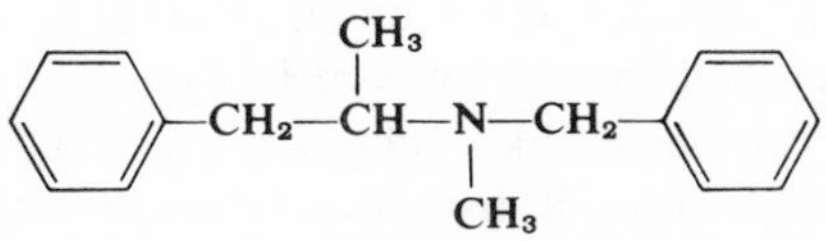

$$CH_3$$
$$-CH_2-CH-N-CH_2-$$
$$CH_3$$

Synonym: (+)-*N*-benzyl-*N*-α-dimethylphenethylamine.
Pharmaceutical Preparations: Didrex[R] (Upjohn)—Tablets: unscored, yellow, labeled "UPJOHN," containing 25 mg benzphetamine; scored, pink, labeled "UPJOHN," containing 50 mg benzphetamine
General Comment: Benzphetamine was added to Schedule III after the Controlled Substances Act was passed when abuse was noted to increase.
Biochemistry: Benzphetamine is chemically related to the amphetamines.

Toxicology–Pharmacology: Benzphetamine, like the other members of the amphetamine group, has sympathomimetic and central nervous system (CNS) stimulant properties. Its only therapeutic indications are as an anorectic agent. Because of the stimulant properties, it is subject to use for this purpose, and may become habit-forming.

Chronic usage may lead to insomnia, irritability, hyperactivity, and personality changes. In severe cases, the abuser may show signs of psychosis similar to those of schizophrenia.

Benzphetamine, as a sympathomimetic amine, is a CNS stimulant with anorexigenic effect that makes it useful as a short-term adjunct in the control of obesity along with caloric restriction.

▶ **BENZQUINAMIDE**
Dangerous Drug

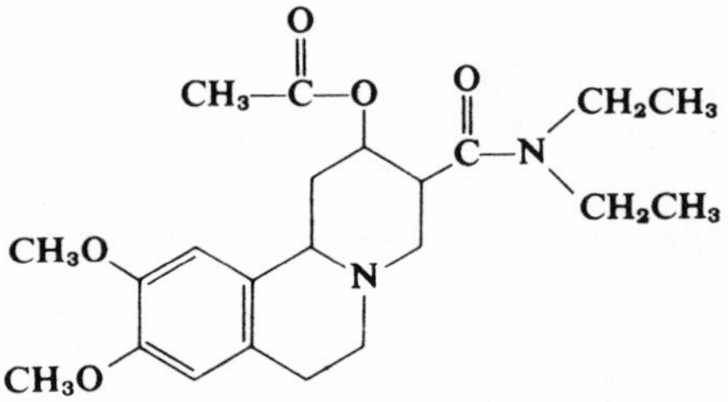

Synonym: 2-Acetoxy-1,3,4,6,7,11-b-hexahydro-9,10-dimethoxy-2*H*-benzo-[α]-quinolizine-3-carboxydiethylamide.
Pharmaceutical Preparations: Benzquinamide is not found in any pharmaceutical preparations sold in the United States.
General Comment: Benzquinamide is classified pharmacologically as a tranquilizer and is therefore classified in this text as a Dangerous Drug.
Biochemistry: Benzquinamide cannot be classified precisely with either the phenothiazines or reserpine on the basis of its biological properties. At low doses, it produces neuroleptic-like actions without affecting monoamine levels. However, at high doses, it displays a relatively weak amine-depleting action. Benzquinamide enhances the behavioral and biochemical effects of reserpine.

Benzquinamide is readily absorbed after oral administration and rapidly distributed throughout the tissues. From animal experiments, the plasma half-life of benzquinamide was determined to be 30–40 minutes. The metabolites are excreted both in the urine and in the bile. The more polar metabolites are not reabsorbed from the bile and are excreted in the feces. The major metabolite is *N*-deethylbenzquinamide (see following page).

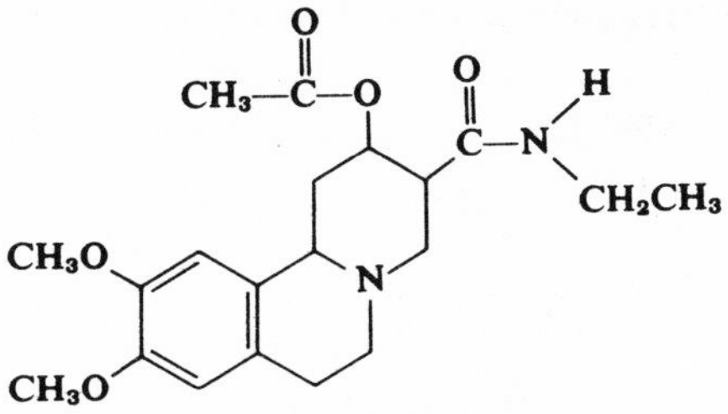

N-Deethylbenzquinamide

Ten other metabolites have also been identified. These are products of N-dealkylation, O-demethylation, and deacetylation (Wiseman *et al.*, 1964; Koe and Pinson, 1964).

Toxicology–Pharmacology: Benzquinamide is rapidly and completely absorbed after oral administration. However, when given rectally, it is slowly absorbed and is eliminated from the body prior to complete absorption.

Benzquinamide resembles the phenothiazine tranquilizers in its ability to depress conditioned avoidance behavior. It has been advocated in the treatment of anxiety in psychoneurotic patients, and has been reported to be helpful in treatment of anxiety in psychotic patients.

No toxicity information or blood levels have been reported.

BENZYLMORPHINE
Schedule I

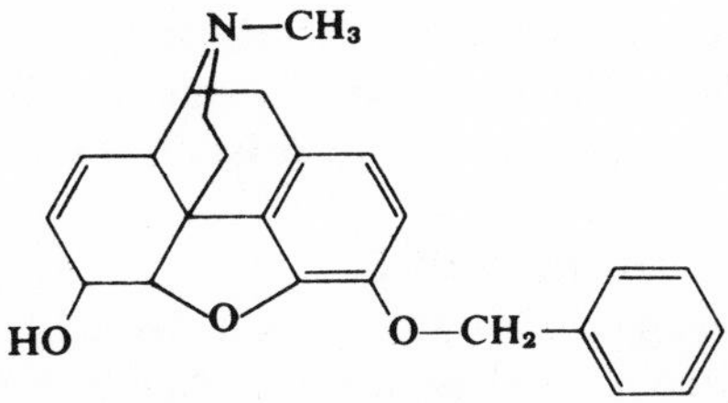

Synonym: 3-Benzyloxy-7,8-dehydro-4,5-epoxy-6-hydroxy-N-methylmorphinan.
Pharmaceutical Preparations: Benzylmorphine is not found in any pharmaceutical preparations sold in the United States.
General Comment: Benzylmorphine is a narcotic analgesic that has not been accepted for medicinal use in the United States because of its high addictive properties.
Biochemistry: Unknown.
Toxicology–Pharmacology: Unknown.

▶ **BETAACETYLMETHADOL**
Schedule I
See **ACETYLMETHADOL**

▶ **BETAMEPRODINE**
Schedule I
See **MEPRODINE**

▶ **BETAMETHADOL**
Schedule I
See **METHADOL**

▶ **BETAPRODINE**
Schedule I

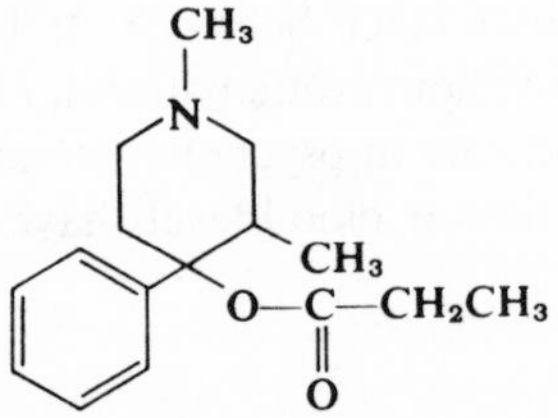

Synonym: β-1,3-Dimethyl-4-phenyl-4-propionyloxypiperidine.
Pharmaceutical Preparations: Unlike its α isomer, β-prodine is not prepared pharmaceutically and is thus placed in Schedule I.
General Comment: β-Prodine and α-prodine must be distinguished from one another by some means, such as optical rotation, to present adequate court evidence.
Biochemistry: See **ALPHAPRODINE.**
Toxicology–Pharmacology: β-Prodine is quite dissimilar chemically to morphine, but has many pharmacological similarities. The mechanism of action is probably the same as that of morphine.

In the nontolerant human, a toxic dose of either α- or β-prodine produces respiratory depression. This can be treated with nalorphine.

In addicts, large doses, repeated at short intervals, produce tremors, muscle twitches, dilated pupils, hyperactive reflexes, and convulsions.

Tolerance to the isomers of prodine develops slowly, probably due to the short duration of action, which is 1–2 hours.

The pattern of withdrawal symptoms after abrupt discontinuation of both α- and β-prodine is somewhat different than that caused by the use of morphine. The autonomic nervous system is affected less, but the symptoms develop more rapidly and are of shorter duration.

An effective dosage range for analgesia is estimated to be 30–40 mg for α-prodine. However, considering that the physiological action of the β isomer is much greater, one should consider these numbers somewhat large.

▶ **BIPERIDEN**
Dangerous Drug

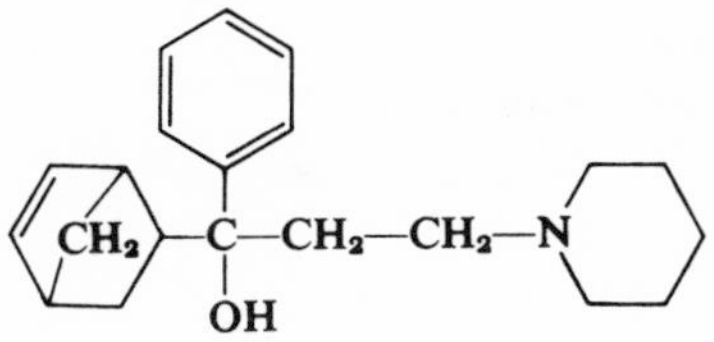

Synonym: 1-(Bicyclo-[2,2,1]-hept-5-5-en-2-yl)-1-phenyl-3-piperidine-propanol.
Pharmaceutical Preparations: Akineton^R (Knoll)—Ampules: 1 ml, containing 5 mg biperiden as lactate salt. Tablets: white, single-scored, with identification mark "△," containing 2 mg biperiden as hydrochloride salt.
General Comment: Since all pharmaceutical preparations containing biperiden require a prescription, and thus bear the label "Caution: Federal law prohibits dispensing without a prescription," it is classified in this text as a Dangerous Drug.
Biochemistry: Unknown.
Toxicology–Pharmacology: Biperiden is a parasympatholytic drug that has anticholinergic activity useful in treating drug-induced parkinsonism.

A therapeutic dose of biperiden is considered to be about 2.0–5.0 mg; however, the toxicity of this drug is relatively low.

▶ **4-BROMO-2,5-DIMETHOXYAMPHETAMINE**
Schedule I

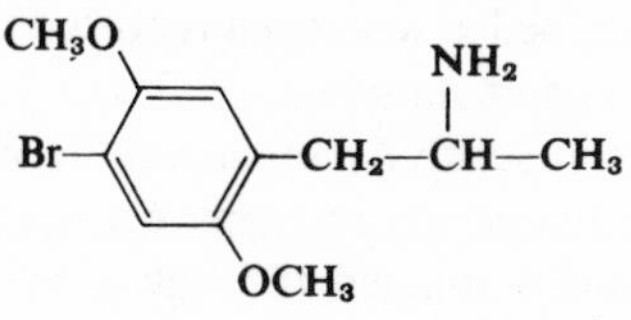

Synonyms: 4-Bromo-2,5-dimethoxy-α-methylphenethyl-amine; 4-bromo-2,5-DMA.

Pharmaceutical Preparations: This drug is not found in any pharmaceutical preparations sold in the United States.

General Comments: 4-Bromo-2,5-dimethoxyamphetamine has appeared to a limited extent on the illicit market in the past. It has been found in tablet form sold illicitly under the name "100X." It is chemically prepared by bromination of 2,5-dimethoxyamphetamine.

4-Bromo-2,5-dimethoxyamphetamine is one of the "psychotomimetic amphetamines" that produce many of the effects of amphetamine but have the added capability of producing hallucinations. Therefore, it is controlled under Schedule I as a hallucinogen.

Biochemistry: Unknown.

Toxicology–Pharmacology: Unknown.

▶ **BUFOTENINE**
Schedule I

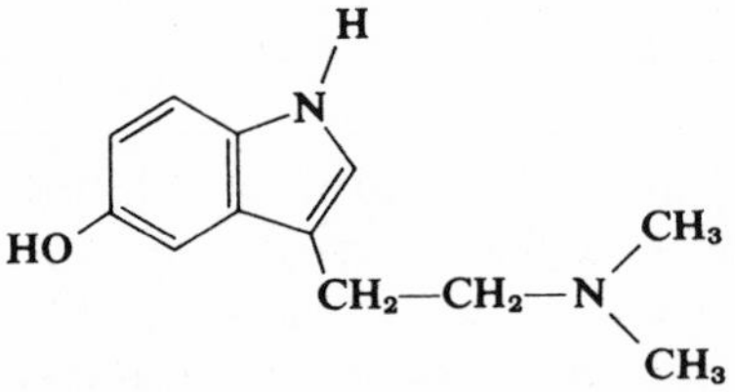

Synonyms: Bufotenine is a derivative of 5-hydroxytryptamine and has the chemical names of N,N-dimethylserotonin, 5-hydroxy-N-dimethyltryptamine, mappine, and 3-(2-dimethylaminoethyl)-5-hydroxyindole.

Bufotenine received its name because it was first discovered in skin and glands of toads (*Bufo* sp.). It is now known to be widely distributed in higher plants and animals.

Pharmaceutical Preparations: Bufotenine is not found in any pharmaceutical preparations sold in the United States.

General Comments: The genus *Anadenanthera* has been shown to contain bufotenine. It has also been found as a minor component in the plant *Banisteriopsis rusbyana*. Bufotenine has also been reported in some species of *Piptadenia phalaris* (the fungus) and *Amanita*.

Certain Indian tribes in South America and the West Indies use the seeds and pods from the plant *Piptadenia* to prepare a snuff called cohobo, niopo, parica, or yopo. The snuff is inhaled through a bifurcated tube fitting the nose. The Indians believe the snuff makes them fearless and insensitive to pain.

Biochemistry: Bufotenine is a 5-hydroxytryptamine derivative. Serotonin,

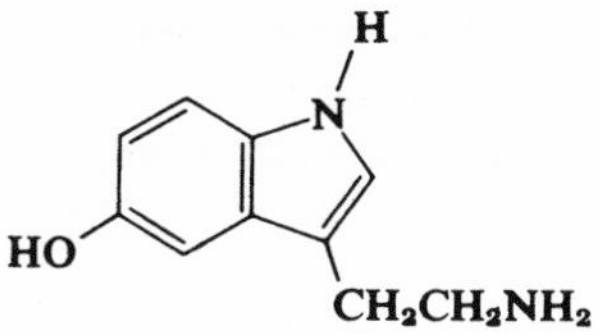

Serotonin

which is 5-hydroxytryptamine, is a neurohumoral factor that is widely distributed in warm-blooded animals. It accumulates in the brain, where it plays a role in the biochemistry of central nervous regulations. Thus, by this comparison, one can see the properties that bufotenine has in producing psychotomimetic symptoms.

Toxicology–Pharmacology: Bufotenine has pharmacological activity similar to that of dimethyltryptamine. Intravenous doses of 8–70 mg have been reported to produce hallucinations. However, there have been reports of 20-mg intravenous doses and 50-mg oral doses not producing a hallucinogenic effect.

After doses of 4–16 mg intravenously, subjects experienced placiditis, lightheadedness, seeing colored spots, visual hallucinations, and nausea. The effects were reported to be similar to those of lysergic acid diethyl amide, but of shorter duration (Fabig and Hawkins, 1956).

▶ **BUTABARBITAL**
Schedule III

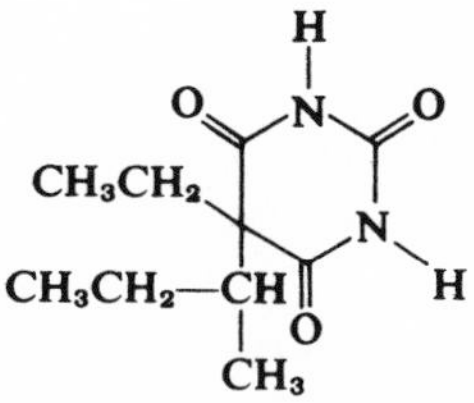

Synonyms: Secbutobarbitone, secbutabarbital, secumalum, 5-ethyl-5-S-butylbarbituric acid.

Pharmaceutical Preparations

Butiserpazide[R] (McNeil)—Schedule III, Penalty Group 3, preparation: Tablets: green, containing 30 mg butabarbital, 25 mg hydrochlorothiazide, and 0.1 mg reserpine; orange, containing 30 mg butabarbital, 50 mg hydrochlorothiazide, and 0.1 mg reserpine

Cystopaz[R] (Webcon)—Capsule: opaque blue and clear yellow, containing 45 mg butabarbital and 35 μg hyoscyamine

Decholin-BB[R] (Dome)—Tablet: tan, single-scored, containing 15 mg butabarbital, 250 mg dehydrocholic acid, and 10 mg belladonna extract

Quibron^R Plus (Mead Johnson)—Capsule: light green, labeled "MJ," liquid-filled soft gelatin. Elixir. Each capsule or 15 ml elixir contains 20 mg butabarbital, 150 mg theophylline, 100 mg glyceryl guaiacolate, and 25 mg ephedrine.

Sedapap-10^R (Mayrand)—Tablet containing 16 mg butabarbital and 648 mg acetaminophen

Sidonna^R (Reed & Carnrick)—Tablet: single-scored, labeled "R-C," light green, containing 16 mg butabarbital, 25 mg simethicone, and belladonna alkaloids of 0.1037 mg hyoscyamine, 0.0194 mg atropine, and 0.0065 mg scopolamine

Also see Chapter 6.

General Comments: Butabarbital is an intermediate-acting barbiturate. It is listed under Schedule III of the Controlled Substances Act under "derivatives of barbituric acid."

Biochemistry: Similar to that of pentobarbital.

Toxicology–Pharmacology: Butabarbital is an intermediate-acting barbiturate. Overdosage with butabarbital will cause central nervous system depression. One may see the symptoms of depression of respiration, reflexes, and constriction of the pupils (however, in severe poisoning, the pupils may dilate). Urine formation may decrease, as may the body temperature. The patient may be comatose. Death may result from respiratory depression. Lethal blood concentrations are probably greater than 3.0 mg/dl.

▶ **BUTALBITAL**
Schedule III

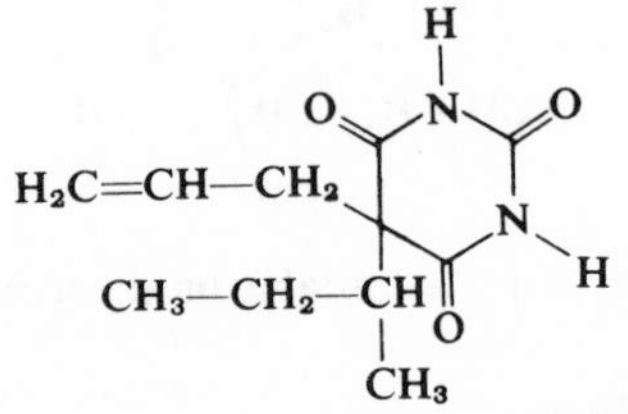

Synonyms: Allylbarbituric acid, itobarbital, tetrallobarbital, 5-allyl-5-iso-butylbarbituric acid.

Pharmaceutical Preparations

Buff-A-Comp^R (Mayrand)—Tablet: labeled "M/R," containing 648 mg aspirin, 130 mg phenacetin, 43.2 mg caffeine, 48.6 mg butalbital

Fiorinal^R (Sandoz)—Tablets: labeled "SANDOZ." Capsules: Kelly green and lime green, labeled "SANDOZ." Each tablet and capsule contains

50 mg butalbital, 40 mg caffeine, 200 mg aspirin, and 130 mg phenacetin.

Fiorinal^R w/Codeine (Sandoz)—Capsules: Nos. 1, 2, and 3, each containing 50 mg butalbital, 40 mg caffeine, 200 mg aspirin, and 130 mg phenacetin; No. 1 capsule, red and yellow, containing 7.5 mg codeine; No. 2 capsule, gray and yellow, containing 15 mg codeine; No. 3 capsule, blue and yellow, containing 30 mg codeine

Plexonal^R (Sandoz)—Tablet: white, triangular, sugar-coated, labeled "-57," containing 45 mg barbital, 15 mg phenobarbital, 25 mg butalbital, 0.08 mg scopolamine, and 0.16 mg dihydroergotamine

Rengesin^R (Kenwood)—Tablet containing 30 mg butalbital, 60 mg caffeine, 450 mg aspirin, and 150 mg aluminum hydroxide

Repan^R (Everett)—Tablet containing 50 mg butalbital, 40 mg caffeine, 130 mg phenacetin, and 300 mg acetaminophen

General Comments: Butalbital is an intermediate-acting barbiturate. It is listed under Schedule III of the Controlled Substances Act under "derivatives of barbituric acid."

Biochemistry: Similar to that of pentobarbital.

Toxicology–Pharmacology: Butalbital is an intermediate-acting barbiturate. Overdosage will cause central nervous system depression. One may see the symptoms of depression of respiration, reflexes, and constriction of the pupils (however, in severe poisoning, the pupils may dilate). Urine formation may decrease, as may the body temperature. The patient may be comatose.

▶ **BUTALLYLONAL**
Schedule III

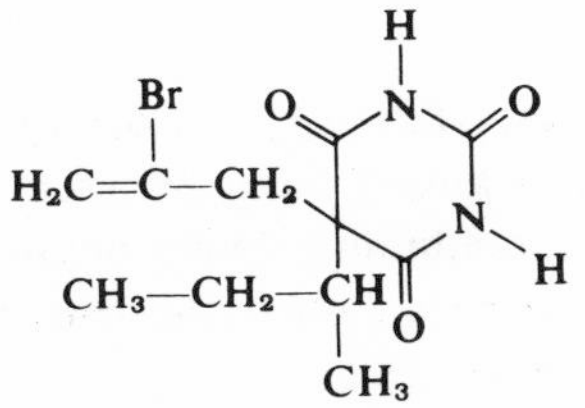

Synonyms: Butyl-bromallyl-barbituric acid, 5-(2-bromallyl)-5-S-butyl-barbituric acid.

Pharmaceutical Preparations: Butallylonal is not found in any pharmaceutical preparations sold in the United States.

General Comments: Butallylonal is an intermediate-acting barbiturate. It is listed under Schedule III of the Controlled Substances Act under "derivatives of barbituric acid."

Biochemistry: The ketone product, ketobutallylonal, is the major metabolite of the 2-bromoalkylbarbiturate, butallylonal (Williams, 1959):

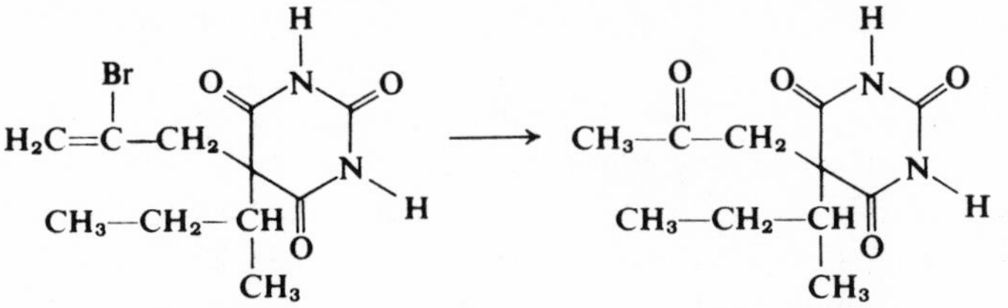

Butallylonal   Ketobutallylonal

Toxicology–Pharmacology: Butallylonal is an intermediate-acting barbiturate. Its pharmacological and toxicological actions will be similar to those of other intermediate-acting barbiturates such as butabarbital.

▶ **BUTAPERAZINE**
Dangerous Drug
Prescription Drug

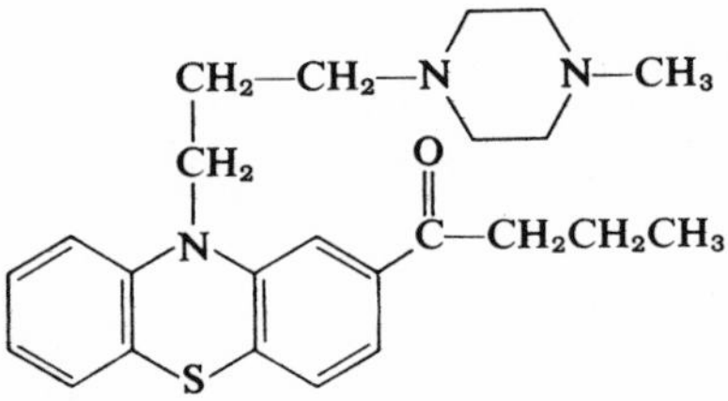

Synonyms: Butyrylperazine, 2-butyryl-10-[3-(4-methylpiperazine-lyl)-propyl]-phenothiazine.
Pharmaceutical Preparations: Repoise^R (Robins)—Tablets, film-coated, labeled "AHR": yellow, containing 5 mg butaperazine; green, containing 10 mg butaperazine; orange, containing 25 mg butaperazine
General Comment: Butaperazine is a phenothiazine tranquilizer. As such, it is listed in this text as a Dangerous Drug.
Biochemistry: The biochemistry of butaperazine is more complex than that of other phenothiazines due to the structural complexity of the molecule.
Toxicology–Pharmacology: An overdose of butaperazine may produce a Parkinson-like effect exhibited by tremors, rigidity, shuffling gait, and excessive salivation. Symptoms of central nervous system depression or agitation and restlessness may be observed. Chills, fever, gastrointestinal disturbances, shock, and coma may occur.

▶ **BUTHALITAL**
Schedule III

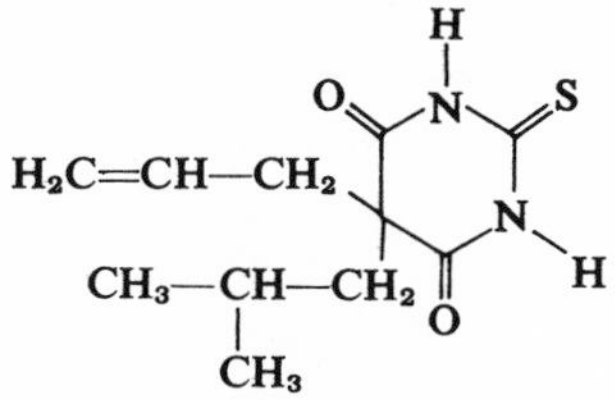

$H_2C{=}CH{-}CH_2$
$CH_3{-}CH{-}CH_2$
CH_3

Synonym: Buthalitone 5-allyl-5-isobutyl-2-thiobarbituric acid.
Pharmaceutical Preparations: Buthalital is not found in any pharmaceutical preparations sold in the United States.
General Comments: Buthalital is a short-acting barbiturate. It is listed under Schedule III of the Controlled Substances Act under "derivatives of barbituric acid."
Biochemistry: Similar to that of secobarbital.
Toxicology–Pharmacology: Buthalital is a short-acting barbiturate. Its pharmacological and toxicological actions are similar to those of secobarbital.

▶ **BUTOBARBITAL**
Schedule III

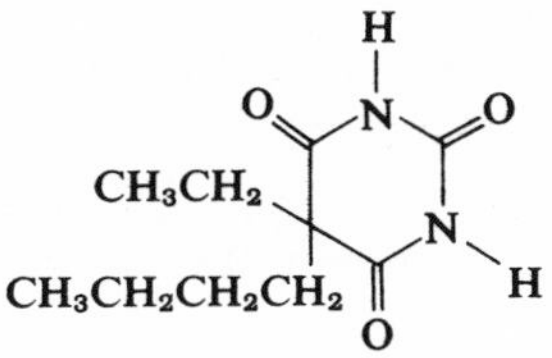

CH_3CH_2
$CH_3CH_2CH_2CH_2$

Synonyms: Butobarbitone, butethal, 5-butyl-5-ethylbarbituric acid.
Pharmaceutical Preparations: Butobarbital is not found in any pharmaceutical preparations sold in the United States.
General Comments: Butobarbital is an intermediate-acting barbiturate. It is listed under Schedule III of the Controlled Substances Act under "derivatives of barbituric acid."
Biochemistry: Similar to that of secobarbital.
Toxicology–Pharmacology: Butobarbital is an intermediate-acting barbiturate that has pharmacological and toxicological actions similar to those of butabarbital.

▶ **CAFFEINE**
Noncontrolled Substance

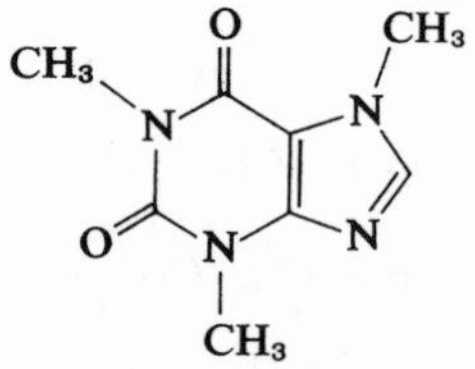

General Comments: Caffeine, a xanthine derivative, is found as an ingredient of several pharmaceutical preparations, as well as several illicit preparations. It is not a controlled substance and may be purchased "over the counter."

Toxicology–Pharmacology: Caffeine is one of a group of alkaloids known as xanthines. It is a component of coffee beans, tea leaves, colas, and chocolate. Its primary pharmacological actions are from central nervous system stimulation, stimulation of the heart muscle and general circulation, and increase in the production of urine (diuresis).

It is used primarily for its general stimulant actions, and is consumed most popularly in the beverages coffee, tea, and colas. It may be used medicinally in the treatment of sedative drug intoxication, such as that from barbiturates, and as a cardiac stimulant.

Toxicity is uncommon, but fatal reactions have occurred from ingestion or injection of large doses of caffeine. A lethal dose is estimated at 10 g in adults. Ingestion of about 5 g has been fatal to a 5-year-old child (Di Maio and Garriott, 1974). Insomnia, restlessness, and excitement occur after overdose. Death may result from cardiac arrhythmia.

Usual blood levels of caffeine after ingestion of two cups of strong coffee are around 0.50 mg/dl. Fatal levels reach 15.0 mg/dl or higher. The plasma half-life is about 3.0–3.5 hours in man (Peters, 1967).

▶ **CAPTODIAME**
Dangerous Drug

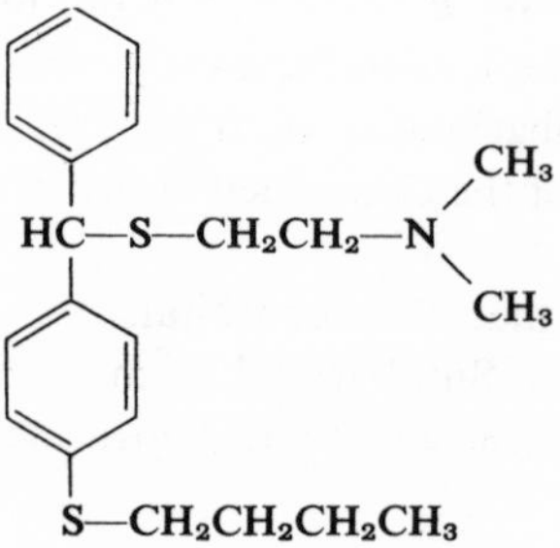

Synonym: *p*-Butylthiodiphenylmethyl-2-dimethylaminoethyl sulfide.

Pharmaceutical Preparations: Captodiame is not found in any pharmaceutical preparations sold in the United States.

General Comment: Captodiame is a tranquilizer and is therefore classified in this text as a Dangerous Drug.

Biochemistry: Unknown.

Toxicology–Pharmacology: The estimated lethal dose in man is 25–250 mg/kg.

▶ **CARBROMAL**
Noncontrolled Substance

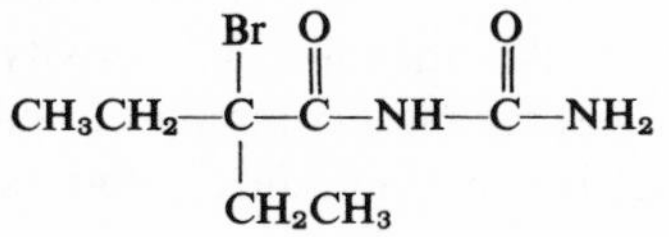

$$CH_3CH_2-\overset{\displaystyle Br}{\underset{\displaystyle CH_2CH_3}{C}}-\overset{\displaystyle O}{C}-NH-\overset{\displaystyle O}{C}-NH_2$$

Synonyms: Bromadal, bromodiethylacetylurea, uradal, *N*-(α-bromo-α-ethyl-butyryl) urea.

General Comments: Carbromal has been regarded as a "safe" sedative–hypnotic drug and may be found in preparations sold over the counter, and thus is controlled by law only under FDA regulations governing OTC preparations.

Carbromal is hydrolyzed in the body to release free bromide ions. Thus, patients chronically intoxicated with this drug may show high serum bromide levels. Characteristic symptoms of bromism may be observed in these cases, such as mental confusion and muscular incoordination.

▶ **CARISOPRODOL**
Dangerous Drug

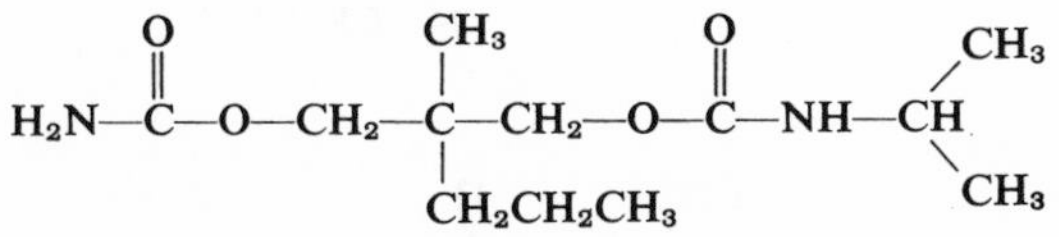

$$H_2N-\overset{\displaystyle O}{C}-O-CH_2-\overset{\displaystyle CH_3}{\underset{\displaystyle CH_2CH_2CH_3}{C}}-CH_2-O-\overset{\displaystyle O}{C}-NH-CH\overset{\displaystyle CH_3}{\underset{\displaystyle CH_3}{}}$$

Synonyms: *N*-isopropylmeprobamate, 2-carbamoyloxymethyl-2-isopropyl-carbamoyl-oxymethylpentane.

Pharmaceutical Preparations

Rela^R (Schering)—Tablet: round, sugar-coated, pink, labeled "SCHERING," containing 350 mg carisoprodol

Soma^R (Wallace)—Tablet: white, labeled "WALLACE 37-2001," containing 350 carisoprodol. Capsule: yellow and orange, containing 250 mg carisoprodol.

Soma^R Compound (Wallace)—Tablet: orange, scored, labeled "WALLACE 37-2101," containing 200 mg carisoprodol, 160 mg phenacetin, and 32 mg caffeine

Soma^R Compound with Codeine (Wallace)—This preparation is a Schedule III drug. See **CODEINE.**

General Comments: Carisoprodol is included in this text because it is encountered in cases of abuse of drugs. It is classified in this text as a Dangerous Drug under the legend "drugs which bear the label 'Caution: Federal law prohibits dispensing without a prescription.'"

Biochemistry: Similar to that of meprobamate.

Toxicology–Pharmacology: Carisoprodol is the *N*-isopropyl derivative of meprobamate. It exhibits weak anticholinergic activity and is an antipyretic. The acute toxicity is low, and the most common side effect is drowsiness. It is commonly used as a sedative or tranquilizer, and as a muscle relaxant in treatment of muscular spasm or rigidity.

An acute overdose may produce stupor, coma, shock, and/or respiratory depression. It may, on rare occasions, produce death. However, in most commonly observed cases in which carisoprodol is involved in a death, other central nervous system depressants, such as alcohol, will also be involved, producing a combined depressant effect. Treatment is both symptomatic and supportive. Since carisoprodol is dialyzable, diuresis, osmotic diuresis, peritoneal dialysis, and hemodialysis may be useful in some cases.

Therapeutic blood concentrations are between 0.10 and 0.50 mg/dl. Serious toxicity may occur with greater than 3.00 mg/dl.

▶ **CARPHENAZINE**
Dangerous Drug

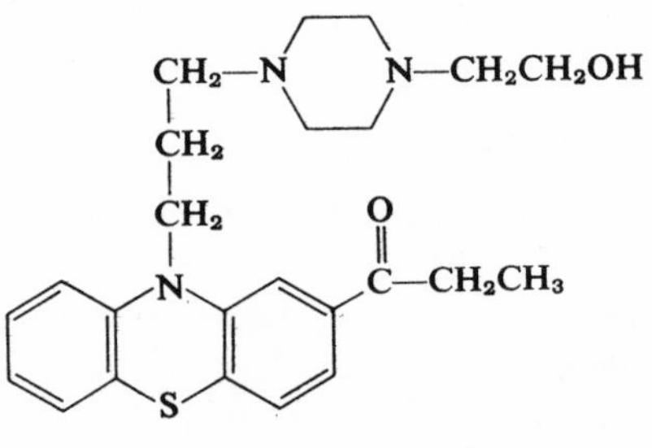

Synonyms: Carfenazine, 10-(3-[4-(2-hydroxyethyl)piperazine-1-yl]propyl)-2-propionyl-phenothiazine.

Pharmaceutical Preparations: Carphenazine is not found in any pharmaceutical preparations sold in the United States.

General Comment: Carphenazine is a phenothiazine tranquilizer and is therefore classified in this text as a Dangerous Drug.

Biochemistry: Unknown.

Toxicology–Pharmacology: Carphenazine is over 100 times more potent as an antiemetic than chlorpromazine. The acute lethal dose of carphenazine in man is believed to be toward the lower end of the range of phenothiazine tranquilizers, which is 15–150 mg/kg.

▶ **CHLORAL BETAINE**

Schedule IV

General Comments: Chloral betaine is a complex of chloral hydrate that slowly hydrolyzes in the gastric contents, forming chloral hydrate and an inactive product.

Pharmaceutical Preparations: Beta-Chlor^R (Mead-Johnson)—Tablet: orange, football-shaped, labeled "MJ," containing 870 mg chloral betaine (equivalent to 500 mg chloral hydrate)

▶ **CHLORAL HYDRATE**

Schedule IV

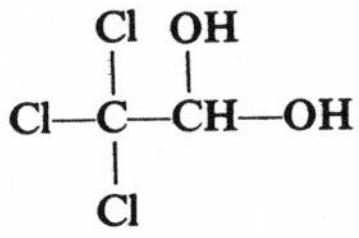

$$Cl-\underset{\underset{Cl}{|}}{\overset{\overset{Cl}{|}}{C}}-\underset{}{\overset{\overset{OH}{|}}{C}}H-OH$$

Synonyms: Chloral, 2,2,2-trichloroethane-1,1-diol.

Pharmaceutical Preparations

Aquachloral^R Supprettes (Webcon)—Suppositories, scored: green, containing 325 mg chloral hydrate; blue, containing 648 mg chloral hydrate; yellow, containing 970 mg chloral hydrate

Felsules^R (Fellows)—Capsules: blue and white, containing 250 mg chloral hydrate; blue, labeled "FELLOWS," containing 500 mg chloral hydrate; yellow, labeled "FELLOWS," containing 1 g chloral hydrate

Kessodrate^R (McKesson)—Capsules, labeled "McKESSON": Red (smaller), containing 250 mg chloral hydrate; red (larger), containing 500 mg chloral hydrate. Syrup, containing 500 mg/5 ml.

Rectules^R (Fellows)—Suppositories, yellow, two strengths: 650 mg chloral hydrate and 1.3 g chloral hydrate

General Comments: Chloral hydrate is the oldest known hypnotic, having been first discovered in 1823. However, it was the late 1800s before its pharmacological properties were realized.

Chronic use of chloral hydrate may result in the development of tolerance, physical dependance, and addiction similar to that of alcohol.

Biochemistry: See Toxicology–Pharmacology below.

Toxicology–Pharmacology: Chloral hydrate is a general depressant, similar in action to the barbiturates. In therapeutic doses, it produces sleep, although not deep hypnosis, and without analgesia. Toxic doses induce severe respiratory depression and hypotension. It depresses contractility of the myocardium.

The actions of chloral hydrate are due to trichlorethanol, to which it is rapidly converted in the body. Therapeutic blood concentrations of trichlorethanol are around 1.00 mg/dl, while fatalities may occur at about 10.00 mg/dl.

The minimum acute lethal dose of chloral hydrate is considered to be 10 g. However, deaths have been recorded with as little as 4 g, and recoveries have been recorded with as much as 30 g. Chloral hydrate poisoning resembles acute barbiturate intoxication.

▶ **CHLORDIAZEPOXIDE**
Schedule IV

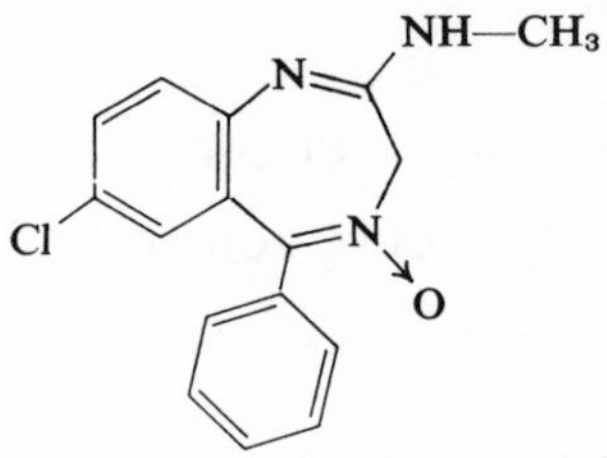

Synonyms: Methaminodiazepoxide, 7-chloro-2-methylamine-5-phenyl-3H-1, 4-benzodiazepine 4-oxide.

Pharmaceutical Preparations

Librax^R (Roche)—Capsules: green, labeled "ROCHE 7," containing 5 mg chlordiazepoxide and 2.5 mg clidinium bromide (see Chapter 6)

Libritabs^R (Roche)—Tablets, green: labeled "13," containing 5 mg chlordiazepoxide; labeled "14," containing 10 mg chlordiazepoxide; labeled "15," containing 25 mg chlordiazepoxide

Librium^R (Roche)—Capsules: yellow and green, labeled "ROCHE 1," containing 5 mg chlordiazepoxide; green and black, labeled "ROCHE 2," containing 10 mg chlordiazepoxide; white and green, labeled "ROCHE 3," containing 25 mg chlordiazepoxide

Menrium^R (Roche)—Tablets: light green, labeled "23," containing 5 mg chlordiazepoxide and 0.2 mg water-soluble esterified estrogens; dark green, labeled "24," containing 5 mg chlordiazepoxide and 0.4 mg water-soluble esterified estrogens; purple, labeled "25," containing 10 mg chlordiazepoxide and 0.4 mg water-soluble esterified estrogens (see Chapter 6)

General Comments: Chlordiazepoxide is one of the benzodiazepine derivatives currently used medically in the United States. These compounds are used primarily for treatment of anxiety, but they are employed in some cases for skeletal muscle relaxation and in the treatment of alcoholism.

Biochemistry: Chlordiazepoxide was the first benzodiazepine to be studied metabolically. Many metabolites are currently known; however, there are several metabolites yet to be identified. One important metabolitic pathway is shown below:

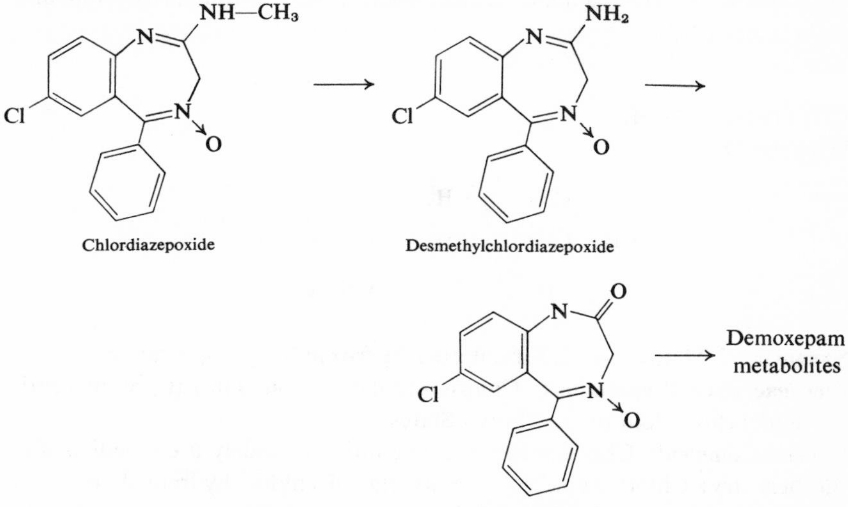

Chlordiazepoxide

Desmethylchlordiazepoxide

Demoxepam

Demoxepam metabolites

Toxicology–Pharmacology: The toxicity of chlordiazepoxide is relatively low. It may be slightly greater than that of meprobamate. It is rapidly absorbed after ingestion and has a plasma half-life in man of 22–24 hours. Chlordiazepoxide is metabolised yielding a major lactam derivative probably via the *N*-demethyl derivative.

The signs and symptoms of overdosage of chlordiazepoxide include those of central nervous system depression, primarily drowsiness and lethargy.

Physical dependence on chlordiazepoxide may develop with chronic use. This dependence resembles that seen with the barbiturates and meprobamates. Withdrawal seizures may occur after discontinuance. Other symptoms of withdrawal may be depression, agitation, insomnia, loss of appetite, and aggravation of the psychopathological state.

Therapeutic blood concentrations of up to 1.00 mg/dl may be seen in patients taking high regular doses. The usual therapeutic blood concentrations are less than 0.20 mg/dl, however (Koechlin and D'Arconte, 1963). Overdose symptoms may occur at levels greater than this in nontolerant patients. Death from overdose of this drug alone is extremely rare. Overdose with chlordiazepoxide in combination with alcohol or other depressant drug medications is more commonly seen. In 22 patients who had taken overdoses up to 2250 mg, sedation, ataxia, and dysarthria, and, in rare instances, sleep and coma were produced. Recovery was uneventful in all cases (Zbinden *et al.*, 1961).

The plasma half-life of chlordiazepoxide after a single oral dose may range from 6.6 to 28 hours (Schwartz *et al.*, 1971). After an overdose of 500 mg, a blood level of 2.53 mg/dl of chlordiazepoxide was found (Koechlin and D'Arconte, 1963).

▶ **CHLORHEXADOL**
Schedule III

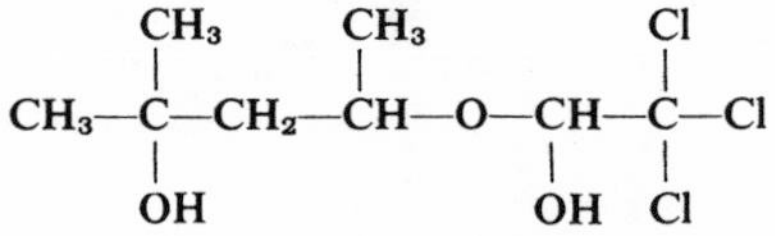

Synonym: 2-Methyl-4-(2,2,2-trichloro-1-hydroxyethoxy)-2-pentanol.
Pharmaceutical Preparations: Chlorhexadol is not found in any pharmaceutical preparations sold in the United States.
General Comment: Chlorhexadol is a hypnotic not widely used medicinally.
Biochemistry: Chlorhexadol is a hemiacetal of chloral hydrate. It is $\frac{1}{32}$ as potent as secobarbital in terms of duration of sleep (Condouris and Bonnycastle, 1961). However, it has a hypnotic effect equal to that of chloral hydrate (Degerholm *et al.*, 1964).
Toxicology–Pharmacology: Similar to that of chloral hydrate.

▶ **CHLORMEZANONE**
Dangerous Drug

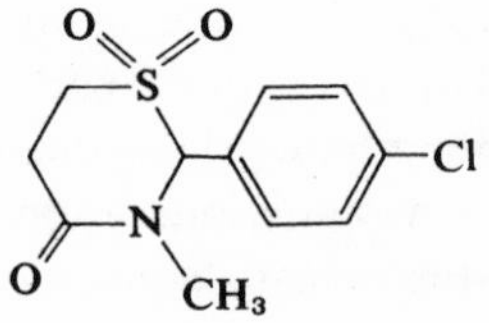

Synonyms: Chlormethazanone, 2-*p*-chlorophenyltetrahydro-3-methyl-2*H*-1,
3-thiazin-4-one-1,1-dioxide.
Pharmaceutical Preparations: Trancopal[R] (Winthrop)—Tablets, scored, oblong, labeled "W": peach-colored, containing 100 mg chlormezanone; green-
colored, containing 200 mg chlormezanone
General Comments: Chlormezanone is a tranquilizer; therefore, it is classified
in this text as a Dangerous Drug. Chlormezanone is a drug that produces
sedation and possesses muscle relaxant properties. It is thus used in the treatment of muscle tension and pains associated with anxiety states and psychosomatic disorders, and as a minor tranquilizer for treatment of neuroses.
Biochemistry: Chlormezanone is a thiazone derivative. It was synthesized in
1958 (Surrey *et al.*, 1958).
Toxicology–Pharmacology: See General Comments above.

▶ **CHLORPHENIRAMINE**
Noncontrolled Substance

Toxicology–Pharmacology: Chlorpheniramine is an effective histamine antagonist, being of most use in the treatment of various allergenic diseases.The
respiratory congestion, sneezing, rhinorrhea, and other symptoms of hay
fever, and other allergies due to the release of histamines, can be counteracted
effectively by the use of chlorpheniramine and other antihistamines.

Side effects of chlorpheniramine include drowsiness, sedation, dizziness,
euphoria, and incoordination. Due to these central nervous system effects, the
antihistamine may be abused.

Overdose from antihistamines is characterized by hallucinations, excitement, ataxia, incoordination, and convulsions. Fixed, dilated pupils with a
flushed face are common.

Blood concentrations after a 12-mg oral dose were 0.003 mg/dl in 2 hours.
The plasma half-life after an oral dose was 12–15 hours (Peets *et al.*, 1972).
Toxic or lethal blood concentrations are unknown.

▶ **CHLORPHENTERMINE**
Schedule III

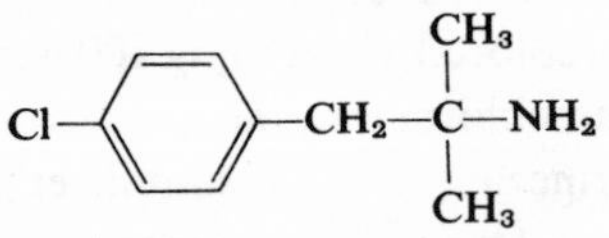

Synonym: *p*-Chloro-α,α-dimethylphenethylamine.
Pharmaceutical Preparations: Pre-Sate^R (Warner/Chilcott)—Tablet: blue, labeled "W/C," containing 65 mg chlorphentermine hydrochloride
General Comment: Chlorphentermine is a sympathomimetic amine, related to amphetamine, used in the treatment of obesity.
Biochemistry: Similar to that of amphetamine.
Toxicology–Pharmacology: Chlorphentermine is one of a group of drugs known as "sympathomimetic amines." These drugs mimic the actions of the sympathoadrenal system of the body, having chiefly the effects of increasing blood pressure and heart rate, stimulation of the central nervous system (CNS), and decreasing motility and actions of the digestive tract. The chief therapeutic use is in suppression of appetite in obese or overweight individuals. Chlorphentermine has a minimal CNS effect in comparison with the amphetamines, but is effective in appetite suppression. The recommended adult dosage is 65 mg per day.

Therapeutic blood concentrations are probably not in excess of 0.02 mg/dl. Toxic or lethal blood concentrations are unknown.

▶ **CHLORPROMAZINE**
Dangerous Drug

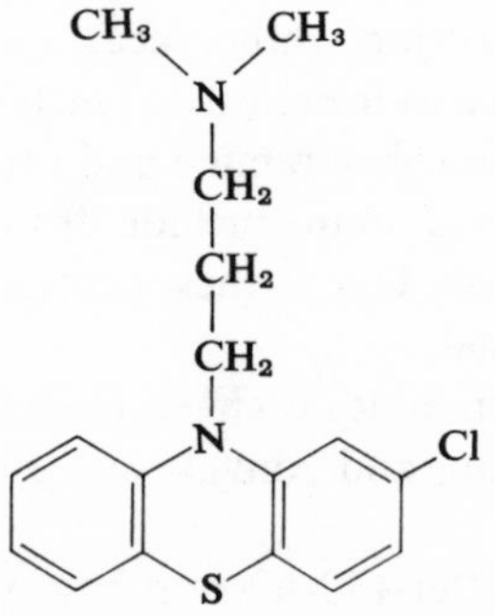

Synonym: 2-Chloro-10-(3-dimethylaminopropyl) phenothiazine.

Pharmaceutical Preparations

Chlor-PZ[R] (USV Pharmaceutical)—Tablets: red, coated, labeled "USV," containing 10, 25, 50, 100, or 200 mg chlorpromazine hydrochloride

Thorazine[R] (Smith Kline & French)—Tablets, orange, coated: labeled "SKF T73," containing 10 mg chlorpromazine hydrochloride; labeled "SKF T74," containing 25 mg chlorpromazine hydrochloride; labeled "SKF T76," containing 50 mg chlorpromazine hydrochloride; labeled "SKF T77," containing 100 mg chlorpromazine hydrochloride; labeled "SKF T79," containing 200 mg chlorpromazine hydrochloride. Capsules, orange and clear: labeled "SKF T63," containing 30 mg chlorpromazine hydrochloride; labeled "SKF T64," containing 75 mg chlorpromazine hydrochloride; labeled "SKF T66," containing 150 mg chlorpromazine hydrochloride; labeled "SKF T67," containing 200 mg chlorpromazine hydrochloride; labeled "SKF T69," containing 300 mg chlorpromazine hydrochloride. Vials: 10 ml, containing 25 mg/ml chlorpromazine hydrochloride, 2 mg/ml ascorbic acid, 1 mg/ml sodium bisulfite, 1 mg/ml sodium sulfite, and 1 mg/ml sodium chloride. Ampules: 1 or 2 ml, containing 25 mg/ml chlorpromazine hydrochloride, 2 mg/ml ascorbic acid, 1 mg/ml sodium bisulfite, 1 mg/ml sodium sulfite, and 6 mg/ml sodium chloride. Syrup: Each 5 ml (one teaspoonful) containing 10 mg chlorpromazine hydrochloride. Suppositories: Labeled "SKF T70," containing 25 mg chlorpromazine hydrochloride, glycerin, glyceryl-monopalmitate, glyceryl monostearate, and fatty acids; labeled "SKF T71," containing 100 mg chlorpromazine hydrochloride.

General Comments: Chlorpromazine is a phenothiazine tranquilizer. As a tranquilizer, it is classified in this text as a Dangerous Drug.

Chlorpromazine was synthesized in 1950 by Charpentier (Charpentier, 1950). In 1952, Delay and co-workers discovered the effectiveness of chlorpromazine in the treatment of psychiatric disorders (Delay *et al.*, 1952). In 1954, chlorpromazine was marketed in the United States as an antiemetic. However, it was not long before chlorpromazine was recognized in the United States as having greater usefulness in the treatment of psychotic states.

Biochemistry: In man, chlorpromazine produces a state in which motor functions are depressed and spontaneous movements are decreased and slow. However, all spinal reflexes remain essentially intact. Response to external stimuli is slow.

Chlorpromazine antagonizes the stimulatory and toxic effects of amphetamine and certain other sympathomimetic amines. At high dose levels, this drug characteristically induces a state of catalepsy. Other properties of chlorpromazine include sympatholytic and α-adrenergic-blocking action. This drug reverses the pressor effects of epinephrine, reduces the pressor response to norepinephrine, and produces vasodilation, postural hypotension, and tachycardia. In addition, chlorpromazine has antihistaminic, local anesthetic, and anticholinergic activity. It also has the property of lowering body temperature.

Toxicology–Pharmacology: Chlorpromazine is of major value in the treatment of psychotic disorders. It exerts a quieting effect on excited or hyperactive psychotic patients, making them more amenable to treatment. Some patients are so benefited that psychopathology is no longer detectable. It can be used to treat a wide variety of schizophrenic symptoms, including thought disturbance, paranoia, delusions, scoial withdrawal, loss of self-care, anxiety, and agitation. Many patients require phenothiazine treatment of anxiety and tension, and are effective antiemetic agents.

The phenothiazines have a high therapeutic index, and chlorpromazine may be given in doses up to 5000 mg per day. The most dangerous effects are those resulting from hypersensitivity reactions, particularly blood dyscrasias, jaundice, and dermatological reactions. Conventional doses may cause faintness, palpitation, nasal stuffiness, and dry mouth, and low blood pressure or orthostatic hypotension may occur.

Death from overdose of chlorpromazine, alone, is rare. It is more dangerous when combined with other depressant medications. Therapeutic blood concentrations may reach 0.30 mg/dl. Toxic concentrations are probably in excess of 0.70 mg/dl.

There have been over 20 metabolites of chlorpromazine found. The two main metabolites are chlorpromazine sulfoxide and N-methyl-chlorpromazine sulfoxide. The action of chlorpromazine may last up to 12 hours. This drug is distributed in the body for a long time. Following cessation of chronic use, the drug or its metabolites or both may be detected in the body up to 12 months.

▶ **CHLORPROTHIXENE**
Dangerous Drug

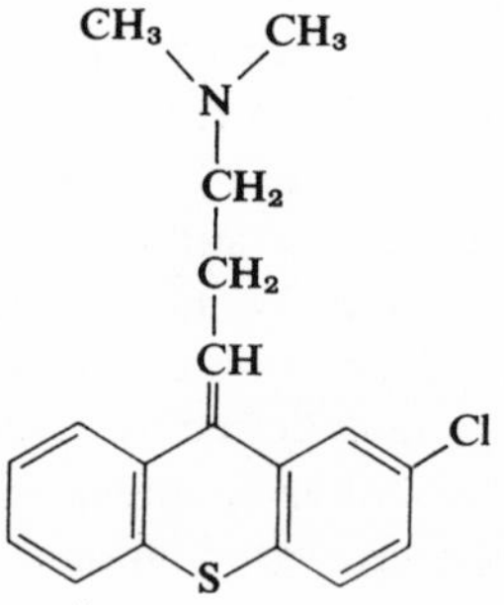

$$CH_3 \quad CH_3$$
$$\diagdown \quad \diagup$$
$$N$$
$$|$$
$$CH_2$$
$$|$$
$$CH_2$$
$$|$$
$$CH$$

Synonyms: Chlorprothixen, α-2-chloro-9-(3-dimethylaminopropylidine)-thiaxanthen.

Pharmaceutical Preparations

Taractan[R] (Roche)—Tablets, orange, coated: labeled "46," containing 25 mg chlorprothixene; labeled "47," containing 50 mg chlorprothixene; labeled "49," containing 100 mg chlorprothixene. Concentrate (20 mg/ml) proprothixene ampules, containing 12.5 mg/ml chlorprothixene.

General Comment: Chlorprothixene is a tranquilizer and is therefore classified in this text as a Dangerous Drug.

Biochemistry: The distribution, metabolism, and basic structure–activity relationship resemble those of chlorpromazine and other corresponding phenothiazine derivatives. Chlorprothixene undergoes sulfoxidation and N-demethylation (Huus and Khan, 1967).

Toxicology–Pharmacology: Chlorprothixene resembles chlorpromazine, structurally, but is a thioxanthine derivative. This drug is advocated for treatment of mild to severe anxiety, various psychotic states, and depressions, and is used as an antiemetic. Side effects include hepatic dysfunction, extrapyramidal symptoms, drowsiness, convulsions, dermatitis, and hematological disorders. It is slightly less potent than chlorpromazine.

A single dose of 50 mg chlorprothixene has given 0.004 mg/dl (blood) after 8 hours. Doses of 100 mg chlorprothixene every 3 hours have produced blood levels as high as 0.3 mg/dl. Chlorprothixene has a blood half-life of 17–24 hours. Approximately 6% of a dose of chlorprothixene is excreted in the urine unchanged and as the sulfoxide derivative within 24 hours.

After ingestion of 7.5 g, a blood concentration of 0.08 mg/dl was found on the fifth day of hospitalization. The patient was comatose for several days. If extrapolated to time zero, the plasma concentration would have been 0.54 mg/dl (DeSilva and D'Arconte, 1969).

▶ **CHLORZOXAZONE**
Dangerous Drug

Synonyms: Chlorobenzoxazolinone, 5-chloro-2,3-dihydro-2-oxobenzoxazole.

Pharmaceutical Preparations: Parafon[R] Forte (McNeil)—Tablets: green, scored (hexagon cap), labeled "McNeil," containing 250 mg chlorzoxazone and 300 mg acetaminophen

General Comments: Chlorzoxazone is a centrally acting skeletal muscle relaxant. Since all pharmaceutical preparations containing chlorzoxazone require a prescription, this drug is classified in this text as a Dangerous Drug.
Biochemistry: A compound was introduced in 1955 and used clinically as a muscle relaxant prior to chlorzoxazone. This compound, zoxazolamine, was

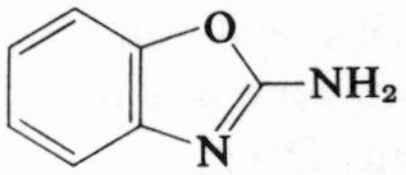

Zoxazolamine

later withdrawn because of its toxicity (Marsh, 1955). Chlorzoxazone was discovered to be a metabolite of zoxazolamine (Conney *et al.*, 1960). It was also determined that chlorzoxazone had the same order of activity as zoxazolamine, but was less toxic (Roszkowski, 1960). Thus, chlorzoxazone was introduced into the market to replace zoxazolamine.
Toxicology–Pharmacology: Chlorzoxazone is a centrally acting muscle relaxant. Little sedation is induced by doses that are effective for muscular relaxation. Minor side effects such as gastrointestinal irritation, headache, and lethargy have been observed.

Chlorzoxazone is rapidly metabolized to 6-hydroxychlorzoxazone and is excreted in the urine as the glucuronide. Peak plasma levels of about 0.7 mg/dl have been obtained in about 120–180 minutes after an oral dose of 500 mg. The half-life of chlorzoxazone is about 170 minutes (Poole and Gardocki, 1963).

▶ **CLONAZEPAM**
Schedule IV

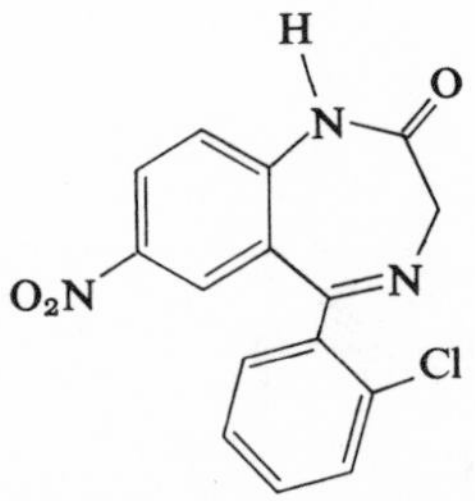

Synonym: 5-(2-Chlorophenyl)-1,3-dihydro-7-nitro-2H-1,4-benzodiazepin-2-one.
Pharmaceutical Preparations: Clonopin[R] (Roche)—Tablets, scored: orange, containing 0.5 mg clonazepam; blue, containing 1.0 mg clonazepam; white, containing 2.0 mg clonazepam

General Comment: Clonazepam is a benzodiazepine related to diazepam.
Biochemistry: The differences between clonazepam and diazepam are: (1) NO_2 group instead of Cl in position 7 or ring A, and (2) Cl group instead of H in the *ortho*-position of ring C. The electron-withdrawing NO_2 group increases sedative and muscle-relaxant properties slightly over Cl (Sternbach, 1971). Likewise, with Cl at the *ortho*-position, the activity and potency increase substantially as compared with the unsubstituted compound. Clonazepam has a much greater margin of safety than diazepam.

The metabolitic pathways of clonazepam are similar to those of chlordiazepoxide and diazepam.

Toxicology–Pharmacology: Muscle-relaxant figures show that diazepam is the most potent of the 7-chloro compounds, with the highest margin of safety between the effective muscle-relaxant dose and the dose that caused loss of righting reflex and death. Of the 7-nitro compounds, clonazepam was more potent than diazepam while having the highest safety margin (Zbinden and Randall, 1967). The safety margin between muscle-relaxant and lethal doses of the benzodiazepine ranges from 100 to 20,000, compared with 2 for phenobarbital.

A 2-mg single dose exhibited peak blood levels from 0.65 to 1.35 $\mu g/dl$ in 1–2 hours after administration. The half-life of elimination ranged from 18.7 to 39.0 hours (Roche, 1975).

Symptoms of overdose include somnolence, confusion, coma, and diminished reflexes. Methyl phenidate or caffeine may be given to control central nervous system depression.

▶ **CLONITAZENE**
Schedule I

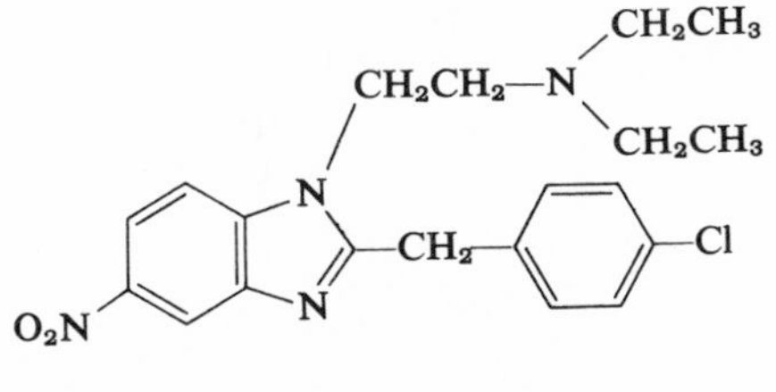

Synonym: 2-(*p*-Chlorobenzl)-1-(2-diethylaminoethyl)-5-nitrobenzinidazole.
Pharmaceutical Preparations: Clonitazene is not found in any pharmaceutical preparations sold in the United States.
General Comment: Clonitazene is a synthetic narcotic analgesic with no accepted medicinal use in the United States.
Biochemistry: Unknown.
Toxicology–Pharmacology: Unknown.

▶ **CLOPENTHIXOL**
Dangerous Drug

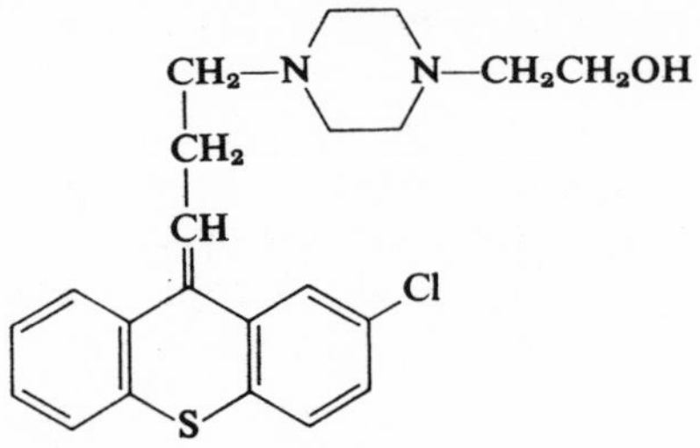

Synonyms: Cloperphenthixan, 2-chloro-9-(3-[4-(2-hydroxyethyl) piperazin-1-yl]-propylidene)thixanthen.

Pharmaceutical Preparations: Clopenthixol is not found in any pharmaceutical preparations sold in the United States.

General Comments: Clopenthixol is a tranquilizer and is therefore classified in this text as a Dangerous Drug. Clopenthixol is congeneric with thiothixene and chlorprothixene.

Biochemistry: Clopenthixol is a hydroxyethylpiperazine that is slightly less potent than its phenothiazine analogue, perphenazine. In addition, the antiemetic effect of clopenthixol is comparable to that of perphenazine.

Toxicology–Pharmacology: The toxicology data of clopenthixol are unknown.

▶ **CLORAZEPATE**
Schedule IV

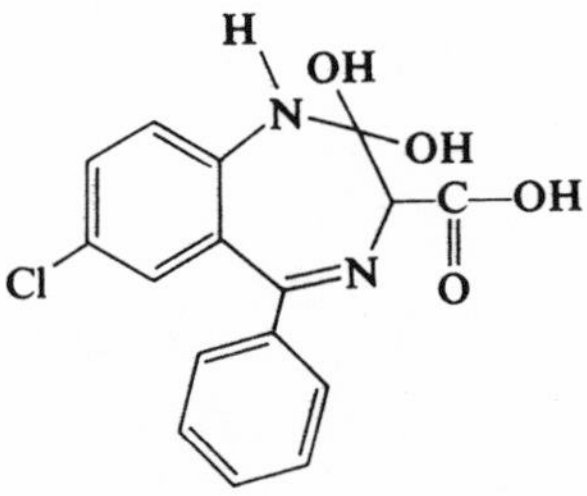

Synonym: 7-Chloro-2,3-dihydro-2,2-dihydroxy-5-phenyl-1H-1,4-benzodiazepine-3-carboxylic acid.

Pharmaceutical Preparations

Tranxene[R] (Abbott)—Capsules, labeled "a": gray and white, containing 7.5 mg clorazepate; gray, containing 15 mg clorazepate

Tranxene[R] (Abbott)—Tablets: tan, containing 22.5 mg clorazepate

General Comments: Clorazepate is a benzodiazepine tranquilizer that has been added to Schedule IV along with the other benzodiazepines (e.g., diazepam, chlordiazepoxide). Clorazepate was developed in France in 1968 by Etablissements Clin-Bayla.

Biochemistry: Clorazepate is structurally related to diazepam and chlordiazepoxide. It produces depressant effects on the central nervous system, but in recommended doses it does not cause respiratory depression.

The primary metabolite of clorazepate is nordiazepam:

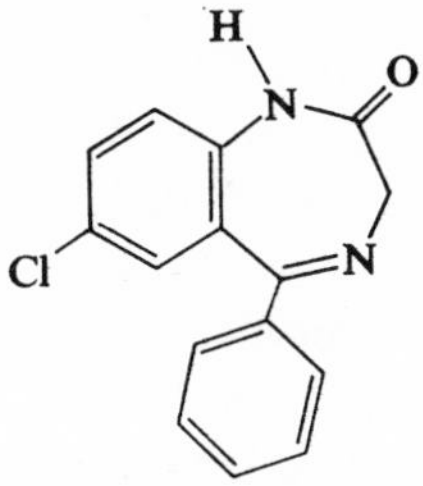

Nordiazepam

Toxicology–Pharmacology: Clorazepate is a benzodiazepine tranquilizer, indicated for the symptomatic relief of anxiety associated with anxiety neurosis, and in disease states in which anxiety is manifested.

It is converted quickly in the blood to nordiazepam, its major metabolite, so that no circulating unchanged drug can be detected.

Nordiazepam reaches a peak blood level in about 1 hour. The plasma half-life of clorazepate is approximately 1 day. The drug is metabolized in the liver and excreted primarily in the urine (Abbott, 1976).

Clorazepate is a central depressant drug, and can cause toxicity when combined with other depressant drugs or alcohol. Nordiazepam levels in blood of up to 0.05 mg/dl may be detected after therapeutic administration.

▶ **CLORTERMINE**
Schedule III

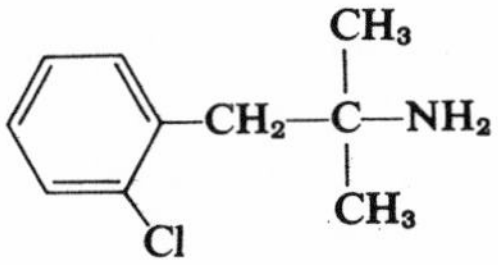

Synonym: o-Chloro-α,α-dimethyl-phenylethylamine.
Pharmaceutical Preparations: Varanil[R] (USV)—Tablets: yellow, containing 50 mg clortermine
General Comments: Clortermine is a sympathomimetic amine used as an anorectic drug. It was added to Schedule III in 1973.

Biochemistry: Clortermine is a sympathomimetic amine with pharmacological activity similar to that of the amphetamines. Actions include stimulation of the central nervous system and increase in blood pressure. It is indicated as an anorectic in treatment of obesity, as an adjunct to dietary restrictions.

Psychological dependence can occur from prolonged use as with the amphetamines.

▶ **COCA**
Schedule II
General Comments: Under the Controlled Substances Act, coca is defined as a "narcotic drug," whether produced directly or indirectly by extraction from substances of vegetable origin, or independently by means of chemical synthesis, or by a combination of extraction and chemical synthesis including, specifically, coca leaves and any salt, compound, derivative, or preparation of coca leaves and any salt, compound, isomer, derivative, or preparation thereof that is chemically equivalent or identical to any of these substances. However, this does not include decocainized coca leaves or extractions of coca leaves that do not contain cocaine or ecgonine.

Coca, scientifically known as *Erythroxylon coca* Lamarck, is the primary source of the alkaloid, cocaine. This plant grows mainly on the western side of South America.

In the Andean highlands, where the coca plant has been cultivated since prehistoric times, the leaf is chewed for refreshment and relief from fatigue, much as North Americans once chewed tobacco. The bulk of the crop serves the needs of a domestic subsistence economy. Bolivia and Peru legally export to the United States a relatively small amount of coca compared with the illicit market. The decocainized leaves are used for flavoring extracts in the beverage industry. The cocaine produced from this process supplies the world market for medical and illicit purposes. While the United States demand for medicinal cocaine has been decreasing, the supply in the clandestine market has been rising.

Cocaine is extracted with base from the plant, producing the naturally occurring *levo* isomer. After harvesting, the coca leaf is converted to coca paste. This process is carried out in mobile laboratories that are widely dispersed geographically. Most of these laboratories have small production capacities, producing quantities of coca paste of about 2–3 kg at a time.

While the manufacture of cocaine paste is apparently carried out by small independent operators, the next stages of operation are controlled by well-organized groups in Chile, Colombia, and Ecuador. The activity of these groups consists of collecting the coca paste, converting it to crystalline cocaine, and delivering it to the United States. The production capability of these operations is estimated to be from 50 to 100 kg of cocaine per month.

► **COCAINE**
Schedule II

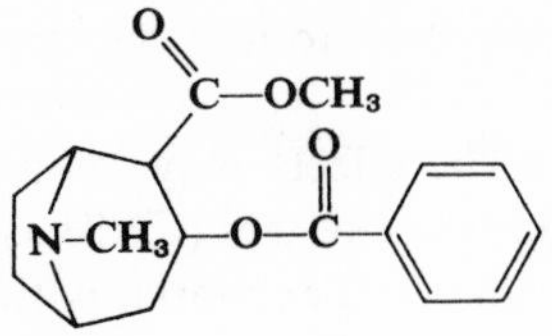

Synonyms: Neurocaine, methylbenzoylecgonine.
Pharmaceutical Preparations
Cocaina—Veterinary preparation
Cocaine—Hospital preparation
General Comments: Cocaine is an alkaloid obtained in the *levo* isomer form from coca, which is the dried leaves of the plant *Erythroxylum coca* and other species within the genus *Erythroxylum*. Cocaine may also be obtained by synthesis from ecgonine. Prepared in this manner, it produces both the *dextro* and the *levo* isomer.

Since the middle of the 19th century, there has been continuous evidence in the literature of its abuse. Cocaine was used as a treatment for fatigue in 1876. It was tried as an antidote for morphinism by Sigmund Freud in 1884 (Musto, 1968; Clark, 1973).

Cocaine is not specifically listed in the Controlled Substances Act, but is controlled through the control of coca. Therefore, only the *levo* isomer (specific rotation = $-35°$), which is the only naturally occurring isomer, is controlled.

Biochemistry: Cocaine is structurally related to atropine and scopolamine. $(-)$ Cocaine has the structure

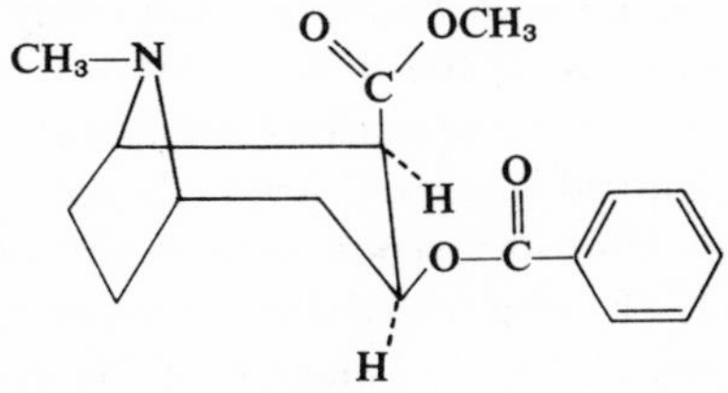

whereas $(+)$ cocaine has the structure

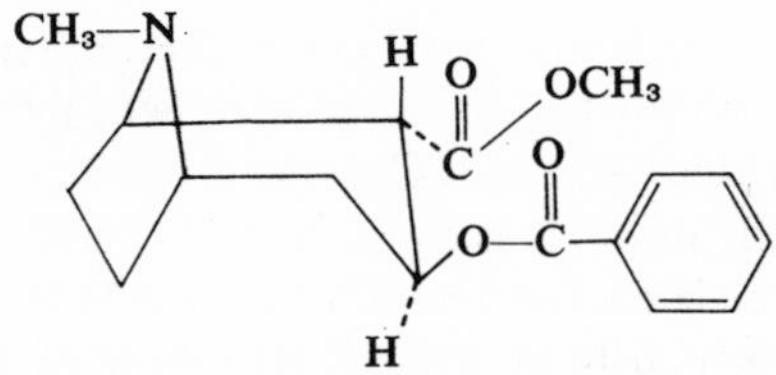

The plasma levels of cocaine depend on the route of administration. This influences both the peak values and the rate of clearance. The metabolism of cocaine involves esterase hydrolysis to form benzoate and ecgonine (Woods, L. A., et al., 1951).

Toxicology–Pharmacology: The effects may be summarized by noting the stimulation of the central nervous system (CNS) as evidenced by increase in mental activity, lack of fatigue, and euphoria, with increased pulse and rate of breathing. Locally, it acts as an effective anesthetic, and may be applied to the nasal membranes for minor surgical procedures. Aftereffects include headache, cardiac and respiratory disturbance, and postdrug depression characterized by indisposition to mental or physical exertion and difficulty in concentration. Modifications of this symptomatology appear related to the route of administration, total dose taken, and rate of administration.

If cocaine use becomes chronic, the initial mental stimulation may be followed by hallucinations, insomnia, failure of appetite, decrease in interest in work, failure of ambition and willpower, and reckless, aimless thought and work. A paranoid psychosis may develop.

There are two distinct types of poisoning from the drug: one characterized by circulatory collapse, the other by symptoms of CNS toxicity. The first type occurs in people after relatively small doses and is due to idiosyncrasy. It is recognized by pallor, dizziness, nausea, failure of pulse, and loss of consciousness. The second type of poisoning by cocaine is characterized by delirium, increased reflexes, convulsions, and violent manic behavior. Respiration is at first stimulated and then depressed. Death is due to respiratory failure.

Cocaine can be administered by mouth, but the preferred routes of administration are through the nose, called "sniffing" or "snorting," or by intravenous injection, referred to as "mainlining." If the drug is "mainlined," all the infections associated with heroin use are likely to occur, including local abscesses and hepatitis. If the drug is sniffed, the small crystals are abrasive to the blood vessels in the mucous membranes lining the nose, and these membranes become reddened and irritated, often resulting in bleeding.

Cocaine, especially after intravenous administration, is alleged to be a potent sexual stimulant. The pleasure of sexual activity is reported to be both enhanced and prolonged under the influence of the drug. There is neither physical dependence nor tolerance developed to cocaine. However, due to its intense pleasurable effects, a strong psychic dependency may develop.

Cocaine is extensively metabolized in the liver, possibly by hydrolysis of the two ester groups producing ecgonine and benzoic acid, with benzoyl-ecgonine as an intermediate product. Cocaine is excreted slowly, the quantity dependent on pH of the urine. It is estimated that between 1 and 12% of an injected dose of cocaine is excreted within the first 24 hours.

Cocaine, acting primarily as a CNS stimulant, is rarely lethal. When overdoses occur, they are due to massive ingestion or intravenous administration. Often, hypersensitivity reactions occur in which minimal or no detectable blood concentration are observed. After death from acute overdose, from 0.8 to 2.1 mg/dl may be found in blood (Lundberg *et al.*, 1977; Di Maio and Garriott, 1978).

Plasma levels after therapeutic use may vary from 0.018 to 0.030 mg/dl (Van Dyke *et al.*, 1976).

▶ **CODEINE**
Schedule II
or
Schedule III if the preparation contains not more than 1.8 g codeine per 100
   ml or not more than 90 mg per dosage unit, with an equal or greater
   quantity of isoquinoline alkaloids of opium
   or
   if the preparation contains not more than 1.8 g codeine per 100 ml or not
   more than 90 mg per dosage unit, with one or more active, nonnarcotic
   ingredients in recognized therapeutic amounts
or
Schedule V if the preparation contains not more than 200 mg codeine per 100
   ml or per 100 g

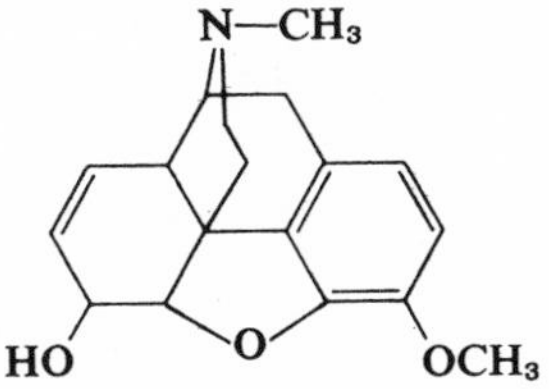

Synonyms: Methylmorphine, morphine methyl ether, 7-8-dehydro-4,5-epoxy-6-hydroxy-3-methyoxy-*N*-methylmorphinan.
Pharmaceutical Preparations
Schedule II
Codeine^R Phosphate 60 (Lilly)—Tablet: hypodermic tablet, white, containing
   60 mg codeine phosphate
Schedule III
Ascodeen-30^R (Burroughs-Wellcome)—Tablet: labeled "BW&CO 30," containing 30 mg codeine phosphate and 325 mg aspirin
Bancaps-C^R (Westerfield)—Capsule containing 32.4 mg codeine phosphate,
   300 mg acetaminophen, and 200 mg salicylamide
Capital^R with Codeine (Carnrick)—Tablet: pale blue, labeled "8644" with a
   sunburst on scored side, containing 30 mg codeine phosphate and 325
   mg acetaminophen

Codalan^R (Lannett)—Tablet: orange, labeled "1," containing $\frac{1}{8}$ gr codeine phosphate, $2\frac{1}{2}$ gr acetaminophen, $3\frac{1}{2}$ gr salicylamide, and $\frac{1}{2}$ gr caffeine; white, labeled "2," containing $\frac{1}{4}$ gr codeine phosphate, $2\frac{1}{2}$ gr caffeine; green, labeled "3," containing $\frac{1}{2}$ gr codeine phosphate, $2\frac{1}{2}$ gr acetaminophen, $3\frac{1}{2}$ gr salicylamide, and $\frac{1}{2}$ gr caffeine

Codasa^R (Stayner)—Capsules: Red, containing $\frac{1}{4}$ gr codeine phosphate and 5 gr aspirin; red and white, containing $\frac{1}{2}$ gr codeine phosphate and 5 gr aspirin; pink and grey, containing $\frac{1}{2}$ gr codeine phosphate and 10 gr aspirin. Tablet: white, containing $\frac{1}{2}$ or $\frac{1}{2}$ gr codeine phosphate and 5 gr aspirin.

Colrex^R (Rowell)—Capsule: yellow, labeled "ROWELL 0840," containing 16 mg codeine phosphate, 16 mg papaverine HCl, 300 mg acetaminophen, 10 mg phenylephrine HCl, 2 mg chlorpheniramine maleate, and 100 mg ascorbic acid

Empirin^R with Codeine (Burroughs-Wellcome)—Tablets: labeled "TABLOID BRAND," containing $3\frac{1}{2}$ gr aspirin, $2\frac{1}{2}$ gr phenacetin, and $\frac{1}{2}$ gr caffeine; labeled "1," containing $\frac{1}{8}$ gr codeine phosphate; labeled "2," containing $\frac{1}{4}$ gr codeine phosphate; labeled "3," containing $\frac{1}{2}$ gr codeine phosphate; labeled "4," containing 1 gr codeine phosphate

Emprazil-C^R (Burroughs-Wellcome)—Tablet: orange and white, labeled "TABLOID BRAND" on orange side, containing 15 mg codeine phosphate, 20 mg pseudoephedrine HCl, 150 mg phenacetin, 200 mg aspirin, and 30 mg caffeine

Fiorinal^R (Sandoz)—See **BUTALBITAL**

Percogesic^R with Codeine (Endo)—Tablet: white, scored, containing 32.4 mg codeine phosphate, 325 mg acetaminophen, and 30 mg phenyltoloxamine citrate

Phenaphen^R with Codeine (Robins)*—Tablets, each containing 194 mg phenacetin, 162 mg aspirin, and 16.2 mg phenobarbital: No. 2, containing 16.2 mg codeine phosphate; No. 3, containing 32.4 mg codeine phosphate; No. 4, containing 64.8 mg codeine phosphate. Capsules, labeled "AHR," each containing 194 mg phenacetin, 162 mg aspirin, and 16.2 mg phenobarbital: No. 2, black and yellow, containing 16.2 mg codeine phosphate; No. 3, black and green, containing 32.4 mg codeine phosphate; No. 4, containing 64.8 mg codeine phosphate

Sinutab^R with Codeine (Warner-Chilcott)—Tablet: pink and white, double-layered, containing 15 mg codeine phosphate, 150 mg acetaminophen, 150 mg phenacetin, 25 mg phenylpropanolamine HCl, and 22 mg phenyltoloxamine citrate

---

* Formulation change in 1977 to tablets containing acetaminophen and codeine.

Soma[R] Compound with Codeine (Wallace)—Tablet: white, capsule-shaped, containing 16 mg codeine phosphate, 200 mg carisoprodol, 160 mg phenacetin, and 32 mg caffeine

Tylenol[R] with Codeine (McNeil)—Tablets, white, containing 300 mg acetaminophen: labeled "1," containing 7.5 mg codeine phosphate; labeled "2," containing 15 mg codeine phosphate; labeled "3," containing 30 mg codeine phosphate; labeled "4," containing 60 mg codeine phosphate

Schedule V

Actifed-C[R] (Burroughs-Wellcome)—Expectorant: each 5 ml (one teaspoonful) containing 10 mg codeine phosphate, 2 mg triprolidine HCl, 30 mg pseudoephedrine HCl, and 100 mg glyceryl guaiacolate

Ambenyl[R] (Parke-Davis)—Expectorant: each 5 ml (one teaspoonful) containing 10 mg codeine sulfate, 3.75 mg bromodiphenhydramine HCl, 8.75 mg diphenhydramine, 80 mg ammonium chloride, 80 mg potassium guaiacosulfonate, and 0.5 mg menthol

Coldex[R] (Rowell)—Elixir: containing 8 mg codeine phosphate, 8 mg papaverine HCl, 120 mg acetaminophen, 1 mg chlorpheniramine maleate, and 5 mg phenylephrine HCl

Dimetane-DC[R] (Robins)—Expectorant: each 5 ml (one teaspoonful) containing 10 mg codeine phosphate, 2 mg brompheniramine maleate, 100 mg glyceryl guaiacolate, 5 mg phenylephrine HCl, and 5 mg phenylpropanolamine HCl

Fedahist-C[R] (Dooner)—Expectorant: each 5 ml (one teaspoonful) containing 10 mg codeine phosphate, 2 mg chlorpheniramine maleate, 100 mg glyceryl guaiacolate, and 30 mg pseudoephedrine HCl

Isoclor[R] (Arnar-Stone)—Expectorant: each 5 ml (one teaspoonful) containing 10 mg codeine phosphate, 2 mg chlorpheniramine maleate, 12.5 mg pseudoephedrine HCl, and 83.3 mg glyceryl guaiacolate

Novahistine-DR[R] (Dow)—Expectorant: each 5 ml (one teaspoonful) containing 10 mg codeine phosphate, 10 mg phenylephrine HCl, and 2 mg chlorpheniramine maleate

Omni-Tuss[R] (Pennwalt)—Suspension: each 5 ml (one teaspoonful) containing 10 mg codeine (base), 5 mg phenyltoloxamine, 3 mg chlorpheniramine, 25 mg ephedrine, and 20 mg guaiacol carbonate

Pediacof[R] (Winthrop)—Syrup: each 5 ml (one teaspoonful) containing 5 mg codeine phosphate, 2.5 mg phenylephrine HCl, and 0.75 mg chlorpheniramine maleate

Phenergan[R] with Codeine (Wyeth)—Expectorant: containing promethazine and codeine

Phenergan-VC[R] with Codeine (Wyeth)—Expectorant: containing promethazine and codeine

Robitussin[R] A-C (Robins)—Syrup: each 5 ml (one teaspoonful) containing 10 mg codeine and 100 mg glyceryl guaiacolate

Triaminic[R] with Codeine (Dorsey)—Expectorant: each 5 ml (one teaspoonful) containing 10 mg codeine phosphate, 12.5 mg phenylpropanolamine HCl, 6.25 mg pheniramine maleate, 6.25 mg pyrilamine maleate, and 100 mg glyceryl guaiacolate

Tussar-2[R] (Armour)—Syrup: each 5 ml (one teaspoonful) containing 10 mg codeine phosphate, 7.5 mg carbetapentane citrate, 2 mg chlorpheniramine maleate, 50 mg glyceryl guaiacolate, 130 mg sodium citrate, and 20 mg citric acid

Tussar[R] SF (Armour)—Syrup: each 5 ml (one teaspoonful) contains 10 mg codeine phosphate, 7.5 mg carbetapentane citrate, 2 mg chlorpheniramine, maleate, 50 mg glyceryl guaiacolate, 130 mg sodium citrate, and 20 mg citrate acid

Tussi-Organidin[R] (Wampole)—Expectorant: each 5 ml (one teaspoonful) containing 10 mg codeine phosphate, 30 mg iodinated glycerol, and 2 mg chlorpheniramine maleate

Exempted (Over-the-Counter)

Chlor-Trimeton[R] with Codeine (Schering)—Expectorant: each 5 ml (one teaspoonful) containing 10 mg codeine phosphate, 2 mg chlorpheniramine maleate, 10 mg phenylephrine HCl, 100 mg ammonium chloride, 50 mg sodium citrate, and 50 mg glyceryl guaiacolate

General Comments: Codeine is an opiate alkaloid that has narcotic analgesic properties. It may be noted that the legal control is based primarily on codeine weight per medicinal unit. This does not specify whether codeine weight is the free base or a particular salt. This has not been brought out in court as yet.

Biochemistry: Codeine is one of the 25 naturally occurring alkaloids found in opium that has medicinal importance (see **OPIUM**).

Codeine is metabolized by undergoing O-demethylation to form morphine.

Toxicology–Pharmacology: Codeine is distinct from morphine in having a high efficacy when administered orally. Thus, it is usually given in oral doses for treatment of pain. It is also used extensively to suppress the cough reflex in cases of uncontrolled coughing.

Codeine is much less toxic than morphine, and even large overdoses do not produce the central and respiratory depression characteristics of morphine; death directly attributable to codeine is very rare. Both tolerance and addiction to codeine can occur, although it has only a feeble euphoric action when taken by mouth in comparison with that of morphine. The estimated lethal dose in man is 800 mg, and more than 200 mg in one dose is dangerous.

Therapeutic blood concentrations may reach 0.05 mg/dl with high doses. Lethal concentrations may range from 0.12 to 0.50 mg/dl (Wright *et al.*, 1975). Most fatalities involving codeine have other drugs present as well.

▶ **CODEINE METHYLBROMIDE**
Schedule I

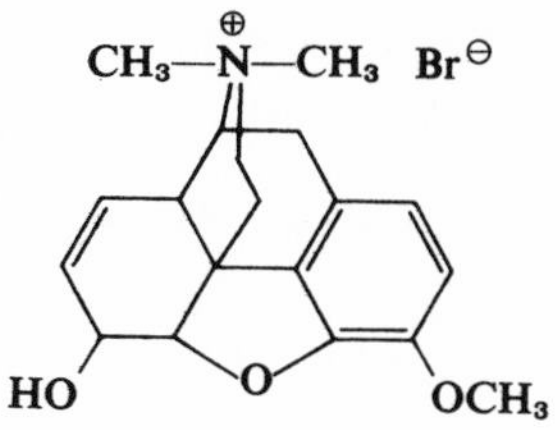

Synonym: Eucodin.
Pharmaceutical Preparations: Codeine methylbromide is not found in any pharmaceutical preparations sold in the United States.
General Comments: Codeine methylbromide is a quaternary compound resulting from treating codeine with methylbromide. It has no accepted medicinal value in the United States and is not recognized by any official compendium.
Biochemistry: Same as that of codeine.
Toxicology–Pharmacology: Same as that of codeine.

▶ **CODEINE-N-OXIDE**
Schedule I

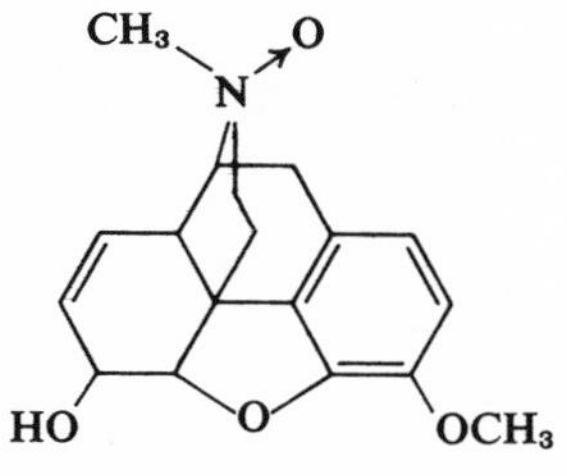

Synonyms: Genocodeine, gencodein, codeigene.
Pharmaceutical Preparations: Codeine-N-oxide is not found in any pharmaceutical preparations sold in the United States.
General Comments: Codeine-N-oxide is the N-oxide prepared by oxidation of codeine with peroxides. This drug has the same pharmacological properties as codeine, but has not been accepted for medicinal use.
Biochemistry: Same as that of codeine.
Toxicology–Pharmacology: Unknown.

▶ **4-CYANO-2-DIMETHYLAMINO-4,4-DIPHENYL BUTANE**
Schedule II

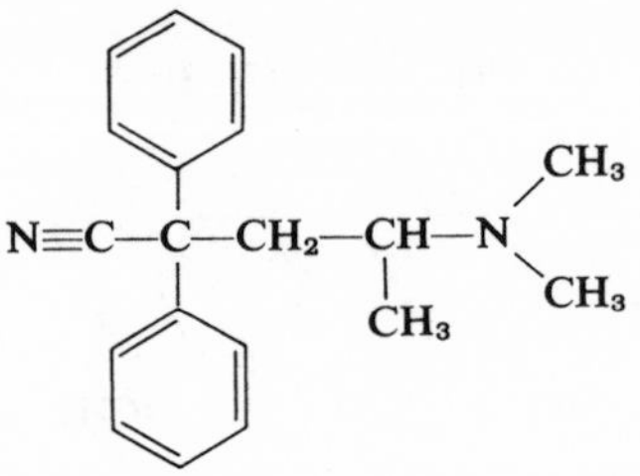

Synonym: 2,2-Diphenyl-4-dimethylaminovaleronitrite.
Pharmaceutical Preparations: This drug is not found in any pharmaceutical preparations sold in the United States.
General Comments: 4-Cyano-2-dimethylamino-4,4-diphenyl butane is an "immediate precursor" in the synthesis of pethidine. It is formed as the result of the condensation of *N*-bis-(chloroethyl)-methylamine with benzyl cyanide. Under Section 201 of the Controlled Substances Act, an immediate precursor may be placed in the same schedule as the controlled substance to which it is a precursor, or in any other schedule with a higher numerical designation (i.e., Schedule III, IV, or V). Since pethidine is a Schedule II drug, Schedule II was a logical choice in which to place 4-cyano-2-dimethylamino-4,4-diphenyl butane.
Biochemistry: Unknown.
Toxicology–Pharmacology: Unknown.

▶ **4-CYANO-1-METHYL-4-PHENYLPIPERIDINE**
Schedule II

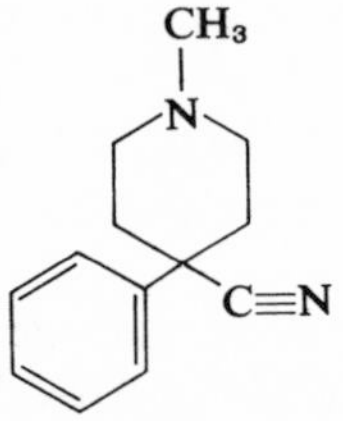

Synonyms: None.
Pharmaceutical Preparations: This drug is not found in any pharmaceutical preparations sold in the United States.
General Comments: 4-Cyano-1-methyl-4-phenylpiperidine is an "immediate precursor" in the synthesis of pethidine. It is formed as the result of the con-

densation of *N*-bis-(chloroethyl)-methylamine with benzyl cyanide. Under Section 201 of the Controlled Substances Act, an immediate precursor may be placed in the same schedule as the controlled substance to which it is a precursor, or in any other schedule with a higher numerical designation (i.e., Schedule III, IV, or V). Since pethidine is a Schedule II drug, 4-Cyano-1-methyl-4-phenylpiperidine was also placed in Schedule II.
Biochemistry: Unknown.
Toxicology–Pharmacology: Unknown.

► **CYCLOBARBITAL**
Schedule III

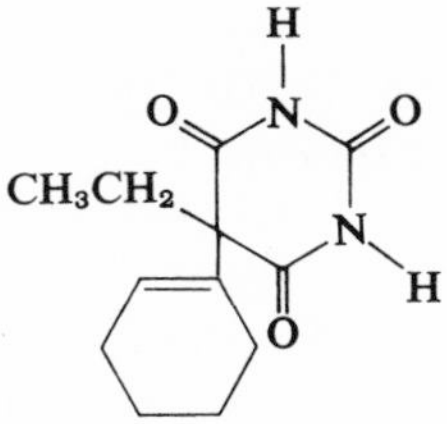

Synonyms: Cyclobarbitone, ethylhexabital, hexemalum, 5-cyclohexl-enyl-5-ethyl-barbituric acid.
Pharmaceutical Preparations: Cyclobarbital is not found in any pharmaceutical preparations sold in the United States.
General Comments: Cyclobarbital is a short-acting barbiturate with pharmacological and toxicological properties similar to those of secobarbital. It is placed in Schedule III because it is a "derivative of barbituric acid."
Biochemistry: Cyclobarbital is metabolized by man to a cyclohexenone derivative, ketocyclobarbital [5-ethyl-5-(3'-oxo-1'-cyclohexenyl) barbituric acid], which is pharmacologically inactive (Tsukamoto *et al.*, 1955). In man, 18–22% of a dose of cyclobarbital is excreted in the urine as ketocyclobarbital together with 2–7% as the unchanged drug (Fretwurst *et al.*, 1932). Metabolism in man is slow, for ketocyclobarbital has been detected in human urine even 5 or 6 days after a dose of cyclobarbital (Frey *et al.*, 1959).

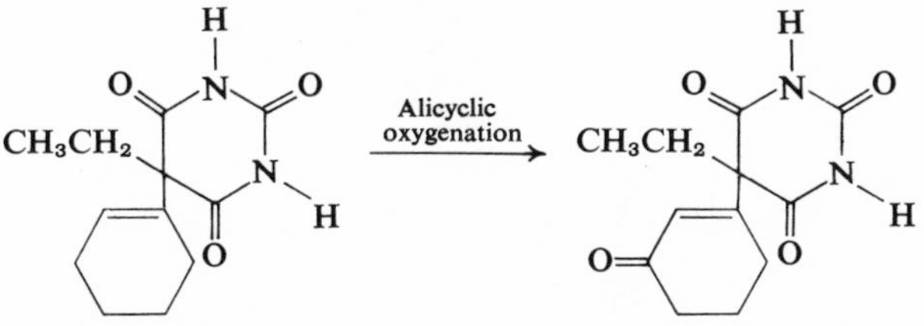

Cyclobarbital   Ketocyclobarbital

Toxicology–Pharmacology: As a short-acting derivative of barbituric acid, cyclobarbital is a general depressant, depressing the activity of nerve, skeletal muscle, smooth muscle, and cardiac muscle. Depression of the central nervous system ranges from mild sedation to coma. The primary use of the short-acting barbiturates is to induce sleep.

Blood levels associated with severe poisoning range from 1 to 3 mg/dl. The estimated lethal dose is about 2 g.

▶ **CYCLOPENTENYLALLYLBARBITURIC ACID**
Schedule III

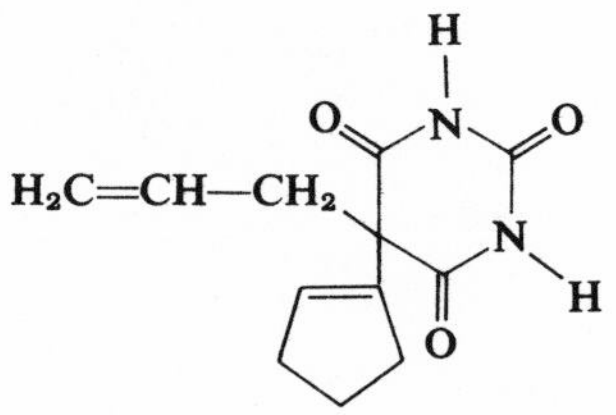

Synonym: 5-Allyl-5-(2-cyclopenten-1-yl)barbituric acid.
Pharmaceutical Preparations: Zantrate[R] (Upjohn)—See Chapter 6.
General Comments: Cyclopentenylallylbarbituric acid is an intermediate-acting barbiturate. It may be compared in actions as being between those of allobarbital and hexobarbital. Cyclopentenylallylbarbituric acid is listed under Schedule III of the Controlled Substances Act as being a "derivative of barbituric acid."
Biochemistry: See **CYCLOBARBITAL.**
Toxicology–Pharmacology: As an intermediate-acting derivative of barbituric acid, cyclopentenylallylbarbituric acid has general depressant actions. Intermediate-acting barbiturates may be used for daytime sedation.

Therapeutic and toxic blood levels are unknown.

▶ **CYPRENORPHINE**
Schedule I

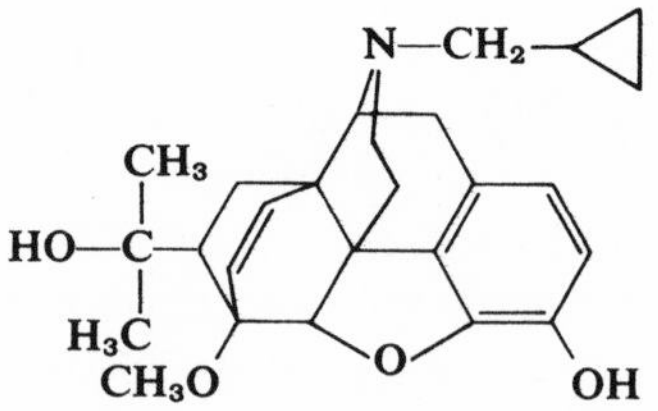

Synonyms: *N*-cyclopropylmethyl-19-methylvororvinol and *N*-cyclopropyl-methyl-7,8-dihydro-7α-(1-hydroxy-1-methylethyl)-O^6-methyl-6,14-endo-etheno-normorphine.

Pharmaceutical Preparations: Cyprenorphine is not found in any pharmaceutical preparations sold in the United States.

General Comments: Cyprenorphine is a highly potent narcotic antagonist with actions many times those of nalorphine. However, this drug has hallucinogenic properties with doses of 1 mg. It is therefore not accepted for medicinal use.

Biochemistry: Unknown.

Toxicology–Pharmacology: Narcotic antagonists compete with narcotic drugs at the receptor sites, counteracting the effects of respiratory and central nervous system depression, euphoria, and analgesia. They can be used for emergency treatment of narcotic overdoses.

Toxicity or concentrations in biological fluids are unknown.

▶ **CYPROHEPTADINE**
Noncontrolled Substance

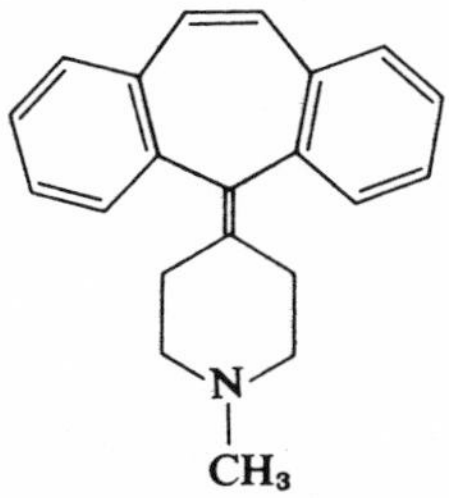

General Comments: Cyproheptadine is an antihistamine found frequently in cases of drug abuse. However, unless it is contained in a pharmaceutical preparation requiring a prescription, it is not subject to control.

Toxicology–Pharmacology: Cyproheptadine is a potent antihistaminic agent. It has been found to be of use in various diseases of allergy. It is also of value in the treatment of pruritic dermatoses. Since it also antagonizes the action of serotonin, it reportedly has beneficial effects in intestinal hypermotility. Side effects may include drowsiness, dry mouth, anorexia, dizziness, and with high doses, confusion and ataxia. In one case of death from overdose, 50–60 tablets were taken prior to death. The blood concentration was 0.09 mg/dl, and the liver concentration was 2.65 mg/100 g (Jones, 1973).

▶ **DESIPRAMINE**
Dangerous Drug

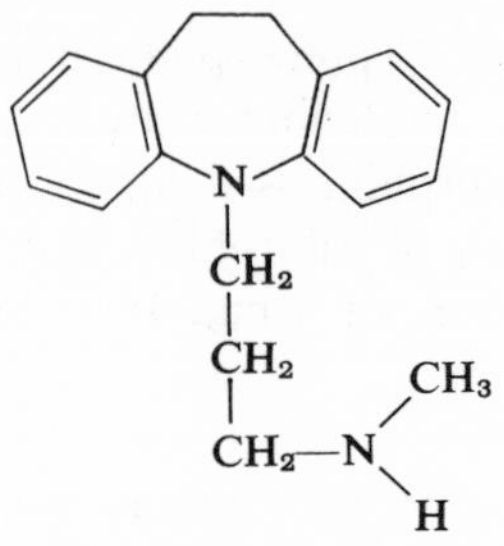

$$N$$
$$CH_2$$
$$CH_2 \quad CH_3$$
$$CH_2—N$$
$$H$$

Synonyms: Desmethylimipramine, 10,11-dihydro-5-(3-methylaminopropyl)-5H-dibenz[b,f]azepine.

Pharmaceutical Preparations

Norpramine[R] (Lakeside)—Tablets: yellow, sugar-coated, labeled "L11," containing 25 mg desipramine hydrochloride; green, sugar coated, labeled "L12," containing 50 mg desipramine hydrochloride

Pertofrane[R] (USV)—Capsules: pink, labeled "USV," containing 25 mg desipramine hydrochloride; maroon and pink, labeled "USV," containing 50 mg desipramine hydrochloride

General Comments: All pharmaceutical preparations containing desipramine require a prescription. It is therefore classified in this text as a Dangerous Drug.

Desipramine is a dibenzazepine antidepressant and is chemically related to imipramine, amitriptyline, and desmethylamitriptyline.

Biochemistry: Desipramine is more potent in antagonizing reserpine sedation, with a faster onset of action, than imipramine. It may be noted that desipramine is also a metabolite of imipramine. Thus, for medical–legal purposes, one must be careful in the interpretation of the parent drug.

Toxicology–Pharmacology: Desipramine is effective in the treatment of depressed patients suffering from a variety of depressive syndromes. Euphoria is not produced in normal individuals, however. In these circumstances, feelings of fatigue accompanied by dryness of the mouth, palpitations, blurred vision, and urinary retention are produced.

Chronic use of desipramine may be comparable to that of chlorpromazine. Euphoria is not produced, but dryness of the mouth, palpitations, blurred vision, and urinary retention may be experienced. In addition, chronic use may lead to difficulty in concentrating and thinking.

Acute overdose of desipramine is characterized by hyperpyrexia (elevated body temperature), hypertension (high arterial blood pressure), seizures, and coma. In some poisoning cases, desipramine has caused cardiac conduction defects and arrhythmias.

The normal daily dose is up to 200 mg per day. Doses of 150 mg per day may show plasma levels of up to 0.14 mg/dl. Normal half-life of desipramine is in the range of 4 to 35 hours, depending on individual metabolism rate.

▶ DESOMORPHINE
Schedule I

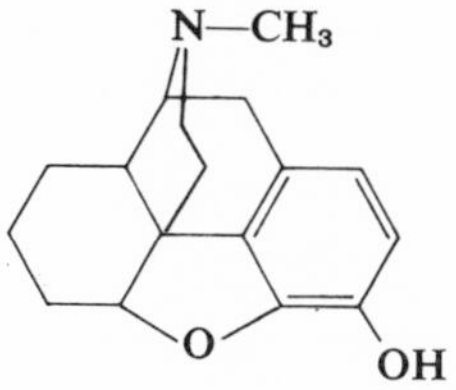

Synonyms: Dihydrodeoxymorphine, 4,5-epoxy-3-hydroxy-N-methylmorphinan.

Pharmaceutical Preparations: Desomorphine is not found in any pharmaceutical preparations sold in the United States.

General Comments: Desomorphine is a synthetic narcotic analgesic that has no accepted medicinal use in the United States. The estimated minimum lethal dose is about 200 mg. It has been reported that desomorphine has greater addiction-producing properties than morphine.

Biochemistry: The alcoholic hydroxyl group in morphine has been modified in several ways with varying effects on analgetic activity. In the case of desomorphine, the replacement by hydrogen produces a drug nearly ten times as potent as morphine with little emetic or gastrointestinal effects.

Toxicology–Pharmacology: Desomorphine is effective when given intramuscularly in 1-mg doses for postoperative pain. This is equivalent in analgesic potency to 10 mg morphine. The onset of action of desomorphine is quicker than that of morphine, but its duration of action is shorter, and it has a less marked sedative effect.

▶ DEXTROMETHORPHAN
Noncontrolled Substance

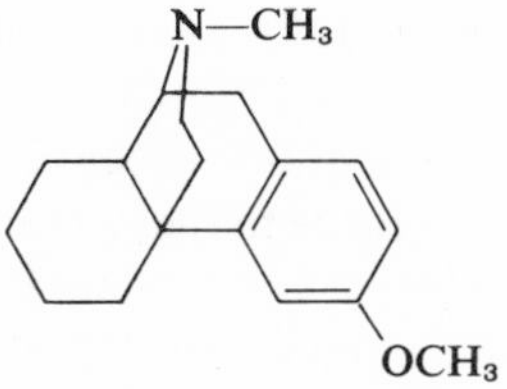

General Comments: Dextromethorphan, an antitussive, is not subject to control; however, its ($-$)-isomer, levomethorphan, and the ($\pm$)-form, racemethorphan, are. Dextromethorphan is available in over-the-counter cough preparations.

Toxicology–Pharmacology: Dextromethorphan has no analgesic or addictive properties. It acts centrally to elevate the threshold for coughing. It has been found to be about equal to codeine in effectiveness for this purpose. However, unlike codeine, it does not produce drowsiness or gastrointestinal disturbances. Toxicity is quite low, but extremely high doses may produce respiratory depression.

▶ **DEXTROMORAMIDE**
Schedule I

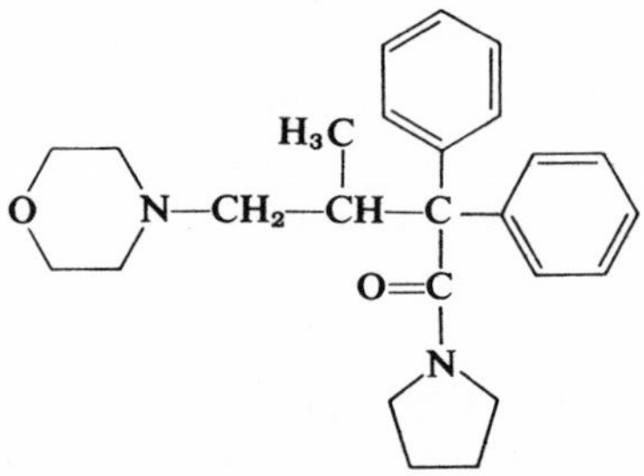

Synonyms: Dextrodiphenopyrine, D-moramid, pyrrolamidol, ($+$)-1-(3-methyl-4-morpholino-2, 2-diphenylbutyryl).

Pharmaceutical Preparations: Dextromoramide is not found in any pharmaceutical preparations sold in the United States.

General Comment: Dextromoramide has no accepted medicinal value in the United States.

Biochemistry: It has been found that methadone analogues with a tertiary amide moiety replacing the alkylketone group are highly potent, morphine-like analgetics. Dextromoramide is such a compound. It is more potent than morphine and retains similar side effects. Thus, it has no particular clinical advantage (Janssen and Jageneau, 1957; Janssen, 1956, 1960).

Toxicology–Pharmacology: Dextromoramide is a synthetic narcotic analgesic chemically related to isomethadone. It is effective as an analgesic when given orally in doses of 5–20 mg. Tolerance to the narcotic effects may enable much larger doses to be taken. Addictive and withdrawal symptoms are similar to those of methadone (Goodman and Gilman, 1971).

The estimated lethal dose is 500 mg.

▶ **DEXTRORPHAN**
Noncontrolled Substance (Removed from Schedule I in 1976)

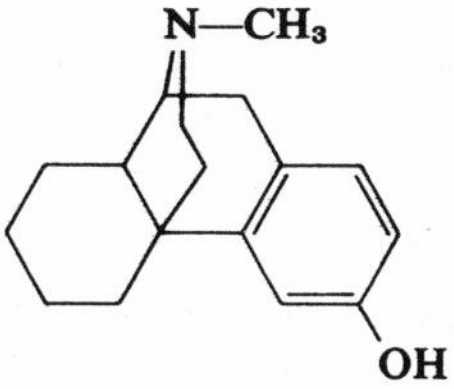

General Comments: Dextrorphan, also called (+)-3-hydroxy-N-methyl-morphinan, is an antitussive. It is the major metabolite of dextromethorphan, but is less active as an antitussive. It is relatively devoid of analgesic action and makes little contribution to the activity of the racemate, racemorphan.

▶ **DIAMPROMIDE**
Schedule I

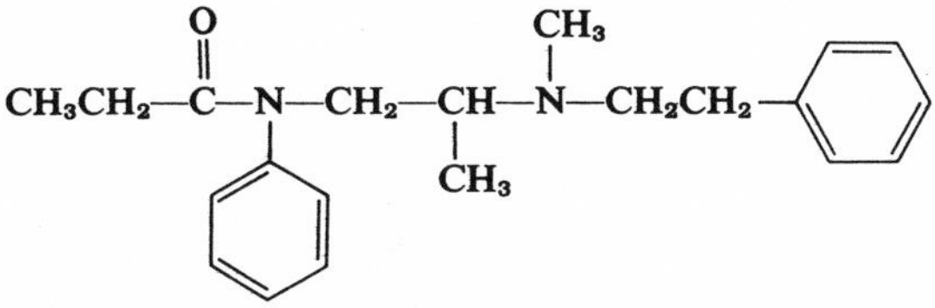

Synonyms: N-[2-(methylphenethylamine)propyl]propionanilide.
Pharmaceutical Preparations: Diampromide is not found in any pharmaceutical preparations sold in the United States.
General Comment: Diampromide is a synthetic narcotic analgesic that has no accepted medicinal value in the United States.
Biochemistry: Wright *et al.* (1959) synthesized this nitrogen analogue of methadone in which the quaternary carbon atom with one attached phenyl group was replaced by nitrogen.
Toxicology–Pharmacology: The basic anilide, diampromide, has a potency comparable to that of pethidine and possesses dependence liability.

▶ **DIAZEPAM**
Schedule IV

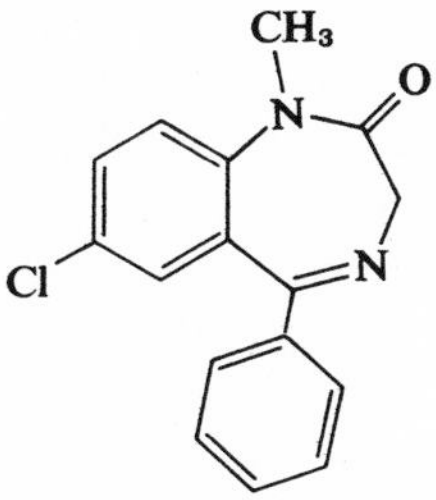

Synonym: 7-Chloro-1,2-dihydro-1-methyl-2-oxo-5-phenyl-3*H*-1,4-benzodiazepine.

Pharmaceutical Preparations

Valium^R (Roche)—Injectable: each 1 ml contains 5 mg diazepam compounded with 40% propylene glycol, 10% ethyl alcohol, 5% sodium benzoate and benzoic acid. Tablets: white, labeled "ROCHE-VALIUM 2," containing 2 mg diazepam; yellow, labeled "ROCHE-VALIUM 5," containing 5 mg diazepam; blue, labeled "ROCHE-VALIUM 10," containing 10 mg diazepam.

General Comment: Diazepam is a benzodiazepine tranquilizer that, along with the other benzodiazepines on the market, was added to Schedule IV of the Controlled Substances Act in 1975.

Biochemistry: Diazepam has been shown to be metabolized in man by:

1. *N*-demethylation to "A":

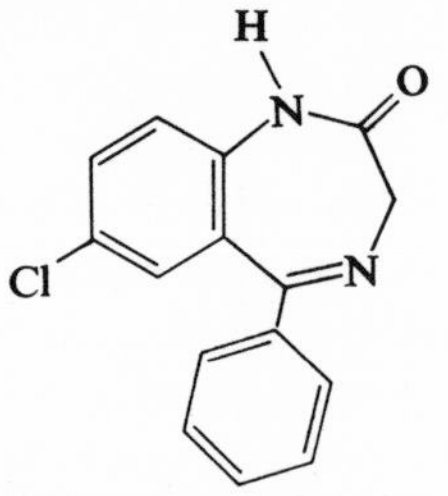

2. Hydroxylation in the 3-position to "B":

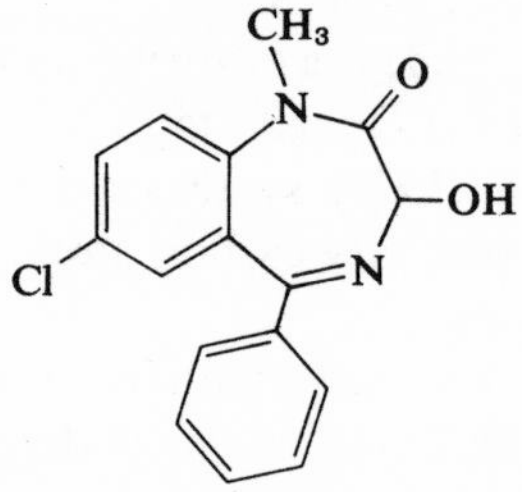

3. *N*-demethylation plus 3-hydroxylation to oxazepam, "C":

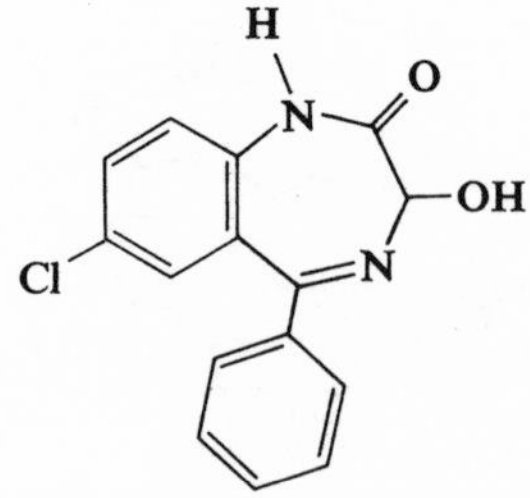

Toxicology–Pharmacology: Diazepam is a widely used benzodiazepine tranquilizer, classified as a "minor" tranquilizer due to its primary usefulness to treat minor psychological disorders, such as neuroses, anxiety, and fear. It is used as a skeletal muscle relaxant, anticonvulsant in epilepsy, and for sedation and sleep in cases of nervous tension.

Its actions are primarily depressant on the central nervous system (CNS), and caution should be used when it is prescribed with other CNS depressants, including alcohol, barbiturate, phenothiazine, monoamine oxidase (MAO) inhibition, and dibenzazepine antidepressants.

Therapeutic blood levels may reach 0.20 mg/dl if high doses of up to 100 mg are given, but the more usual 15- to 20-mg oral dose leads to blood levels not exceeding 0.02 mg/dl (DeSilva, 1964). Intravenous injection of 20 mg in a 170-lb, 16-year-old male led to a blood concentration of 0.10 mg/dl in 30 minutes. After 60 minutes, this had dropped to 0.03 mg/dl (Garriott, 1975).

The half-life after oral dosing is about 10 hours (Roche).

The toxicity of diazepam alone appears to be relatively low. There have been no recorded deaths due to overdose of diazepam alone. However, there have been numerous reports of deaths due to multiple-drug overdoses that include diazepam.

Toxic blood levels, or those in which marked adverse effects occur, are in excess of 0.20 mg/dl. Overdoses with levels up to 1.50 mg/dl have been successfully treated. A lethal blood concentration has not been established for diazepam because of lack of known fatal cases. After intravenous use, respiratory arrest may occur, however.

The *N*-desmethyl metabolite (A above) is the major metabolite that appears in measurable levels after 24 hours and gradually rises with daily doses and persists in the blood longer than diazepam after discontinuing dose.

▶ **DICYCLOMINE**
Dangerous Drug

$$\text{C}-\text{O}-\text{CH}_2\text{CH}_2-\text{N}\begin{cases}\text{CH}_2\text{CH}_3\\\text{CH}_2\text{CH}_3\end{cases}$$

Synonyms: Dicycloverine, 2-diethylaminoethyl bi(cyclohexyl)-1-carboxylate.
Pharmaceutical Preparations
Bendectin[R] (Merrell-National)—Tablets: white, containing 10 mg dicyclomine hydrochloride, 10 mg doxylamine succinate, and 10 mg pyridoxine hydrochloride

Bentyl[R] (Merrell-National)—Capsules: blue, containing 10 mg dicyclomine hydrochloride. Tablets: blue, labeled "M," containing 20 mg dicyclomine hydrochloride. Ampule (for injection): each 2 ml containing 20 mg dicyclomine hydrochloride. Vial (for injection): each 1 ml containing 10 mg dicyclomine hydrochloride.

Bentyl[R] with Phenobarbital (Merrell-National)—See **PHENOBARBITAL**

Dyspas[R] (Savage)—Tablets: green, containing 10 mg dicyclomine hydrochloride; yellow, containing 20 mg dicyclomine hydrochloride. Oral liquid: each teaspoon (5 ml) containing 10 mg dicyclomine hydrochloride. Vials and ampules: each 1 ml containing 10 mg dicyclomine hydrochloride.

General Comments: Dicyclomine is a parasympatholytic drug. All pharmaceutical preparations containing dicyclomine require a prescription. Therefore, dicyclomine is classified in this text as a Dangerous Drug under the legend drug clause; all preparations bear the legend "Caution: Federal law prohibits dispensing without a prescription."

Biochemistry: All synthetic anticholinergic agents have some structural features in common. In most, the molecule has bulky blocking moieties like the cyclic radicals in dicyclomine. These are linked by way of a chain of atoms of limited length to an amine nitrogen. The length and structure of the main chain have great influence on the anticholinergic activity of the drug.

Toxicology–Pharmacology: Dicyclomine is an antispasmodic parasympatholytic drug that decreases spasms of the gastrointestinal tract, biliary tract, ureter, and uterus, without producing effects on the salivary, sweat, or gastrointestinal glands, the eye, or the cardiovascular system (except in large doses) similar to the belladonna alkaloids. The major action appears to be a nonspecific direct relaxant action on smooth muscle, rather than a competitive antagonism of acetylcholine. Anesthesia of the oral mucosa results when tablets of the drug are chewed.

The action of dicyclomine on the central nervous system is stimulation in low doses and depression in higher, toxic doses. Thus, when dicyclomine is combined with phenobarbital, such as Bentyl[R] with Phenobarbital, the preparation will have a lower abuser potential and be classified as an Excepted Substance.

▶ **DIETHYLPROPION**
Schedule IV

Synonyms: Amfepramone, α-diethylaminopropiophenone.

Pharmaceutical Preparations

Tenuate[R] (Merrell-National)—Tablets: blue, labeled "M," containing 25 mg diethylpropion hydrochloride

Tenuate[R] Dospan (Merrell-National)—Tablet: capsule-shaped, white, labeled "MERRELL," containing 75 mg diethylpropion hydrochloride (time release)

Tepanil[R] (Riker)—Tablet: white, labeled "RIKER," containing 25 mg diethylpropion hydrochloride

Tepanil[R] Ten-Tab (Riker)—Tablet: white, labeled "RIKER," containing 75 mg diethylpropion hydrochloride (time-release)

General Comment: Diethylpropion is similar to amphetamine in most every way except control, and in this latter area, diethylpropion is a Schedule IV drug.

Biochemistry: Similar to that of amphetamine.

Toxicology–Pharmacology: Diethylpropion is structurally similar to amphetamine, and has similar subjective effects, toxicity, and patterns of abuse. It is prescribed for use as an anorectic or appetite-suppressant agent for weight reduction.

It is metabolized by N-alkylation and keto-reduction in N-ethyl amino propiophenone, amino propiophenone, N-diethyl norephedrine, N-ethyl norephedrine, and norephedrine. Only 2 percent of the parent compound is excreted unchanged in 30 hours (Mikailova et al., 1974).

A blood concentration of 0.066 mg/dl was obtained 2 hours after a 75-mg dose (Vesell, 1971).

No data are available on toxic or lethal blood concentrations.

▶ **DIETHYLTHIAMBUTENE**
Schedule I

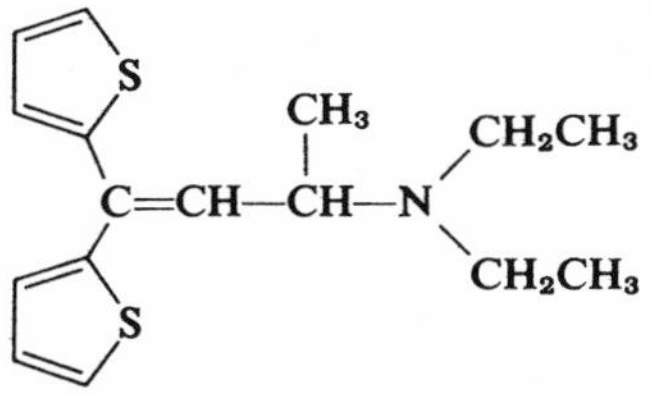

Synonym: 3-Diethylamino-1,1-diethien-2'-ylbut-1-ene.

Pharmaceutical Preparations: Diethylthiambutene is not found in any pharmaceutical preparations sold in the United States.

General Comment: Diethylthiambutene is a synthetic narcotic analgesic that has no accepted medicinal value in the United States.

Biochemistry: Unknown.

Toxicology–Pharmacology: Diethylthiambutene is a synthetic narcotic analgesic that is chemically compared with meperidine (pethidine), and possesses a dependence-producing capability similar to that of morphine. It has been used in veterinary work in the past.

▶ **DIETHYLTRYPTAMINE**
Schedule I

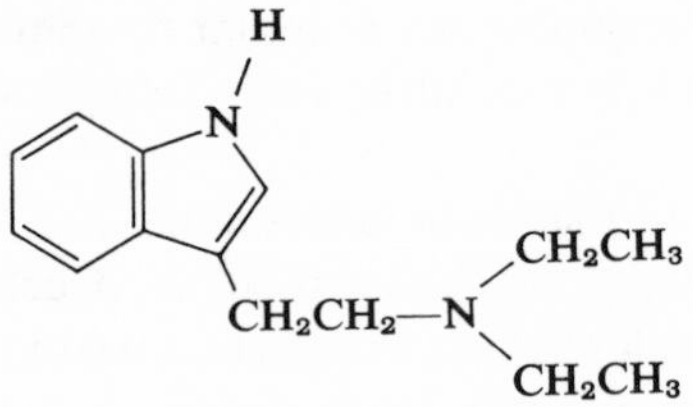

Synonyms: DET, 3(2-diethylaminoethyl)-indole.

Pharmaceutical Preparations: Diethyltryptamine is not found in any pharmaceutical preparation sold in the United States.

General Comment: Diethyltryptamine has been found on the illicit market produced in clandestine laboratories. It is not found naturally occurring.

Biochemistry: Similar to that of bufotenine and dimethyltryptamine.

Toxicology–Pharmacology: Diethyltryptamine is an indole alkaloid classified pharmacologically as a hallucinogen. Structurally, diethyltryptamine is related to LSD, psilocybin, psilocin, and the neurohumoral agent serotonin (5-hydroxytryptamine). Serotonin is present in the brain, where it is involved in central nervous regulations. Thus, it seems that this indole structure is biochemically important in psychic functions.

DIFENOXIN
Schedule I
Synonyms: None located.

Pharmaceutical Preparations: Difenoxin is not found in any pharmaceutical preparation sold in the United States.

General Comment: Difenoxin is a synthetic narcotic analgesic not accepted for medicinal use in the United States.

Biochemistry: Unknown.

Toxicology–Pharmacology: Unknown.

▶ **DIHYDROCODEINE**
Schedule II
or
Schedule III if the preparation contains not more than 1.8 g dihydrocodeine,
    or any of its salts, per 100 ml, or not more than 90 mg per dosage
    unit, with one or more active, nonnarcotic ingredients in recognized
    therapeutic amounts
or
Schedule V if any compound, mixture, or preparation containing not more
    than 100 mg dihydrocodeine, or any of its salts, per 100 ml or per 100 g,
    that also contains one or more nonnarcotic active medicinal ingredients
    in sufficient proportion to confer on the compound, mixture, or prepara-
    tion valuable medicinal qualities other than those possessed by dihydro-
    codeine alone

Synonyms: Morphine 3-methyl ether, 4,5-epoxy-6-hydroxy-3-methoxy-*N*-
methylmorphinan.
Pharmaceutical Preparations
Schedule II
There are no pharmaceutical preparations containing dihydrocodeine located
    listed under Schedule II by these authors.
Schedule III
Synalgos-DC^R (Ives)—Capsule: blue and gray, labeled "IVES 4144," con-
    taining 16.0 mg dihydrocodeine bitartrate, 6.25 mg promethazine hydro-
    chloride, 194.4 mg aspirin, 162.0 mg phenacetin, and 30.0 mg caffeine
Schedule V
There are no pharmaceutical preparations containing dihydrocodeine located
    listed under Schedule V by these authors.
General Comment: The variation in control of dihydrocodeine depends on
formulation specifications. Thus, for adequate admissibility of evidence in
court in criminal cases, complete laboratory screening for all possible medici-
nal substances is necessary.
Biochemistry: Similar to that of codeine.
Toxicology–Pharmacology: Dihydrocodeine is a synthetic narcotic analgesic
with multiple actions qualitatively similar to those of codeine. The principal

actions of therapeutic value are analgesia and sedation, and suppression of the cough reflex. Its analgesic action is between that of morphine and codeine in potency. Dihydrocodeine exerts a greater histamine-releasing effect than other narcotic analgesics.

The estimated lethal dose of dihydrocodeine is 0.5–1.0 g (Gleason *et al.*, 1969). In six fatalities involving overdose of this drug, blood concentrations of 0.08–1.20 mg/dl were found (Peat and Sengupta, 1977).

▶ DIHYDROCODEINONE (HYDROCODONE)

Schedule II
Listed as Hydrocodone
or
Schedule III for any material, compound, mixture, or preparation containing
   not more than 300 mg dihydrocodeinone, or any of its salts, per 100 ml,
   or not more than 15 mg per dosage unit, with a fourfold or greater
   quantity of an isoquinoline alkaloid of opium
   or
   not more than 300 mg dihydrocodeinone, or any of its salts, per 100 ml,
   or not more than 15 mg per dosage unit, with one or more active, nonnarcotic ingredients in recognized therapeutic amounts
Synonyms: Hydrocodone, demethyldihydrothebaine, hydrocone.
Pharmaceutical Preparations
Schedule II
Hydrocodone is not frequently found in pharmaceutical preparations controlled by Schedule II.
Schedule III
Anexsia-D^R (Beecham)—Tablet: white, scored, containing 7 mg hydrocodone
   bitartrate, 150 mg phenacetin, 230 mg aspirin, and 30 mg caffeine
Citra^R Forte (Boyle)—Capsule: containing 5 mg hydrocodone bitartrate, 50
   mg ascorbic acid, 6.25 mg pheniramine, 8.33 mg pyrilamine, 8.33 mg
   methapyrilene, 10 mg phenylephrine, 227 mg salicylamide, 30 mg caffeine,
   and 120 mg phenacetin. Syrup: each 5 ml containing 5 mg hydrocodone
   bitartrate, 30 mg ascorbic acid, 2.5 mg pheniramine, and 3.3 mg pyrilamine.

Codimal[R] DH (Central)—Syrup: each 5 ml containing 1.66 mg hydrocodone bitartrate, 5 mg phenylephrine, and 8.3 mg pyrilamine

Duradyne[R] DHC (O'Neal, Jones & Feldman)—Tablets: green, scored, containing 5 mg hydrocodone bitartrate, 230 mg aspirin, 150 mg acetaminophen, and 30 mg caffeine

Expectico[R] (Coastal)—Expectorant: each fluid ounce containing 30 mg hydrocodone bitartrate, 600 mg glyceryl guaiacolate, 900 mg sodium citrate, and 12 mg chlorpheniramine

Hycodan[R] (Endo)—Tablet and syrup: each tablet or 5 ml syrup containing 5 mg hydrocodone bitartrate and 1.5 mg homatropine methylbromide

Hycomine[R] (Endo)—Compound: tablet, coral pink, scored, containing 5 mg hydrocodone bitartrate, 2 mg chlorpheniramine, 10 mg phenylephrine, 250 mg acetaminophen, and 30 mg caffeine. Pediatric: syrup, each 5 ml containing 2.5 mg hydrocodone bitartrate and 12.5 mg phenylpropanolamine. Syrup: each 5 ml containing 5 mg hydrocodone bitartrate and 25 mg phenylpropanolamine.

Hycotuss[R] Expectorant (Endo)—Syrup: each 5 ml containing 5 mg hydrocodone bitartrate and 100 mg guaifenesin

Triaminic[R] Expectorant DH (Dorsey)—Syrup: each 5 ml containing 1.67 mg hydrocodone bitartrate, 12.5 mg phenylpropanolamine, 6.25 mg pheniramine, 6.25 mg pyrilamine, and 100 mg guaifenesin

Tussend[R] (Dow)—Liquid and tablet: each 5 ml liquid or each tablet containing 5 mg hydrocodone bitartrate and 30 mg pseudoephedrine

Tussend[R] Expectorant (Dow)—Liquid: each 5 ml containing 5 mg hydrocodone bitartrate, 30 mg pseudoephedrine, and 200 mg glycerylguaiacolate

Tussionex[R] (Pennwalt)—Capsule: green and white; tablet: light brown, scored; suspension. Each capsule, tablet, or 5 ml liquid contains 5 mg hydrocodone and 10 mg phenyltoloxamine.

General Comments: Dihydrocodeinone is listed in Schedule II under the name "hydrocodone." However, in Schedule III, under specified formulation requirements, it is listed as "dihydrocodeinone." The variation in names has no bearing on its control. Under the specified formulation requirements, however, a complete quantitative analytical laboratory screen is necessary for evidentiary material in criminal cases.

Biochemistry: Dihydrocodeinone is a strong analgetic that is the result of the catalytic rearrangement of codeine or the hydrolysis of dihydrothebaine. Even though this ketone is roughly three times as effective as its hydroxyl counterpart, its utility is limited due to a higher dependence liability.

Toxicology–Pharmacology: Hydrocodone is essentially similar to codeine in its actions; however, on an equimolar basis, hydrocodone is both more active and more prone to cause addiction. Its primary medicinal use is as an antitussive.

▶ **DIHYDROERGOTAMINE**
Dangerous Drug

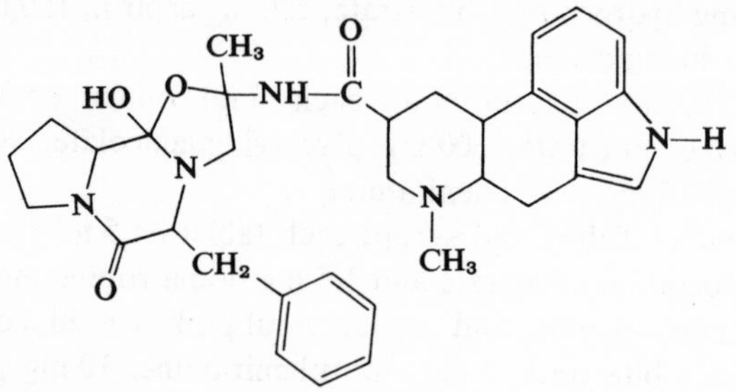

Synonyms: None found.

Pharmaceutical Preparations

DHE-45[R] (Sandoz)—Injection, containing 1.0 mg dihydroergotamine

Plexonal[R] (Sandoz)—See **BARBITAL**

General Comment: Dihydroergotamine is classified in this text as a Dangerous Drug under the "legend drug" definition because all pharmaceutical preparations containing dihydroergotamine bear the legend "Caution: Federal law prohibits dispensing without a prescription."

Biochemistry: Dihydroergotamine is a semisynthetic alkaloid produced from alkaloids found in ergot.

Toxicology–Pharmacology: The ergot alkaloids have three major pharmacological properties: vasoconstrictive actions, stimulant effects on the human uterus (oxytocic), and adrenergic blockade. Their primary clinical applications are to relieve the symptoms of migraine headache and as oxytocic agents (e.g., induction of labor).

Symptoms of poisoning by the ergot alkaloids include vomiting, diarrhea, unquenchable thirst, tingling, itching, rapid, weak pulse, confusion, and unconsciousness.

▶ **DIHYDROERGOTOXINE**
Dangerous Drug

General Comments: Dihydroergotoxine, found in the pharmaceutical preparation Hydergine[R] (Sandoz) (white tablets, no markings, unscored), is a mixture of the methylsulfonates of dihydroergocornine, dihydroergocristine, and dihydroergocryptine, the hydrogenated derivatives of the three ergot alkaloids of ergotoxine. This drug is considered a Dangerous Drug in this text because it requires a prescription.

Toxicology–Pharmacology: The ergot alkaloids, such as dihydroergotoxine, produce an α-adrenergic blockade, and have antagonistic actions to serotonin.

Dihydroergotoxine is also a potent emetic, and as little as 0.3 mg may induce vomiting. The pressor effects of sympathomimetic amines and the sympathetic nervous system are blocked. It also has a vasodilatory action on peripheral blood vessels, producing a fall in venous pressure.

Toxic effects consist of gangrene of the extremities ("ergotism").

▶ **DIHYDROMORPHINE**
Schedule I

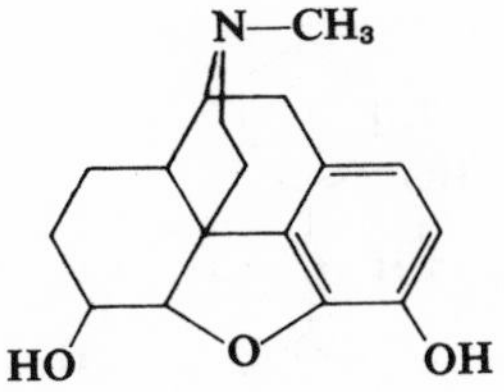

Synonym: 4,5-Epoxy-3,6-dihydroxy-*N*-methylmorphinan.

Pharmaceutical Preparations: Dihydromorphine is not found in any pharmaceutical preparations sold in the United States.

General Comments: Dihydromorphine is a synthetic narcotic analgesic not accepted for medicinal use in the United States. It is prepared by hydrogenation of morphine or by demethylation of tetrahydrothebaine.

Biochemistry: Unknown.

Toxicology–Pharmacology: Unknown.

▶ **DIMENOXADOL**
Schedule I

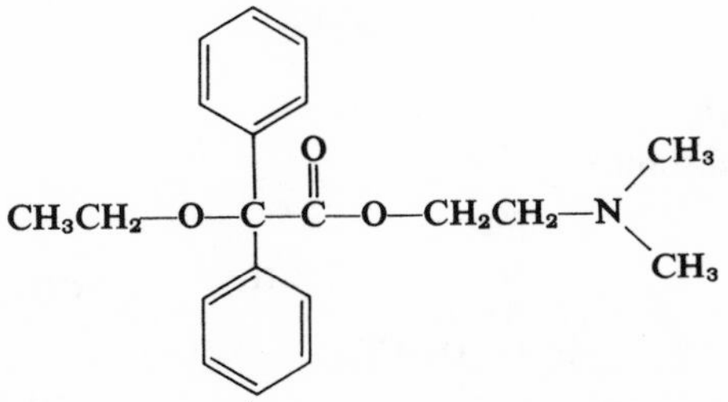

Synonyms: 2-Dimethylaminoethyl α-ethoxy-α,α-diphenylacetate, ethoxydiphenylacetic acid 2-dimethylaminoethyl ester, α,α-diphenyl-α-ethoxyacetic acid β-dimethylaminoethyl ester.

Pharmaceutical Preparations: Dimenoxadol is not found in any pharmaceutical preparations sold in the United States.

General Comment: Dimenoxadol is a synthetic narcotic analgesic that has no accepted medicinal use in the United States.
Biochemistry: Unknown.
Toxicology–Pharmacology: Unknown.

▶ **DIMEPHEPTANOL**
Schedule I

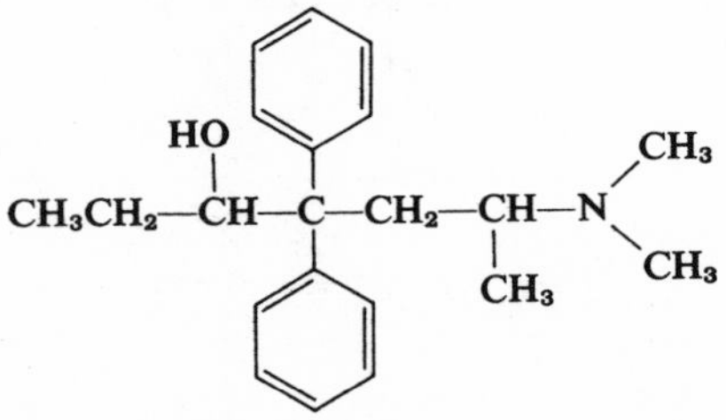

$$CH_3CH_2-\overset{\displaystyle HO}{\underset{}{CH}}-\overset{}{\underset{CH_3}{C}}-CH_2-\overset{}{CH}-N\overset{\displaystyle CH_3}{\underset{CH_3}{}}$$

Synonyms: Bimethadol, 6-(dimethylamino)-4,4-diphenyl-3-heptanol, 2-dimethylamino-4,4-diphenyl-5-heptanol, and 3-hydroxy-4,4-diphenyl-6-dimethylaminoheptane.
Pharmaceutical Preparations: Dimepheptanol is not found in any pharmaceutical preparations sold in the United States.
General Comment: Dimepheptanol is a synthetic narcotic analgesic that has no accepted medicinal use in the United States.
Biochemistry: Unknown.
Toxicology–Pharmacology: Unknown.

▶ **DIMETHOCAINE**
Noncontrolled Substance

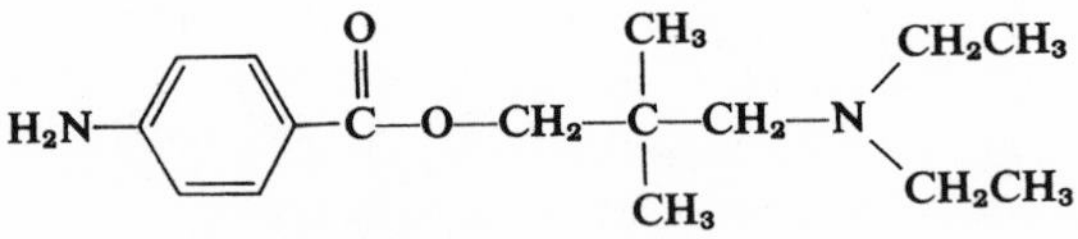

$$H_2N-\!\!\!\!\bigcirc\!\!\!\!-\overset{\displaystyle O}{\underset{}{C}}-O-CH_2-\overset{\displaystyle CH_3}{\underset{CH_3}{C}}-CH_2-N\overset{\displaystyle CH_2CH_3}{\underset{CH_2CH_3}{}}$$

Synonyms and Pharmacology: Dimethocaine, also known as larocaine, 3-(diethylamino)-2,2-dimethyl-1-propanol p-aminobenzoate, 3-diethylamino-2,2-dimethylpropyl p-aminobenzoate, and 1-aminobenzoyl-2,2-dimethyl-3-diethylaminopropanol, is a local anesthetic.

▶ **2,5-DIMETHOXYAMPHETAMINE**
Schedule I

$$OCH_3$$

CH$_3$O—⟨benzene ring⟩—CH$_2$—CH(NH$_2$)—CH$_3$

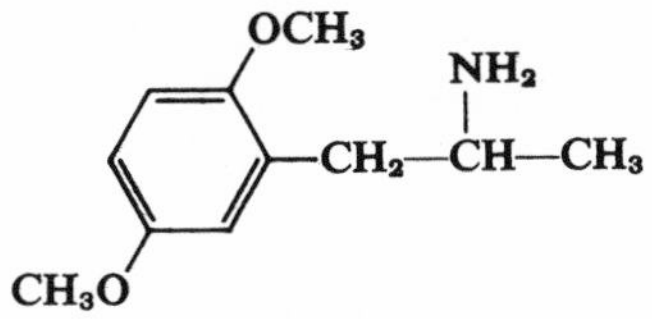

Synonyms: 2,5-Dimethoxy-α-methylphenethylamine, 2,5-DMA.

Pharmaceutical Preparations: 2,5-Dimethoxyamphetamine is not found in any pharmaceutical preparations sold in the United States.

General Comment: 2,5-Dimethoxyamphetamine is one of the dimethoxy series of amphetamine derivatives that have no accepted medicinal use in the United States.

Biochemistry: The dimethoxy series of amphetamine derivatives has been studied for hallucinogenic properties, and it has been found that the 2,3-, 2,5- and 3,5- compounds are relatively inactive, giving only amphetamine profiles at high doses (6.1 and 12.5 mg/kg). However, the 3,4-compound was a highly active hallucinogen, 12.5 mg/kg being roughly equivalent to mescaline in a dose of 25 mg/kg (Smythies *et al.*, 1967).

Toxicology–Pharmacology: Similar to that of amphetamine.

▶ **2,5-DIMETHOXY-4-METHYLAMPHETAMINE**
Schedule I

$$OCH_3$$

CH$_3$—⟨benzene ring⟩—CH$_2$—CH(NH$_2$)—CH$_3$
CH$_3$O

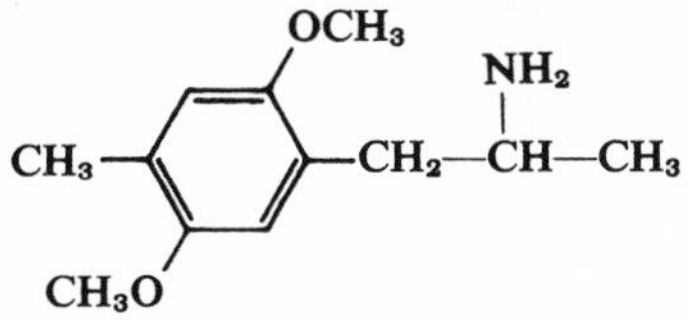

Synonyms: 2,5-Dimethoxy-4-methyl-α-methylphenethylamine, STP, DOM.

Pharmaceutical Preparations: 2,5-Dimethoxy-4-methylamphetamine is not found in any pharmaceutical preparations sold in the United States.

General Comments: 2,5-Dimethoxy-4-methylamphetamine is an amphetamine derivative having central nervous system (CNS) stimulating, as well as hallucinogenic, properties. It is encountered in cases of drug abuse.

In 1967, psychedelic promoter Timothy Leary began a campaign for a "new" hallucinogen that, according to underground newspapers, was stronger than LSD. Leary called this "new" hallucinogen STP, for "Serenity,

Tranquility, and Peace." Shortly after this campaign began, several thousand tablets of STP were distributed free at a "love-in" in San Francisco, resulting in numerous hospitalizations. These tablets were white, blue, or peach color, and were single-scored and biconvex. The excipient in all was lactose monohydrate. The active ingredient was 4-methyl-2,5-dimethoxy amphetamine, also called DOM.

Biochemistry: That the potent psychotomimetic drug 2,5-dimethoxy-4-methylamphetamine possesses a structure similar to those of mescaline, dopamine, and norepinephrine has led to speculations as to whether there is a relationship between hallucinogenic activity and the interaction of a psychotomimetic drug with catecholamines in the CNS. There have been no data to support this theory as yet.

Toxicology–Pharmacology: Low doses produce a mild euphoria. Doses greater than 3 mg may cause pronounced hallucinogenic effects, similar to those of LSD, mescaline, or psilocybin. The effects last up to 8 hours. It is 100 times more potent than mescaline, and 1/30th as potent as LSD (Snyder et al., 1967).

After administration of low doses, an increase in pulse rate and body temperature was observed. Somatic changes included nausea, sweating, paresthesia, and tremors. Perceptual changes included blurred vision, multiple images, distorted shapes, enhancement of details, slowed passage of time, and loss of control of thoughts. About 20% of a dose was excreted in urine within 24 hours (Snyder et al., 1967).

▶ **DIMETHYLTHIAMBUTENE**
Schedule I

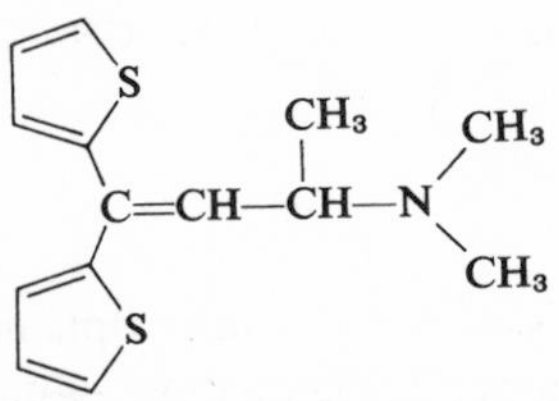

Synonyms: Aminobutene, cobatone, dimethibutin, N,N,1-trimethyl-3,3-di-(thien-2'-yl)allylamine.

Pharmaceutical Preparations: Dimethylthiambutene is not found in any pharmaceutical preparations sold in the United States.

General Comments: Dimethylthiambutene is a synthetic narcotic analgesic not accepted for medicinal use in the United States. It is clinically compared with meperidine (pethidine), but maintains the dependence-producing capability of morphine. It has had illicit use in Japan in the past.

Biochemistry: Unknown.

Toxicology–Pharmacology: Dimethylthiambutene has analgetic effects similar to those of meperidine. However, its dependence-producing capability is like that of morphine.

▶ **DIMETHYLTRYPTAMINE**
Schedule I

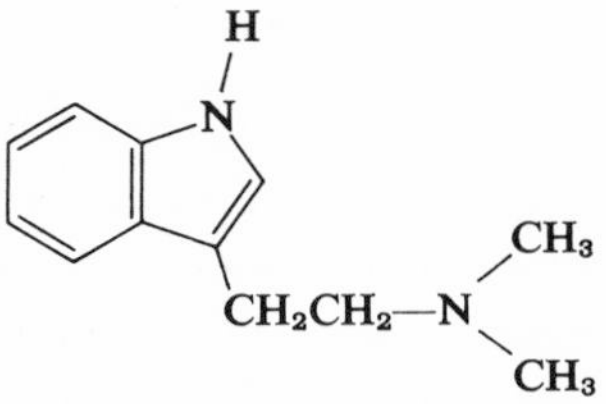

Synonyms: 3-(Dimethylaminoethyl)indole, DMT.

Pharmaceutical Preparations: Dimethyltryptamine is not found in any pharmaceutical preparations sold in the United States.

General Comments: Dimethyltryptamine is an indole alkaloid with hallucinogenic properties. It has no accepted medicinal value in the United States.

Biochemistry: Dimethyltryptamine (DMT) has been identified in a snuff prepared from the shrub *Piptadenia peregrina* (Mimosaceae) as well as from the genus *Virola* (Myristicaceae). Bufotenine was also identified as a component of *Piptadenia* (Fisk *et al.*, 1955; Lewis and Elvin-Lewis, 1977).

Like diethyltryptamine (DET), DMT is not active when administered orally. When abused, it is usually inhaled via smoke vapors when applied to tobacco, parsley, or marijuana, and smoked. When injected the effects begin in less than two minutes. As the effects last less than one hour, the term "businessman's high" has been applied for DMT use (Lewis and Elvin-Lewis, 1977).

Toxicology–Pharmacology: The effective dose for man is about 1 mg/kg injected intramuscularly. The hallucinogenic effects set in rapidly and lessen in intensity and disappear after 50–60 minutes. It is not active orally (Schultes and Hofmann, 1973).

Psychotic effects were elicited by intramuscular injection of 0.70–1.0 mg/kg, beginning in 3–5 minutes and lasting 50–70 minutes. The effects were characterized by intense vegetative phenomena, anxiety, disturbances in mood and perception, visual illusions, and alterations of space and time. The effect was similar to single phases of the LSD effect, but had no resemblance to schizophrenia or endogenous psychotic states (Boszormenyi and Szara, 1958).

▶ **DIOXAPHETYL BUTYRATE**
Schedule I

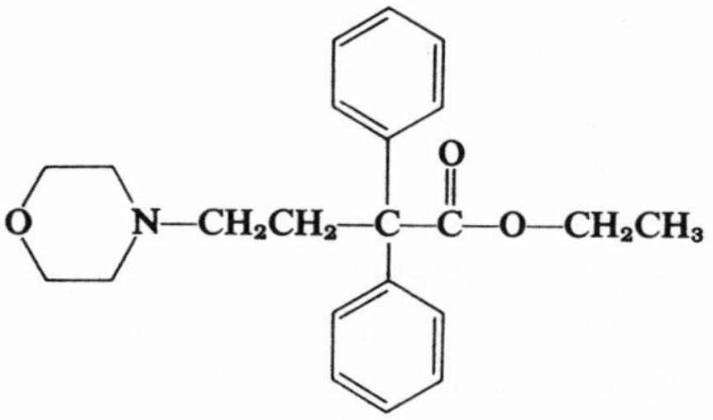

Synonyms: Amidalgon, ethyl-y-morpholine-α,α-diphenylbutyrate.
Pharmaceutical Preparations: Dioxaphetyl butyrate is not found in any pharmaceutical preparations sold in the United States.
General Comments: Dioxaphetyl butyrate is a synthetic narcotic analgesic that has no accepted medicinal value in the United States.
Biochemistry: Unknown.
Toxicology–Pharmacology: Unknown.

▶ **DIPHEMANIL METHYLSULFATE**
Noncontrolled Substance
Found in Excepted Substances

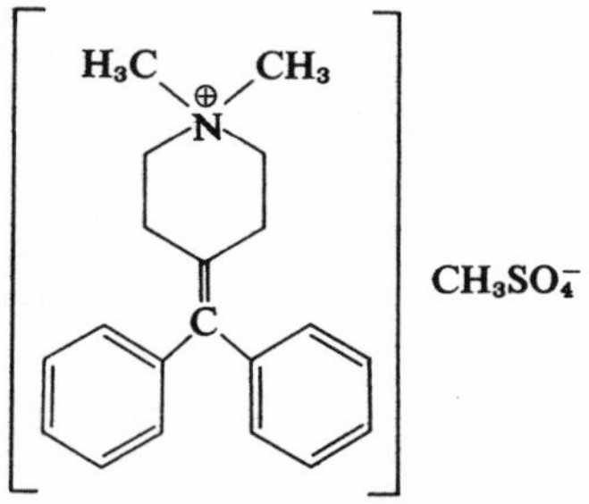

General Comments: Diphemanil methylsulfate, also known as diphenmethanil methylsulfate and 4-diphenylmethylene-1,1-dimethylpiperidinium methylsulfate, is a parasympatholytic drug. It is found in excepted phenobarbital preparations with a phenobarbital/diphenmanil methylsulfate minimum ratio of 1/6.25.

▶ **DIPHENHYDRAMINE**
Noncontrolled Substance

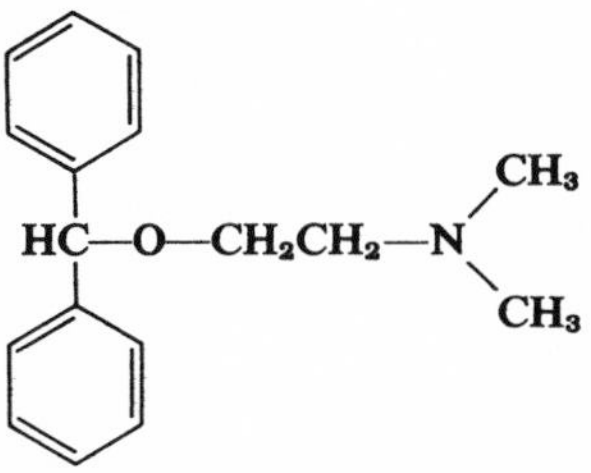

$$HC-O-CH_2CH_2-N \begin{array}{c} CH_3 \\ \\ CH_3 \end{array}$$

General Comments: Diphenhydramine was the first antihistamine to have become available in the United States. Its actions have served as a standard for comparison in the development of many other antihistamines now available.

Toxicology–Pharmacology: Diphenhydramine is an antihistaminic agent widely used in the treatment of allergic syndromes in which histamine release is a major factor. Seasonal hay fever, and certain types of rhinitis, may be treated with antihistamines. They are of little value in treatment or symptomatic relief of the common cold. Thus, antihistamines are of value for the treatment of motion sickness to protect against vertigo, nausea, and vomiting. A prominent side effect of diphenhydramine is drowsiness and sedation, and other central nervous system (CNS) effects may include dizziness, tinnitus, fatigue, ataxia, or blurred vision. Euphoria, dryness of the mouth, and weakness may also be experienced. Overdose is characterized by CNS depression, or sometimes excitement leading to convulsions.

After an oral dose of 400 mg, a blood concentration of about 0.10 mg/dl is attained. After a more usual therapeutic dose of 50 mg, a plasma level of 0.008 mg/dl was observed after 3 hours (Bilzer and Gundert, 1973). Diphenhydramine has a plasma half-life of 6.8 hours after a 100-mg dose (Glazko *et al.*, 1974). In one death of a 13-year-old girl from an overdose of diphenhydramine, a blood concentration of 0.23 mg/dl was found, in combination with a phenobarbital level of 2.25 mg/dl (Garriott, 1977).

▶ **DIPHENOXYLATE**

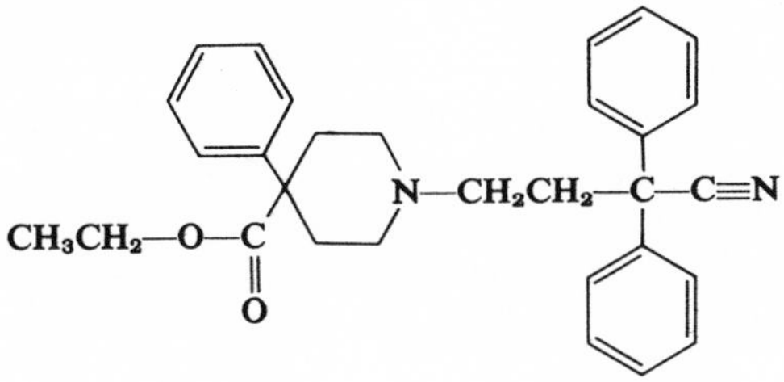

$$CH_3CH_2-O-\underset{\underset{O}{\parallel}}{C} \qquad N-CH_2CH_2-\underset{}{C}-C\equiv N$$

Schedule II
or
Schedule V for any compound, mixture, or preparation containing not more
  than 2.5 mg diphenoxylate and not less than 25 μg atropine sulfate per
  dosage unit.
Synonym: Ethyl-1-(3-cyano-3,3-diphenyl-propyl)-4-phenylpiperidine 4-car-
boxylate.
Pharmaceutical Preparations
Schedule II
None found.
Schedule V
Lomotil[R] (Searle)—Tablet: white, labeled "SEARLE" on one side and
  "61" on the other, containing 2.5 mg diphenoxylate hydrochloride
  and 0.025 mg atropine sulfate. Liquid: each 5 ml (one teaspoon) containing 2.5 mg diphenoxylate hydrochloride and 0.025 mg atropine
  sulfate.
General Comment: As noted above, diphenoxylate varies in control by its
formulation specifications. Thus, when laboratory examinations are conducted for evidentiary material, a complete screen with quantitation for all
medicinal agents is necessary.
Biochemistry: Diphenoxylate has been described as an effective agent for the
symptomatic relief of diarrhea. It acts by inhibiting excessive gastrointestinal
propulsion (Barowsky and Schwartz, 1962).
Toxicology–Pharmacology: Diphenoxylate is chemically and pharmacologically related to meperidine (pethidine), but is essentially devoid of the
central nervous system effects. Diphenoxylate has a definite constipating
effect in man and is used exclusively in the treatment of diarrhea. A single
dose in the therapeutic range does not produce morphine-type effects. However, in higher doses (above 40 mg) the drug begins to exhibit symptoms
similar to morphine.

Diphenoxylate, as the free base or the hydrochloride salt, is insoluble in
aqueous media. Therefore, its abuse potential via the parenteral route is
nonexistent.

A 5-mg dose produces a blood concentration of 0.001–0.012 μg/ml
during the first 8 hours after administration. It has a plasma half-life of 4.38 $\pm$
1.04 hours (Karim *et al.*, 1972).

This drug frequently results in intoxication and death in children,
who may experience severe poisoning with as little as 20 mg (Gleason
et al., 1969). Respiratory difficulty and apnea are characteristic of overdose. Narcotic antagonists such as naloxone can be used to treat such
overdoses.

▶ **DIPIPANONE**
Schedule I

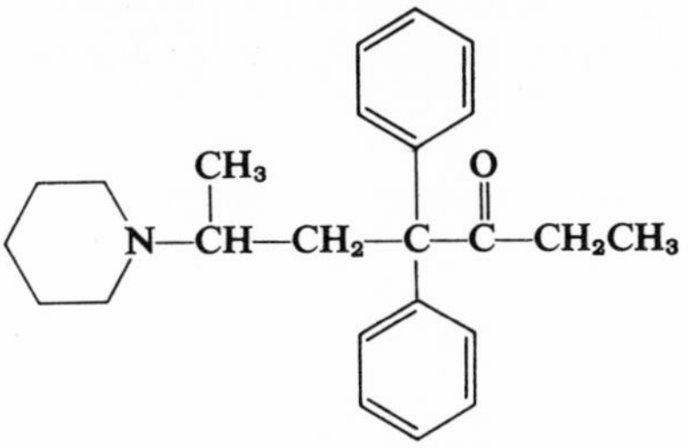

Synonyms: Fenpidon, pamedone, phenylpiperone, piperidyl methadone, piperidylamidone, ($\pm$)-4,4-diphenyl-6-piperidinoheptan-3-one.

Pharmaceutical Preparations: Even though this drug has medicinal use in some countries, dipipanone is not found in any pharmaceutical preparations sold in the United States.

General Comment: Dipipanone is a synthetic narcotic analgesic that has no accepted medicinal value in the United States.

Biochemistry: Unknown.

Toxicology–Pharmacology: The therapeutic dose of dipipanone is considered to be 20–25 mg having a duration of action of 4–5 hours. Like methadone, dipipanone may exhibit cumulative effects with repeated doses and retains most of its analgesic efficacy when given orally. Dipipanone, like phenadoxone, may produce marked irritation at injection sites.

The toxicity of dipipanone is of the same order as that of methadone.

▶ **DIPROPYLTRYPTAMINE**
Noncontrolled Substance

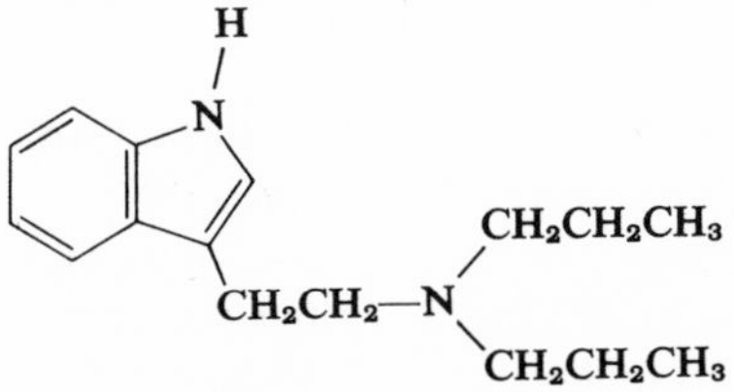

General Comments: Dipropyltryptamine, also known as 3-(2-dipropylamino-ethyl)-indole, is an indole alkaloid with hallucinogenic properties.

Dipropyltryptamine has never been found occurring naturally. Like diethyltryptamine, dipropyltryptamine is not active when administered orally. When abused, it is usually inhaled via smoke vapors when applied to tobacco, parsley, or marijuana, and smoked. Injections of dipropyltryptamine have been carried out by abusers, but are infrequent. There are no commercial pharmaceutical preparations containing dipropyltryptamine.

▶ **DOXAPRAM**
Dangerous Drug

Synonym: 1-Ethyl-4-(2-morpholinoethyl)-2-oxo-3,3-diphenylpyrrolidine.

Pharmaceutical Preparations: Dopram[R] (A. H. Robins)—Vial: each 1 ml containing 20 mg doxapram hydrochloride

General Comment: Doxapram is an analeptic drug that is classified in this text as a Dangerous Drug under the "legend drug" provision because all pharmaceutical preparations containing doxapram require a prescription and thus bear the label "Caution: Federal law prohibits dispensing without a prescription."

Biochemistry: Doxapram was introduced as a nonspecific CNS stimulant with analeptic properties in 1963 (Wasserman and Richardson, 1963). It is used in the treatment of postanesthetic respiratory depression as well as accelerating recovery after general anesthesia. When doxapram is used as a respiratory stimulant, it produces an increase in total volume and respiratory rate. However, at this dosage, there is only a slight increase in blood pressure and pulse rate. Since at this dosage there is little cerebral cortical stimulation, the danger of convulsions is reduced.

It has been postulated that the metabolitic pathway of doxapram involves opening of the morpholine ring (Bruce *et al.*, 1965).

Toxicology–Pharmacology: Doxapram is a nonspecific analeptic used primarily for stimulation of respiration in the postanesthetic period. Although its distribution is not fully documented, its metabolism is rapid.

The margin of safety between therapeutic and toxic levels appears to be greater with doxapram than with other nonspecific analeptics. A dose of doxapram that improves respiration is considerably below the dose that is needed to induce convulsions.

Acute toxicity of doxapram can result in effects such as hypertension, tachycardia, arrhythmias, muscle rigidity, anorexia, nausea, and at higher levels it may produce cardiovascular effects.

► **DOXEPIN**
Dangerous Drug

Synonyms: *N,N*-Dimethyl-3-(dibenz[*b,e*]oxepin-11(6*H*)ylidine)-propylamine.
Pharmaceutical Preparations
Adapin^R (Pennwalt)—Capsules: orange, containing 10 mg doxepin; orange
and green, containing 25 mg doxepin; green, containing 50 mg doxepin
Sinequan^R (Pfizer)—Capsules: red and brown, containing 10 mg doxepin;
blue and red, containing 25 mg doxepin; red and beige, containing 50 mg
doxepin; blue and beige, containing 100 mg doxepin
General Comment: Doxepin is an antidepressant drug that is classified in this
text as a Dangerous Drug under the "legend drug" provision because all
pharmaceutical preparations containing doxepin require a prescription and
thus bear the label "Caution: Federal law prohibits dispensing without a
prescription."
Biochemistry: Doxepin is an amitriptyline analog that is a clinically effective
antidepressant. Both the *cis* and *trans* isomers possess antidepressive actions
(Simpson and Salim, 1965).
   Substitution by appropriate dialkylaminoalkyl groups at the 11 position
of the 11-substituted 6,11-dihydrodibenz[*b,e*]oxepin derivatives produces

additional central stimulating, central depressant, antihistaminic, antispasmodic, and/or adrenolytic activity. In this respect, doxepin possesses antispasmodic, vasodilator, and antihistaminic properties (Witiak, 1970).
Toxicology–Pharmacology: Doxepin acts predominantly on the central
nervous system (CNS). It is neither a monoamine oxidase (MAO) inhibitor
nor a primary stimulant of the CNS; however, it has been utilized in the
treatment of patients with psychotic disorders and endogenous depression.
However, serious side effects and even death may occur if doxepin is used
concomitantly with MAO inhibitors.

Doxepin is used to treat psychoneurotic patients with depression and/or anxiety or various psychotic depressive disorders causing anxiety, tension, sleep disturbance, and other symptoms. It does not induce euphoria or addiction, and therefore has little potential for abuse. The usual dosage range is 75–150 mg per day. The maximum therapeutic blood concentration with this dosage is around 0.03 mg/dl, and fatalities from overdose may occur with levels around 0.70 mg/dl. Symptoms of overdose include respiratory depression, hypotension, coma, convulsions, and cardiac arrhythmias. After a death from an overdose of 3000 mg, a blood level of 0.90 mg/dl was found (Baselt *et al.*, 1975b).

▶ **DROPERIDOL**
Dangerous Drug

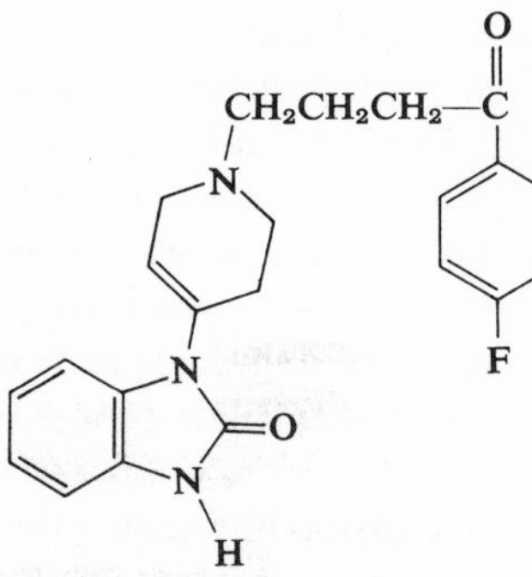

Synonyms: Dehydrobenzperidol, 1-(1,2,3,6-tetrahydro-1-[4-(*p*-fluorophenyl)-4-oxobutyl]pyrid-4-yl)-2-oxobenzimidazoline.
Pharmaceutical Preparations
Inaspine[R] Injection (McNeil)—Ampules: each 1 ml containing 2.5 mg droperidol. Vials: each 1 ml containing 2.5 mg droperidol.
Innovar[R] Injection (McNeil)—Ampules: each 1 ml containing 0.05 mg fentanyl and 2.5 mg droperidol
General Comment: Droperidol is a tranquilizer, and as such is classified in this text as a Dangerous Drug.
Biochemistry: Droperidol is a tetrahydropyridine derivative of butyrophenone. This type of antipsychotic drug has the ability to calm severely disturbed psychiatric patients and to alleviate symptoms of their illness without clouding consciousness or causing other incapacitating neurological effects.
Toxicology–Pharmacology: Droperidol is similar to the phenothiazine tranquilizers. It is usually used in combination with other drugs for intravenous anesthesia. Droperidol, a butyrophenone derivative, has potent neuroleptic activity. Thus, in preoperative therapy, it produces tranquility and decreases

anxiety and pain. Its sedative and tranquilizing effects generally last from 2 to 4 hours, but alteration of consciousness may persist as long as 12 hours. It will have a synergistic effect with other depressant drugs; thus, any other central nervous depressant will be potentiated in effects with concomitant use of droperidol.

Overdose and adverse effects include hypotension, dizziness, bronchospasm or laryngospasm, and postoperative hallucinatory episodes.

▶ **DROTEBANOL**
Schedule I
Synonyms: None found.
Pharmaceutical Preparations: Drotebanol is not found in any pharmaceutical preparations sold in the United States.
General Comment: Drotebanol is a synthetic narcotic analgesic that has no accepted medicinal value in the United States.
Biochemistry: Unknown.
Toxicology–Pharmacology: Unknown.

▶ **DYPHYLLINE**
Encountered in Excepted Substances

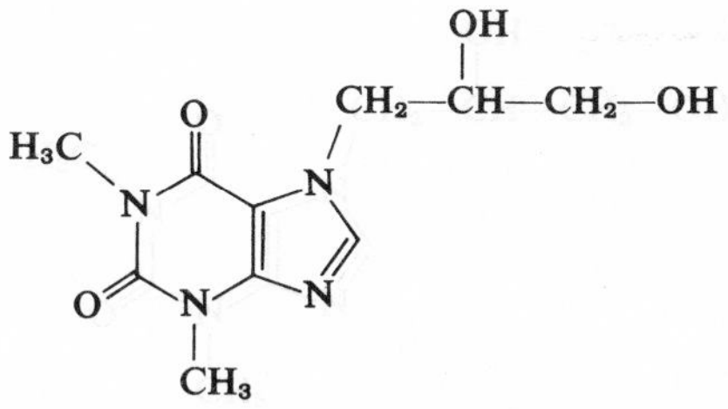

$$H_3C-N \quad O \quad N-CH_2-CH(OH)-CH_2-OH$$
$$O=\quad N(CH_3)\quad N$$

Synonyms and Pharmaceutical Preparations: Dyphylline, also called diprophylline, dihydroxypropyltheophyllinum, glyphyllin, hyphylline, and 7-(2,3-dihydroxypropyl)-1,3-dimethylxanthine, is a xanthine derivative. It has a stimulating effect on the central nervous system (CNS). When combined with a CNS depressant, the pharmaceutical preparation may be classified as an Excepted Substance. It is found in excepted phenobarbital preparations with a phenobarbital/dyphylline/ephedrine ratio of about 1/6.25/1.
Toxicology–Pharmacology: Dyphylline acts as a bronchodilator, myocardial stimulant, diuretic, and smooth muscle relaxant. In human therapeutics, its chief action is bronchodilation for treatment of bronchial asthma and bronchospasm associated with chronic bronchitis and emphysema. Usual dosage for this purpose is 200 mg three or four times a day. Administration of

high doses may result in nausea, vomiting, epigastric or substernal pain, palpitation, dizziness, or headache.

Lethal doses or blood concentrations are not known.

▶ **ECGONINE**
Schedule II

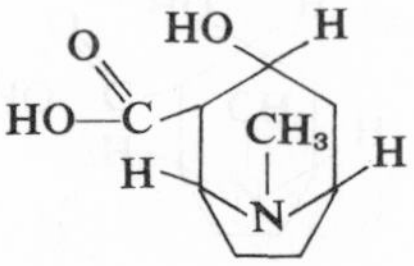

Synonym: 3-Hydroxy-2-tropanecarboxylic acid.

Pharmaceutical Preparations: Ecgonine is not found in any pharmaceutical preparations sold in the United States.

General Comment: Ecgonine is listed under Schedule II as a stimulant. However, the logic behind its control is that of an "immediate precursor" of cocaine. Under Section 201 of the Controlled Substances Act, an immediate precursor may be placed in the same schedule as the controlled substance to which it is a precursor, or in any other schedule with a higher numerical designation (e.g., Schedule III, IV, or V).

Biochemistry: See **COCAINE.**

Toxicology–Pharmacology: Ecgonine probably has little or no pharmacological activity.

▶ **EMYLCAMATE**
Dangerous Drug

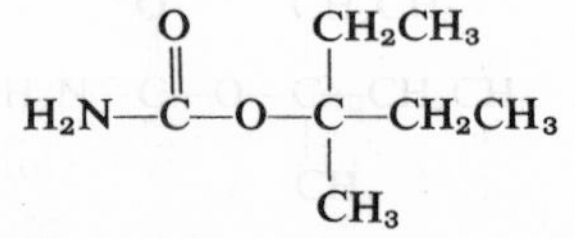

Synonyms: 1-Ethyl-1-methylpropyl carbamate, 2-ethylbut-2-yl carbamate.

Pharmaceutical Preparations: Emylcamate is not found in any pharmaceutical preparations sold in the United States.

General Comment: Emylcamate is classified pharmacologically as a tranquilizer. It is therefore classified in this text as a Dangerous Drug.

Biochemistry: Unknown.

Toxicology–Pharmacology: Emylcamate is structurally and pharmacologically similar to meprobamate. It is rapidly absorbed from the gastrointestinal tract, peak blood levels being obtained in 1–2 hours. It is metabolized in the liver and excreted in the urine.

The lethal dose in man is estimated to be between 100 and 500 mg/kg body weight.

▶ **EPHEDRINE**
Encountered in Excepted Substances

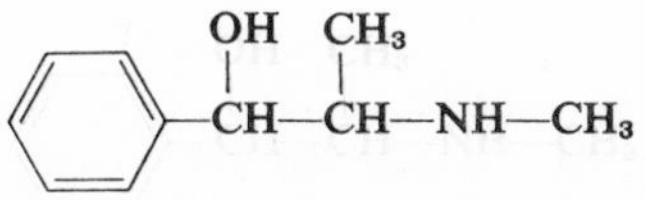

Synonyms and Pharmaceutical Preparations: Ephedrine, also called (−)-2-methylamino-1-phenylpropan-1-ol hemihydrate, is a sympathomimetic drug. It has a stimulating effect on the central nervous system (CNS). When combined with a CNS depressant, a pharmaceutical preparation may be classified as an Excepted Substance. The following ratios of drugs and mixtures are found in pharmaceutical preparations classified as Excepted Substances:

1. Allobarbital/stramonium extract/ephedrine/theophylline, ratio 1/0.5/0.5/6.25
2. Butabarbital/ephedrine/theophylline, ratio 1/0.96/5.2
3. Cyclopentenylallylbarbituric acid; cyclopentenylallylbarbituric acid/ephedrine/theophylline, ratio 1/0.75/4
4. Pentobarbital drug mixture: pentobarbital/aminophylline/ephedrine, ratio 1/1/0.5
5. Phenobarbital:
   a. Drug mixture: phenobarbital/aminophylline/ephedrine, ratio 1/3.33/1
   b. Drug mixture: phenobarbital/dyphylline/ephedrine, ratio 1/6.25/1
   c. Phenobarbital/ephedrine, ratio 1/1.5
   d. Phenobarbital/ephedrine/euphoebia extract, ratio 1/1/4
   e. Phenobarbital/theophylline/ephedrine, ratio 1/3.7/0.74

General Comments: Ephedrine is an alkaloid produced commercially either by the extraction of plant material from the genus *Ephedra* or by a chemical procedure involving a reductive condensation between L-1-phenyl-1-acetyl-carbinol and methylamine. The genus *Ephedra*, also known as "ma huang," is found near the east coast in southern China, and this source formerly supplied most of the American market. At present, northwestern India and west Pakistan represent primary areas from which *Ephedra* is obtained. "Ma huang" is a Chinese term coming from "Ma," meaning astringent, and "huang," meaning yellow, probably referring to the taste and color of the drug. *Ephedra* has been used as a medicinal substance in China for more than 5000 years. Ephedrine was discovered as a medicinal substance in 1923.

Toxicology–Pharmacology: Ephedrine is an adrenergic drug, and simulates the actions of epinephrine, but is effective orally, whereas epinephrine is not. It also has a longer duration of action, and has more pronounced central effects, than epinephrine. The primary effects are on the cardiovascular system and the bronchial smooth muscle. It elevates the systolic and diastolic blood pressure by vasoconstriction and cardiac stimulation. It relaxes the bronchial smooth muscle, aiding in lung ventilation, and dilates the pupils of the eye. It is used in man primarily as treatment for bronchospasm, as a nasal decongestant, as a mydriatic, and in certain allergic disorders. It may also be used as a pressor agent to prevent fall of blood pressure in surgical procedures. It has central stimulant properties similar to those of amphetamines, but is much less potent in this respect.

The estimated lethal dose in children up to 2 years of age is 200 mg and for adults, up to 2 g. Ephedrine is absorbed from the gastrointestinal tract, and after injection, it accumulates in tissues such as liver, lung, kidney, brain, and spleen. About 80% of the dose is excreted unchanged in the urine in 24 hours. Phenylpropanolamine, the demethylated metabolite, has been identified in the urine.

▶ **ERGONOVINE**
Dangerous Drug

Synonyms: Ergometrine, ergobasine, ergometrinine, (+)-*N*-(2-hydroxy-1-methylethyl)lysergamide.

Pharmaceutical Preparations: Ergotrate[R] (Lilly)—Ampules and hyporets: each 1-ml ampule or hyporet containing 0.2 mg ergonovine maleate. Tablets: containing 0.2 mg ergonovine maleate.

General Comments: This alkaloid was discovered almost simultaneously in 1935 by five independent research groups, and four different names were assigned to it. To resolve the conflict, a fifth name, ergonovine, was officially adopted in the United States. Ergometrine is used in practically all other countries, except Switzerland, where ergobasine is preferred.

Biochemistry: Numerous alkaloids have been found to be uterine stimulants. However, only a few are useful therapeutically, since most produce pronounced side effects when administered in therapeutically effective doses. In contrast, ergot alkaloids possess oxytocic activity and have very few undesirable actions at effective dose levels. Of these alkaloids, ergonovine is the most potent and selective oxytocic agent.

Both the *dextro* and *levo* isomers have been isolated from ergot. However, only the levorotatory isomer is pharmacologically active (Sawhney, 1970).

Toxicology–Pharmacology: Ergonovine, as an oxytocic, produces a much faster stimulation of the uterine muscles than other ergot alkaloids. It is used, or indicated, for the prevention and treatment of postpartum hemorrhage due to uterine atony.

Ergonovine is more rapidly absorbed from the gastrointestinal tract than ergotamine. It has been detected unchanged in the urine up to $8\frac{1}{2}$ hours after an injection, a maximum concentration generally occurring 2–3 hours after injection.

Ergonovine is less toxic than ergotamine. In mice, the LD_{50} is considered to be about 145 mg/kg body weight.

▶ **ERGOTAMINE**
Dangerous Drug

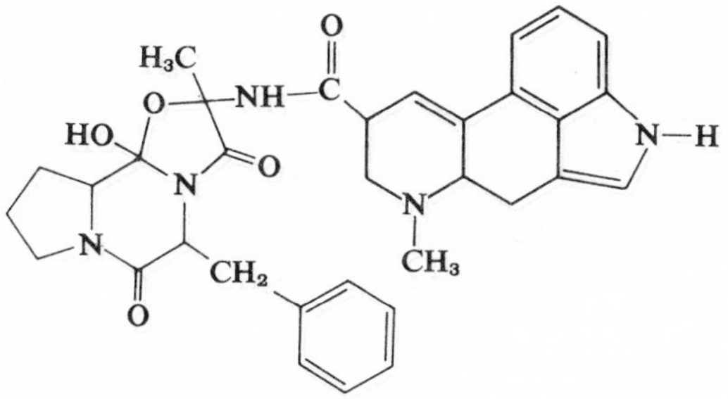

Pharmaceutical Preparations

Cafergot[R] (Sandoz)—Tablet: flesh-pink-colored, sugar-coated, containing 1.0 mg ergotamine tartrate and 100 mg caffeine. Suppository: containing 2.0 mg ergotamine tartrate and 100 mg caffeine.

Cafergot[R] P-B (Sandoz)—Tablet: bright green, sugar-coated, containing 1.0 mg ergotamine tartrate, 100 mg caffeine, 1.25 mg belladonna alkaloids, and 30.0 mg sodium pentobarbital. Suppository: containing 2.0 mg ergotamine tartrate, 100 mg caffeine, 0.25 mg belladonna alkaloids, and 60.0 mg pentobarbital.

Ergomar[R] (Fisons)—Tablet: green, containing 2.0 mg ergotamine tartrate

Gynergen^R (Sandoz)—Tablet: ivory gray, sugar-coated, containing 1.0 mg
   ergotamine tartrate. Injection: each 1 cc containing 0.5 mg ergotamine
   tartrate.
Medihaler-Ergotamine^R (Riker)—A medihaler containing 9.0 mg ergotamine
   tartrate per 1 ml
Migral^R (Burroughs-Wellcome)—Tablet: white, sugar-coated, containing 1.0
   mg ergotamine tartrate, 25 mg cyclizine hydrochloride, and 50 mg
   caffeine

General Comment: Ergotamine is an ergot alkaloid that is classified in this
text as a Dangerous Drug under the "legend drug" provision since all pharmaceutical preparations containing ergotamine require a prescription and bear
the label "Caution: Federal law prohibits dispensing without a prescription."
Biochemistry: Ergotamine has a complex cyclic tripeptide structure attached
to the amide side chain of the lysergic acid moiety as compared with ergonovine.

Although highly effective as an oxytocic, ergotamine has pronounced
side effects such as vasoconstriction and adrenergic blockage in addition to a
prolonged latent period.

Toxicology–Pharmacology: Ergotamine has its primary pharmacological
action on the uterus, the cardiovascular system, and in its antagonism of
5-hydroxytryptamine. The stimulant effect on the uterus (oxytocic effect) is
less than that of other ergot alkaloids, and it is not used for this purpose. It is
very effective in treatment of migraine headache, relieving about 90% of all
patients afflicted. Its effect is only temporary, however, and it does not
decrease the frequency of attacks.

Ergotamine is highly toxic, and results in vomiting, diarrhea, unquenchable thirst, confusion, and unconsciousness. Chronic poisoning (ergotism)
arising from ingestion of grain contaminated with ergot (wheat rust) results
in headache, nausea, vomiting, diarrhea, dizziness, and gangrene from impaired circulation in the extremities.

▶ **ERGOTOXINE**
Noncontrolled Substance
General Comments: Ergotoxine, also called ecboline, was formerly used as a
reference standard in the form of ergotoxine ethane sulfonate. However, this
use was discontinued when it was found to be a variable mixture of three
closely related alkaloids: ergocristine, ergocryptine, and ergocornine.

Formerly marketed as Hydergine, it produced vasorelaxation, increased
blood flow, lowering of systemic blood pressure, and bradycardia. The
usual dose is considered to be 0.3 mg daily, given intramuscularly or intravenously.

▶ **ESTROGENS (CONJUGATED)**
Encountered in Excepted Substances
General Comments and Pharmacology: The designation "conjugated estrogens" refers to a mixture of the sodium salts of the sulfate esters of the estrogenic substances that are the type excreted by pregnant mares. Under U.S.P. standards, this mixture must contain not less than 50% and not more than 65% of sodium estrone sulfate and not less than 20% and not more than 35% of sodium equilin sulfate. Equilin is estra-1,3,5(10),7-tetraene-3-ol-17-one and is one of the estrogens that appear in the urine of pregnant mares in increasing quantities as the stage of pregnancy advances. Equilin is only slightly less potent than estradiol.

Estrogens act to excite or sensitize the uterine muscles and to depress the anterior pituitary function.
Pharmaceutical Preparations: Conjugated estrogens may be found in mixtures of scheduled substances, and these mixtures may render the pharmaceutical preparation as an Excepted Substance under legal provisions. The following drugs and drug mixture ratios are found in excepted preparations:

1. Meprobamate—Drug mixture ratio of meprobamate to conjugated estrogens, 1/0.001
2. Phenobarbital—Phenobarbital having conjugated estrogens ratio of 1/0.2

▶ **ETHAVERINE**
Encountered in Excepted Substances

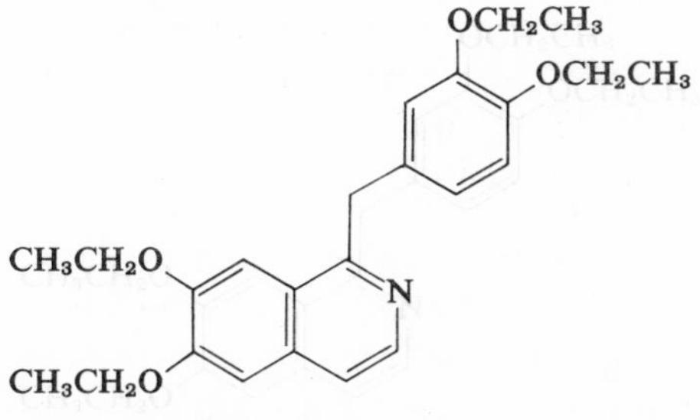

Synonyms: Ethaverine, also known as 6,7-diethoxy-1-(3,4-diethoxybenzyl)-isoquinoline and ethylpapaverine, is a tetraethyl homologue of papaverine.
Pharmaceutical Preparations: Ethaverine may be encountered in numerous preparations that are classified as "Excepted Substances":

1. Mephobarbital—Mephobarbital drug mixture ratio of mephobarbital/pentaerythritol tetranitrate/ethaverine, in a ratio of 1/2/3

2. Phenobarbital—Phenobarbital/ethaverine/theophylline, in a ratio of 1/2/ 13.3

► **ETHCHLORVYNOL**
Schedule IV

$$OH$$
$$HC{\equiv}C{-}\overset{\displaystyle |}{\underset{\displaystyle |}{C}}{-}CH{=}CH{-}Cl$$
$$CH_2CH_3$$

Synonyms: β-Chlorovinyl ethyl ethynyl carbinol, 1-chloro-3-ethylbenz-1-en-4-yn-3-ol.

Pharmaceutical Preparations: Placidyl[R] (Abbott)—Tablets: red (smaller), containing 100 mg ethchlorvynol; red (larger), containing 200 mg ethchlorvynol. Capsules: red, labeled "a KH," containing 500 mg ethchlorvynol; green, labeled "a KN," containing 750 mg ethchlorvynol

General Comments: See Biochemistry and Toxicology–Pharmacology below.

Biochemistry: The observation that ethyl alcohol produces sedation after an initial excitation phase presents the clinical usefulness of alcohol derivatives. The degree of branching at the carbinol carbon is related to sedative and hypnotic activity of the resulting compound. Likewise, the presence of unsaturation, with or without halogenation, in the structure of a tertiary alcohol is also related to the compound's pharmacological activity.

An example of these structural features is seen in ethchlorvynol. This drug, which is as potent as glutethimide, has a rapid onset of action.

Toxicology–Pharmacology: Ethchlorvynol is a halogenated tertiary acetylenic alcohol in which the β chlorovinyl group seems to convey additional hypnotic strength. This drug is an effective hypnotic with a short latency to onset and a short duration to effect. It is used for the induction of sleep in nervous disorders or patients with insomnia. After oral ingestion of 1 g, symptoms of depression appear within half an hour. A maximum blood level is attained in 1–$1\frac{1}{2}$ hours and then rapidly falls. Ethchlorvynol also has anticonvulsant and muscle relaxant properties. Exaggerated reactions may occur if it is taken with alcohol. Habituation and tolerance may occur, and physical dependence may be developed in patients taking ethchlorvynol over a long period of time.

Maximum blood concentrations after ingestion of a high therapeutic dose of 500 mg are up to 0.65 mg/dl after 1 hour, and drop to 0.2 mg/dl at 6 hours (Cummins *et al.*, 1971). After fatal overdose (ingestion of 5 g or more), blood concentrations of greater than 10.0 mg/dl may be present. This drug accumulates in the body fat, and very high concentrations are present in the fat after overdose (Cravey and Baselt, 1968).

▶ **ETHINAMATE**
Schedule IV

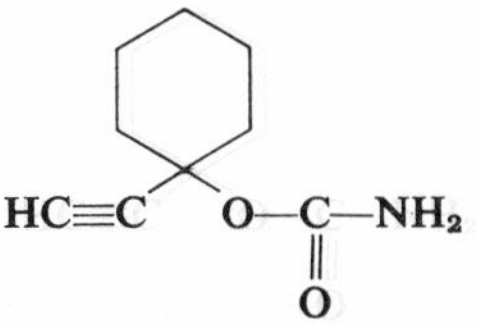

$$HC\equiv C \quad O-\underset{\underset{O}{\|}}{C}-NH_2$$

Synonym: 1-Ethynylcyclohexyl carbonate.
Pharmaceutical Preparations: Valmid[R] Pulvules (Dista)—Capsule: light blue and blue, labeled "Dista H74," containing 500 mg ethinamate
General Comments: See Biochemistry and Toxicology–Pharmacology below.
Biochemistry: Ethinamate is a derivative of urethane. The latter has been abandoned as a sedative and hypnotic because of its toxicity. It has been noted that in the urethane derivatives, with an increase in aliphatic chain length and with branching in the alcohol moiety, potency of the resulting compound increases as well as toxicity. However, replacement of the aliphatic group with a cyclic group results in a compound with increased potency and decreased toxicity. Ethinamate is such an example:

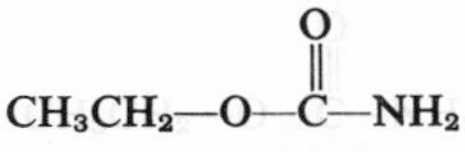

$$CH_3CH_2-O-\overset{\overset{O}{\|}}{C}-NH_2$$
Urethane (ethyl carbamate)

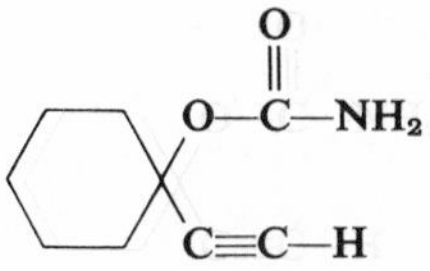

$$O-\overset{\overset{O}{\|}}{C}-NH_2$$
$$C\equiv C-H$$
Ethinamate

Studies in the metabolism of ethinamate have shown hydroxylation to occur, producing *trans*-4-hydroxyethinamate (McMahon, 1959):

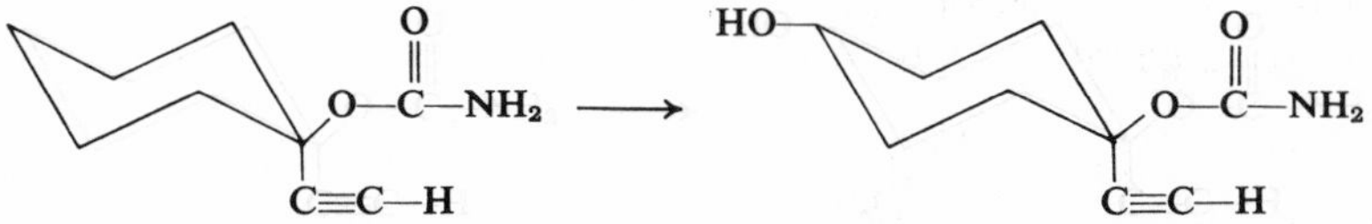

$$O-\overset{\overset{O}{\|}}{C}-NH_2 \longrightarrow O-\overset{\overset{O}{\|}}{C}-NH_2$$
$$C\equiv C-H \qquad\qquad C\equiv C-H$$
Ethinamate   *trans*-4-Hydroxyethinimate

Toxicology–Pharmacology: Ethinamate is a carbamic ester of an alacyclid alcohol. It was introduced in 1953. Ethinamate closely resembles secobarbital, except that it has an even shorter duration of action. Habituation and dependence may occur, and the abstinence syndrome is similar to that which develops when barbiturates are withdrawn.

▶ **ETHOHEPTAZINE**
Noncontrolled Substance

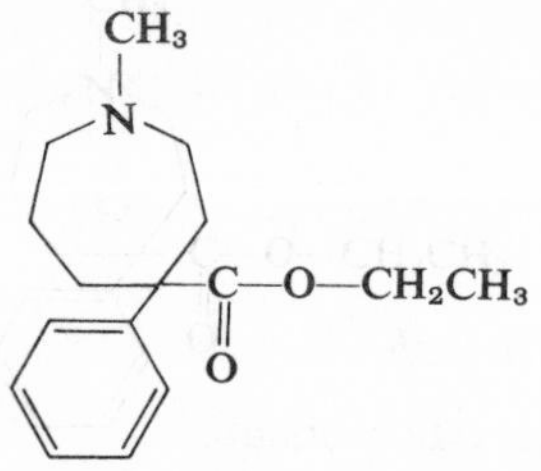

Synonyms, Pharmaceutical Preparations, Biochemistry, and Toxicology–Pharmacology: Ethoheptazine, also known as heptacyclazine, ethyl-1-methyl-4-phenyl-1-azacycloheptane-4-carboxylate, and 1-methyl-4-carbethoxy-4-phenylhexamethyleneimine, is an analgesic structurally related to meperidine. It produces analgesic effects by acting on the central nervous system. The abuse potential of ethoheptazine is extremely low; however, its efficiency as an analgesic is also low. Although official preparations of the citrate salt of ethoheptazine are included in the national formulary, only proprietary compounds ZactirinR and Zactirin Compound-100R (Wyeth), in which ethoheptazine citrate, 100 mg, is combined with aspirin, phenacetin, and caffeine, are generally available.

Studies have shown ethoheptazine to be rapidly absorbed, with peak blood levels being reached within 1 hour of ingestion. Ethoheptazine appears to be extensively metabolized, with very little excreted unchanged in the urine. Metabolic pathways include hydrolysis to the corresponding acid, oxidation to a hydroxy derivative that may further undergo hydrolysis, and possibly in demethylation to the corresponding norderivative, which may subsequently be hydrolyzed.

In a therapeutic trial, 150 mg ethoheptazine was as effective as 65 mg propoxyphene in controlling pain after dental surgery. Both were significantly superior to placebo (Winter *et al.*, 1973).

▶ **ETHOMOXANE**
Dangerous Drug

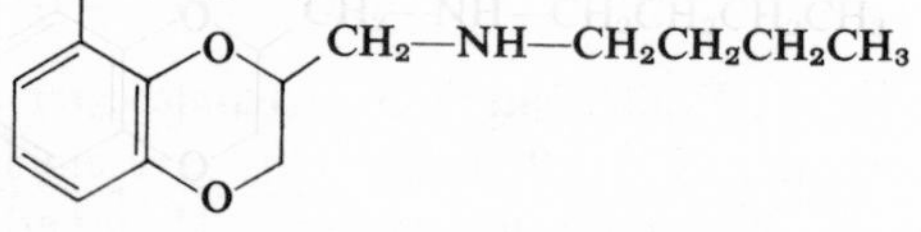

Synonym: 2-Butylaminoethyl-8-ethoxy-1,4-benzodioxan.

Pharmaceutical Preparations: Ethomoxane is not found in any pharmaceutical preparations sold in the United States.

General Comment: Ethomoxane is classified pharmacologically as a tranquilizer. It is therefore classified in this text as a Dangerous Drug.

Biochemistry: Unknown.

Toxicology–Pharmacology: Unknown.

▶ **ETHYLMETHYLTHIAMBUTENE**
Schedule I

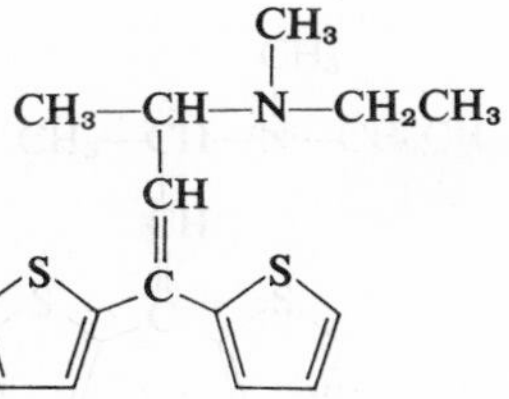

Synonyms: Emethibutin, ethylmethiambutene, N-ethyl-N,1-dimethyl-3,3-di-(thien-2-yl)-allylamine, 3-ethylmethylamino-1,1-di(2-thienyl)but-1-ene.

Pharmaceutical Preparations: Ethylmethylthiambutene is not found in any pharmaceutical preparations sold in the United States.

General Comment: Ethylmethylthiambutene is not accepted for medicinal use in the United States.

Biochemistry: Ethylmethylthiambutene is a dithienylbutenylamine that may possess its narcotic analgetic activity by stereochemically approximating a morphine-like configuration (Beckett *et al.*, 1956):

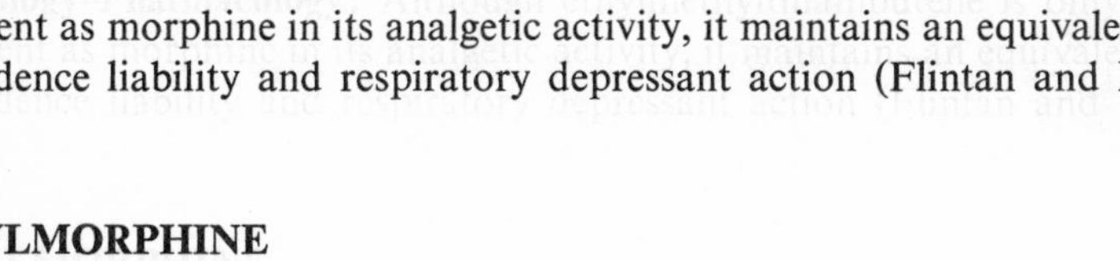

Toxicology–Pharmacology: Although ethylmethylthiambutene is only 1/5th as potent as morphine in its analgetic activity, it maintains an equivalency in dependence liability and respiratory depressant action (Flintan and Keele, 1954).

▶ **ETHYLMORPHINE**
Schedule II
or
Schedule III for any pharmaceutical preparation containing not more than
    300 mg ethylmorphine, or any of its salts, per 100 ml, or not more than

15 mg per dosage unit, with one or more ingredients in recognized therapeutic amounts

or

Schedule V for any compound, mixture, or preparation containing not more
than 100 mg ethylmorphine, or any of its salts, per 100 ml or per 100 g,
that also contains one or more nonnarcotic active medicinal ingredients in
sufficient proportion to confer on the compound, mixture, or preparation
valuable medicinal qualities other than those possessed by the narcotic
drug alone

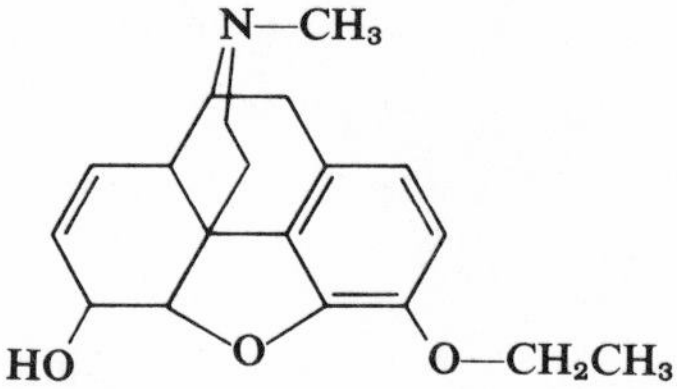

Synonyms: Morphine-3-ethyl ether, 7,8-dehydro-4,5-epoxy-3-ethoxy-6-hy-
droxy-*N*-methylmorphinan.

Pharmaceutical Preparations: Although ethylmorphine is commercially available, it is not commonly prescribed nor found in cases of drug abuse.

General Comment: Since ethylmorphine varies in control depending on its
formulation, any laboratory analysis conducted on a preparation for evidentiary purposes must show both qualitative and quantitative data on
all possible present medicinal substances.

Biochemistry: Ethylmorphine is a narcotic analgesic. It is prepared by treating morphine with ethyl iodide in alkaline solution. Ethylmorphine is
similar to codeine except that the hydrogen of the phenolic group of the
morphine molecule is replaced by an ethyl group.

Toxicology–Pharmacology: The action of ethylmorphine is similar to that of
morphine except that it is less toxic and usually produces no constipation,
nausea, or lassitude. The hydrochloride salt is a chemotic. It may be applied
topically as a 1–5% solution in the eye.

▶ **ETHYL-4-PHENYLPIPERIDINE-4-CARBOXYLATE**
Schedule II

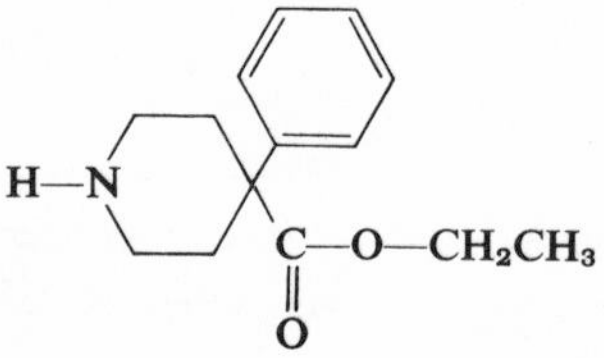

Synonyms: None.

Pharmaceutical Preparations: Ethyl-4-phenylpiperidine-4-carboxylate is not found in any pharmaceutical preparations sold in the United States.

General Comment: Ethyl-4-phenylpiperidine-4-carboxylate is known and controlled for being "pethidine intermediate B." This is an "immediate precursor" in the synthesis of pethidine (meperidine). Under Section 201 of the Controlled Substances Act, an immediate precursor may be placed in the same schedule as the controlled substance to which it is a precursor, or in any other schedule with a higher numerical designation (e.g., Schedule III, IV, or V).

Biochemistry: Unknown.

Toxicology–Pharmacology: Unknown.

▶ *N*-ETHYL-3-PIPERIDYL BENZILATE
Schedule I

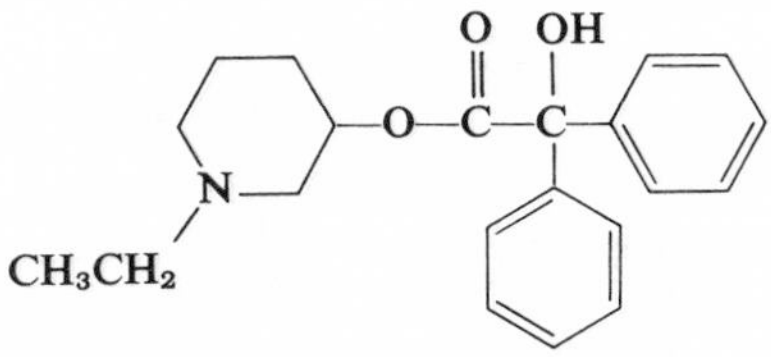

Synonyms: JB-318, TWA.

Pharmaceutical Preparations: *N*-Ethyl-3-piperidyl benzilate is not found in any pharmaceutical preparations sold in the United States.

General Comments: *N*-Ethyl-3-piperidyl benzilate is an experimental drug that proved to have hallucinogenic properties. The drug has no accepted medicinal value in the United States.

Biochemistry: Unknown.

Toxicology–Pharmacology: *N*-Ethyl-3-piperidyl benzilate is an experimental drug synthesized in 1958 for its possible anticholinergic and central nervous system activity. It was found, however, to produce powerful psychotomimetic symptoms and in doses of 1–25 mg produces long-lasting hallucinogenic effects similar in action to LSD. It is also quite toxic, and in larger doses can lead to death through respiratory failure (Biel *et al.*, 1961).

▶ ETONITAZENE
Schedule I

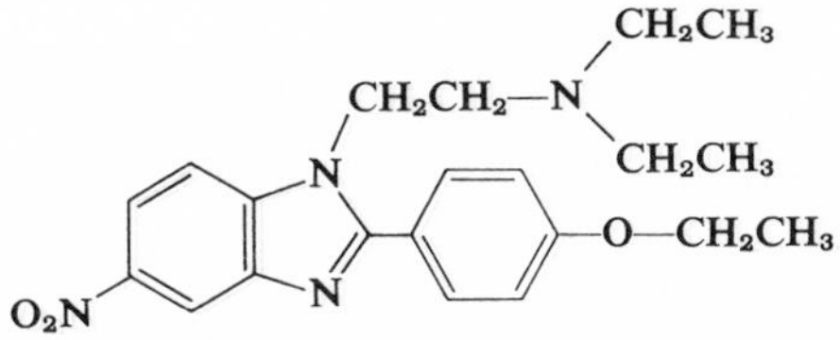

Synonym: 1-(2-Diethylaminoethyl)-2-*p*-ethoxybenzyl-5-nitrobenzimidazole.
Pharmaceutical Preparations: Etonitazene is not found in any pharmaceutical preparations sold in the United States.
General Comment: Etonitazene is a synthetic narcotic analgesic that has no accepted medicinal value in the United States.
Biochemistry: Unknown.
Toxicology–Pharmacology: Etonitazene is a benzimidazole derivative chemically similar to clonitazene and pharmacologically related to morphine. It possesses a high dependence-producing quality.

▶ **ETORPHINE**
Schedule I

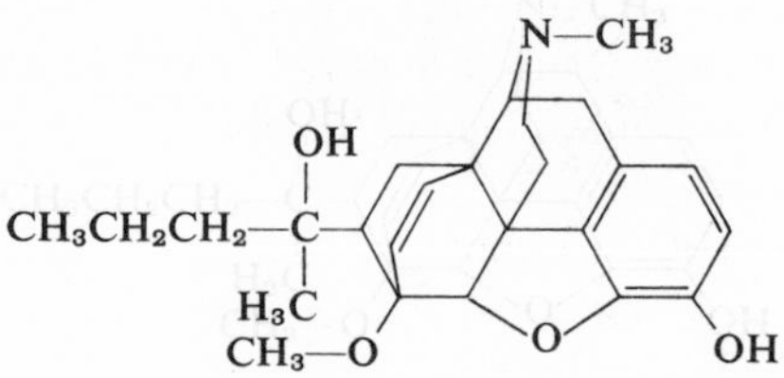

Exception: Etorphine hydrochloride is exempt from Schedule I when it is a hydrochloride salt, this preparation being scheduled under Schedule II.
Synonyms: Tetrahydro-7,α-(1-hydroxy-1-methyl-butyl)-6,14-*endo*-ethenooripavine, 7,8-dihydro-7,α-[1(*R*)-hydroxy-1-methylbutyl]-*O*,6-methyl-6,14-*endo*-ethenomorphine, 19-propylorvinol, tetrahydro-7α-(2-hydroxy-2-pentyl)-6,14-*endo*-ethenooripavine.
Pharmaceutical Preparations: Etorphine hydrochloride is prepared for hospital use only.
General Comment: For evidentiary purposes, a laboratory conducting an analysis for etorphine in a preparation must distinguish between the free base and the hydrochloride salt by suitable techniques.
Biochemistry: Unknown.
Toxicology–Pharmacology: Etorphine is highly potent in both its analgesic properties and its narcotic properties, and has been tried as a sedative to assist in the control of large animals. The effective dose and toxicity range are small and make this substance very dangerous to smell or taste. The effects of etorphine may be antagonized by cyprenorphine or nalorphine.

▶ **ETOXERIDINE**
Schedule I

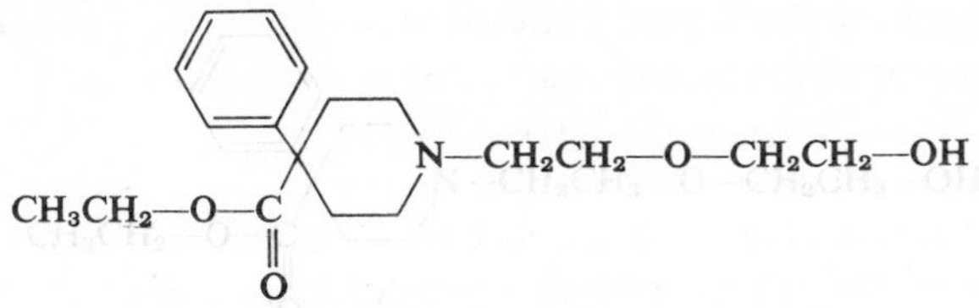

Synonyms: Carbetidine, ethyl-1-[2-(2-hydroxyethoxy)ethyl]-4-phenyl-piperi-dine-4-carboxylate, 1-[2-(2-hydroxyethoxy)-ethoxyl]-4-phenyl-isonipecotic acid ethyl ester, ethyl-1-[2-(2-hydroxyethoxy)ethyl]-4-phenylisonipectate, 1-(2-hydroxyethoxy-ethyl)-4-carbethoxypiperidine.
Pharmaceutical Preparations: Etoxeridine is not found in any pharmaceutical preparations sold in the United States.
General Comment: Etoxeridine is a synthetic narcotic analgesic that has no accepted medicinal value in the United States.
Biochemistry: Unknown.
Toxicology–Pharmacology: Unknown.

▶ **FENCAMFAMIN**
Noncontrolled Substance

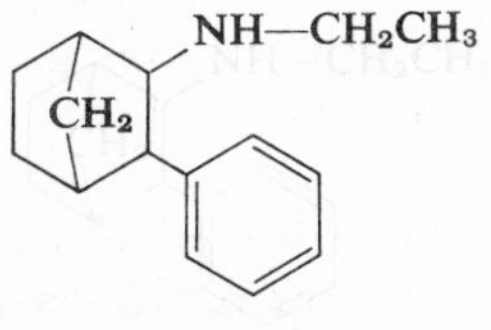

Synonym: 2-Ethylamino-3-phenylnorbanane.
General Comment: Fencamfamin is a central nervous system stimulant that has been encountered in cases of drug abuse.

▶ **FENETHYLLINE**
Noncontrolled Substance

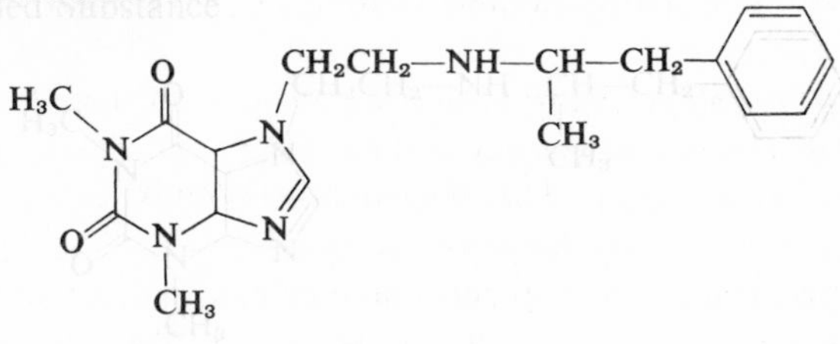

General Comments: Fenethylline, a xanthine derivative, is not a controlled substance. It may be found in preparations frequently abused. It is cleaved metabolically in humans into theophylline and amphetamine. Its action is thus similar to that of amphetamine.

▶ **FENFLURAMINE**
Schedule IV

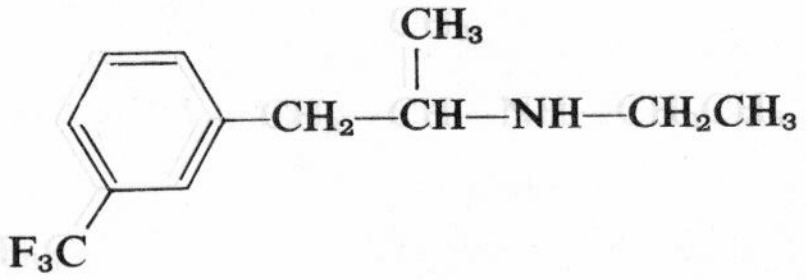

Synonym: N-Ethyl-α-methyl-3-trifluoromethylphenethylamine.
Pharmaceutical Preparations: Pondimin[R] (Robins)—Tablet: orange, scored, labeled "AHR," containing 20 mg fenfluramine hydrochloride
General Comment: Fenfluramine is a sympathomimetic amine used as an anorectic for treating obesity. However, unlike the amphetamines, fenfluramine produces more central nervous system depression than stimulation.
Biochemistry: The parent compound of fenfluramine is β-phenylethylamine. It consists of an aromatic nucleus (benzene ring) and an aliphatic portion (ethylamine). By modifying the structure of β-phenylethylamine, fenfluramine

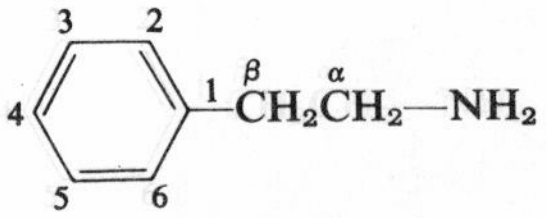

β-Phenylethylamine

is obtained. These modifications consist of substitution of CF_3 at position 3 of the aromatic ring, C_2H_5 on the amine nitrogen, and CH_3 at the α carbon. These modifications alleviate the pressor, local vasoconstriction, bronchodilator, and cardiac activity that β-phenylethylamine possesses and impart anorectic activity.
Toxicology–Pharmacology: Since fenfluramine does not maintain self-injection behavior in rhesus monkeys as does cocaine or methohexital, it is believed not to be subject to abuse in humans (Woods, L. A., and Tessel, 1974).

After a single oral dose of 60 mg, the plasma concentration at 4 hours was 0.007 mg/dl, and at 24 hours was 0.003 mg/dl (Campbell and Moore,

1969). In a death from overdose of 2000 mg, the blood concentration was 0.65 mg/dl, and the norfenfluramine metabolite was found in a concentration of 0.08 mg/dl (Fleisher and Campbell, 1969).

▶ **FENIMIDE**
Dangerous Drug

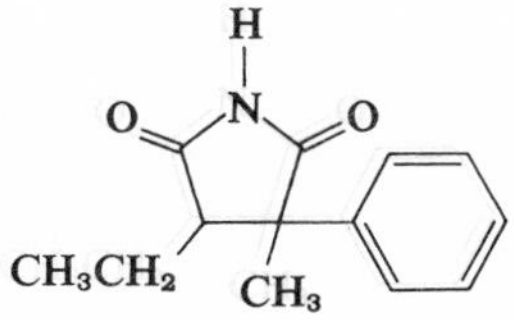

Synonym: α-Ethyl-α'-methyl-α'-phenylsuccinimide.
Pharmaceutical Preparations: Fenimide is not found in any pharmaceutical preparations sold in the United States.
General Comment: Fenimide is classified pharmacologically as a tranquilizer and is therefore classified in this text as a Dangerous Drug.
Biochemistry: Although fenimide is classified pharmacologically as a tranquilizer, it was one of the succimides studied for its anticonvulsant properties. In this study, it was found that fenimide produced a sedative effect prior to deeper central nervous system depression (Chen and Bass, 1964).
Toxicology–Pharmacology: Unknown.

▶ **FENPIPRAMIDE**
Noncontrolled Substance

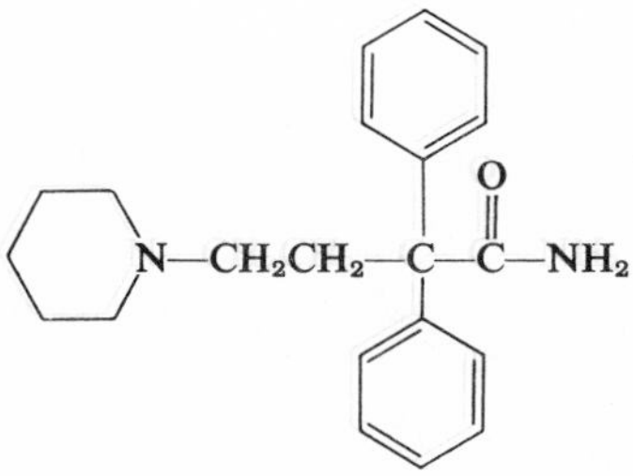

General Comment: Fenpipramide is a parasympatholytic drug not subject to control.

▶ **FENPIPRANE**
Noncontrolled Substance

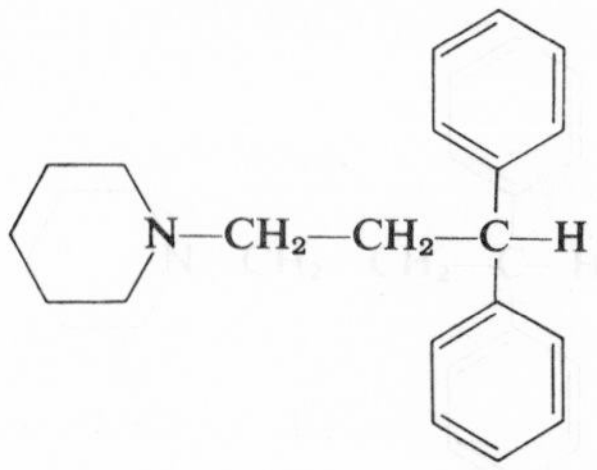

CH structure diagram:

N—CH₂—CH₂—C—H (piperidine ring on left, two phenyl rings attached to the final carbon)

General Comment: Fenpiprane is a parasympatholytic drug not subject to control.

▶ **FENTANYL**
Schedule II

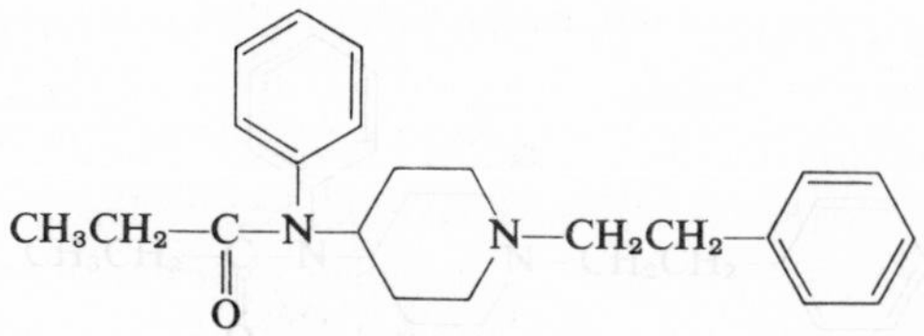

CH₃CH₂—C—N—(piperidine ring)—N—CH₂CH₂—(phenyl)
                    ‖
                    O

Synonyms: Phentanyl, *N*-(1-phenethylpiperid-4-yl)propionanilide.
Pharmaceutical Preparations
Innovar^R (McNeil)—Injection: each 1 ml containing 0.05 mg fentanyl and 2.5 mg droperidol
Sublimaze^R (McNeil)—Injection: each 1 ml containing 0.05 mg fentanyl
General Comment: Fentanyl is a synthetic narcotic analgesic that has accepted medicinal value in the United States.
Biochemistry: Fentanyl was synthesized in Belgium by Janssen Pharmaceutica from propionyl chloride, *N*-(4-piperidyl)aniline, and phenethyl chloride. This compound, which produces morphine-like action at a dose of about 1/100th of that of morphine, is not rigid in its structure. Thus, its stereochemical and metabolic properties are very complex.
Toxicology–Pharmacology: Fentanyl is a synthetic analgesic. A 0.1-mg dose of fentanyl is approximately equivalent to 10 mg morphine or 75 mg meperidine (pethidine) in analgesic activity. Parenterally administered, fentanyl acts faster than morphine, but has a shorter duration of action, beginning in 5–15 minutes and lasting 1–2 hours.

Fentanyl is frequently combined with droperidol as an injectable mixture to induce surgical anesthesia.

▶ **FLUANISONE**
Dangerous Drug

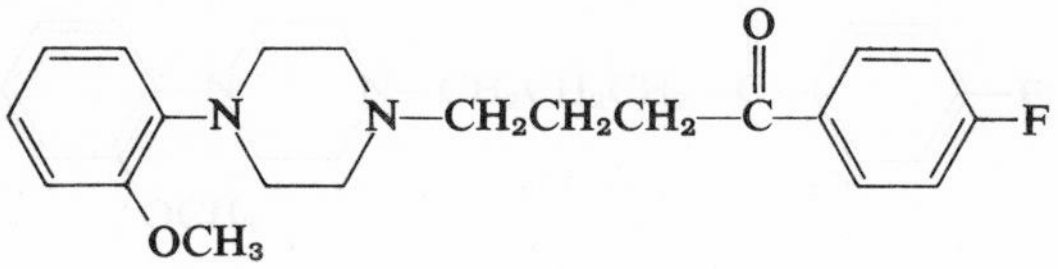

Synonyms: Haloanisone, p-fluoro-8-(4-O-methoxy-phenylpiperazin-1-yl)-buty-rophenone.
Pharmaceutical Preparations: Fluanisone is not found in any pharmaceutical preparations sold in the United States.
General Comment: Fluanisone is indicated pharmacologically as a tranquilizer and is therefore classified in this text as a Dangerous Drug.
Biochemistry: Fluanisone is an antipsychotic drug developed from halo-peridol, the prototype of the butyrophenones. It has been determined among the 4-piperazinobutyrophenone series that for high neuroleptic potency, an aromatic substituent is required in the 4-position of the piperazine ring (Janssen, 1967). This potency is further increased by substitution of a methoxy group in the *ortho* position.
Toxicology–Pharmacology: See **HALOPERIDOL.**

▶ **FLUOPROMAZINE**
Dangerous Drug

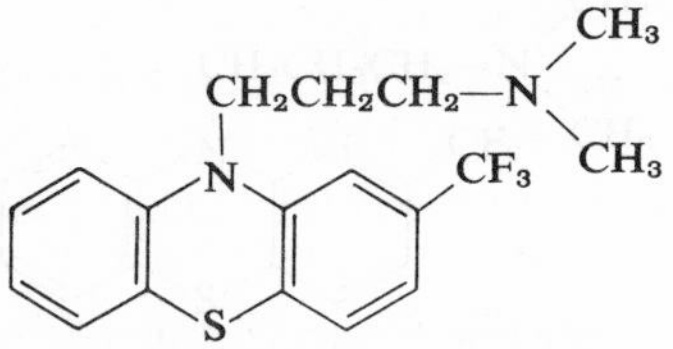

Synonyms: Triflupromazine, 10-(3-dimethylaminopropyl)-2-trifluoromethyl-phenothiazine.
Pharmaceutical Preparations
Vesprin[R] (Squibb)—Injection: containing 10 or 20 mg fluopromazine per 1 ml. Tablet: containing 10, 25, or 50 mg fluopromazine. Suspension: containing 50 mg fluopromazine per 5 ml.
General Comment: Fluopromazine is a phenothiazine tranquilizer and is therefore classified in this text as a Dangerous Drug.

Biochemistry: Similar to that of chlorpromazine.
Toxicology–Pharmacology: Similar to that of chlorpromazine.

▶ **FLUPHENAZINE**
Dangerous Drug

$$CH_2CH_2CH_2-N \diagdown N-CH_2CH_2-OH$$

with phenothiazine ring bearing CF_3 and N, S substituents

Pharmaceutical Preparations

Permitil[R] (Schering)—Tablets: green, sugar-coated, containing 0.25 mg fluphenazine hydrochloride; scored and die-stamped "WL"; light orange, containing 2.5 mg fluphenazine hydrochloride; purple-pink, containing 5 mg fluphenazine hydrochloride; light red, containing 10 mg fluphenazine hydrochloride. Oral concentrate: each 1 ml containing 5 ml fluphenazine hydrochloride.

Permitil[R] Chronotab (Schering)—Tablet: yellow, sugar-coated, containing 1 mg fluphenazine hydrochloride

Prolixin[R] (Squibb)—Injection: each 1 ml containing 2.5 mg fluphenazine hydrochloride. Tablets: Pink, containing 1 mg fluphenazine hydrochloride; yellow, containing 2.5 mg fluphenazine hydrochloride; green, containing 5 mg fluphenazine hydrochloride. Elixir: Orange, each 1 ml containing 5.5 mg fluphenazine hydrochloride.

Prolixir[R] Decanoate (Squibb)—Injection: Each 1 ml containing 25 mg fluphenazine decanoate

Prolixir[R] Enanthate (Squibb)—Injection: Each 1 ml containing 25 mg fluphenazine enanthate

General Comments: Fluphenazine is the 2-trifluoromethyl derivative of perphenazine, a phenothiazine tranquilizer. It is therefore classified in this text as a Dangerous Drug by definition. It is the most potent of the phenothiazine tranquilizers, and is three to five times as potent as perphenazine.

Biochemistry: Similar to that of chlorpromazine.

Toxicology–Pharmacology: Fluphenazine is the most potent phenothiazine available for the treatment of patients with psychiatric problems. It is effective in doses as little as 10 mg, and certain salts may induce effective blood levels for up to 2 weeks in schizophrenic patients.

Plasma levels of 10–25 μg/dl were found 1 hour after administration of 150 mg fluphenazine per day (Viala *et al.*, 1969).

▶ **FLURAZEPAM**
Schedule IV

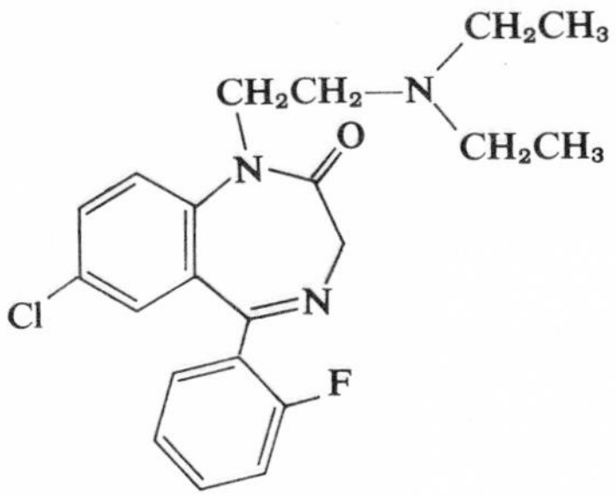

Synonym: 7-Chloro-1,3-dihydro-1-[2-(diethylamino)ethyl]-5-(o-fluorophenyl)-2H-1,4-benzodiazepin-2-one.

Pharmaceutical Preparations: Dalmane[R] (Roche)—Capsules: Yellow and orange, containing 15 mg flurazepam hydrochloride; yellow and red, containing 30 mg flurazepam hydrochloride

General Comments: Like the other benzodiazepines, flurazepam was added to Schedule IV after the Controlled Substances Act became effective.

Flurazepam, related to diazepam, acts on the central nervous system (CNS) to produce sedative, anticonvulsant, and skeletal muscle relaxant effects. Its approved use, however, is as a hypnotic. Flurazepam has potential addictive effects with other CNS depressants (such as alcohol).

Biochemistry: The major urinary metabolite of flurazepam in man has been identified as the conjugated flurazepam, N_1-ethanol (Schwartz and Postma, 1970). Minor metabolites identified are monodesethylflurazepam, didesethylflurazepam, and N_1-desalkyl-3-hydroxyflurazepam (De Silva and Strojny, 1971).

Toxicology–Pharmacology: A blood level of 0.02 μg/ml was detected after a dose of 90 mg, and 0.01 μg/ml was detected at 12 hours. The hydroxyethyl metabolite was detected in concentrations about four times those of the unchanged drug. Approximately 56% of the dose was recovered as metabolites in urine within 48 hours (De Silva and Strojny, 1971). A death from overdose of flurazepam has been reported in which a blood level of 0.18 mg/dl was detected (Baselt and Cravey, 1977).

As a potent sedative–hypnotic, it is enhanced in toxicity when combined with alcohol or other depressant medications, such as barbiturates.

Flurazepam is a hypnotic agent useful in all types of insomnia. It is rapidly absorbed from the gastrointestinal tract. It is rapidly metabolized in man by biotransformation to inactive metabolites (N_1-hydroxyethylflurazepam, N_1-desalkyl flurazepam, and N_1-desalkyl-3-hydroxyflurazepam).

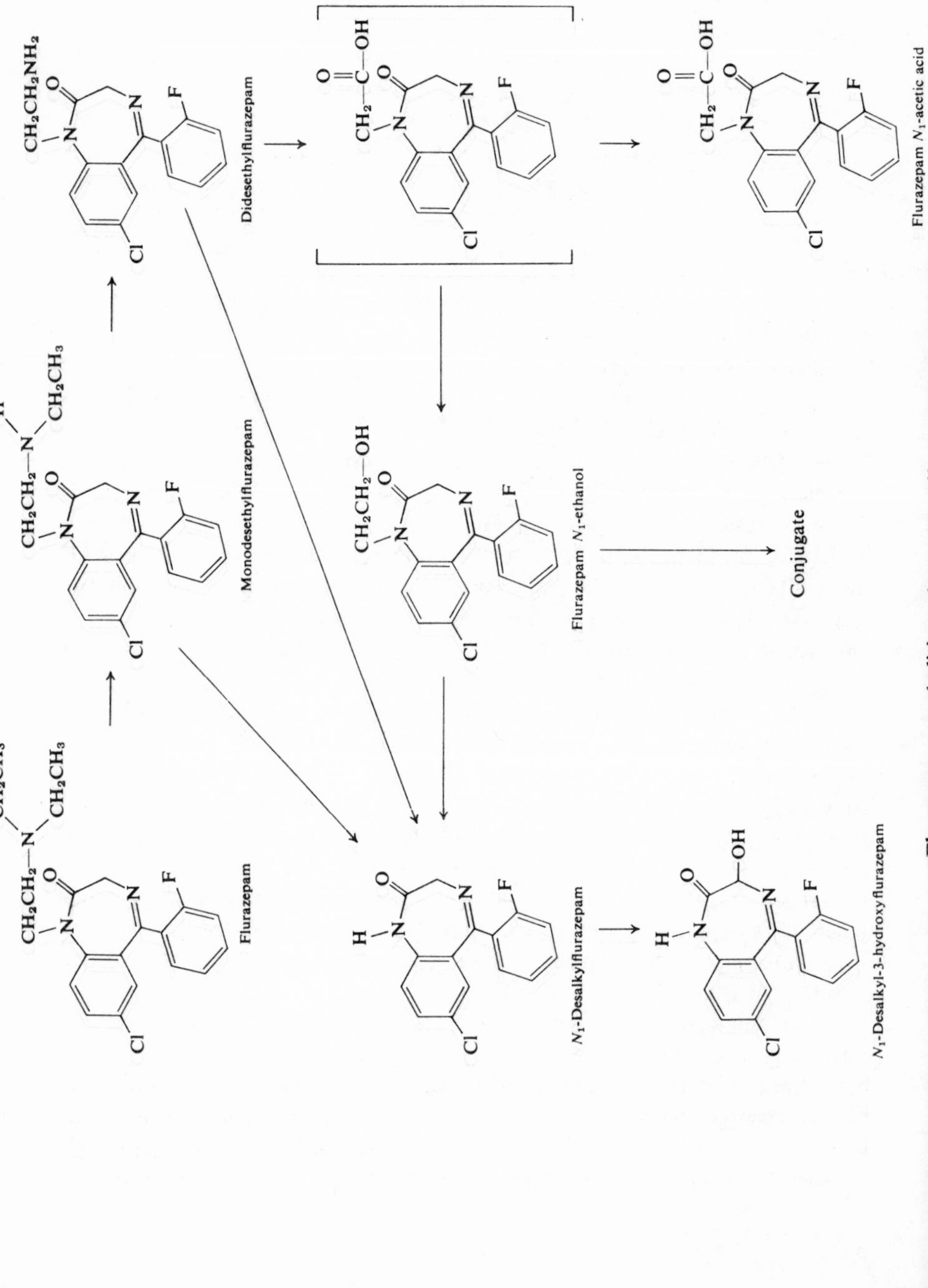

Flurazepam

Monodesethylflurazepam

Didesethylflurazepam

Flurazepam N_1-ethanol

Flurazepam N_1-acetic acid

Conjugate

N_1-Desalkylflurazepam

N_1-Desalkyl-3-hydroxyflurazepam

Flurazepam alone has a high margin of safety, and as much as 7500 mg has been ingested with recovery in an adult (Roche, 1975).

▶ **FURETHIDINE**
Schedule I

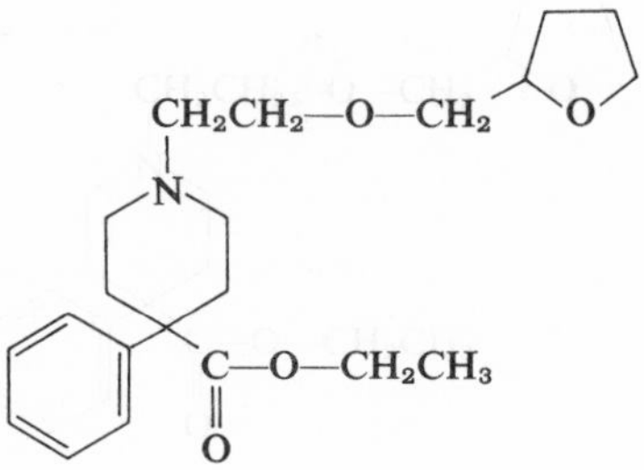

Synonym: 4-Phenyl-1-[2-(tetrahydrofurfuryloxy)ethyl]-isonipecotic acid ethyl ester.
Pharmaceutical Preparations: Furethidine is not found in any pharmaceutical preparations sold in the United States.
General Comment: Furethidine is a synthetic narcotic analgesic that has no accepted medicinal value in the United States.
Biochemistry: Unknown.
Toxicology–Pharmacology: Unknown.

▶ **GLUTETHIMIDE**
Schedule III

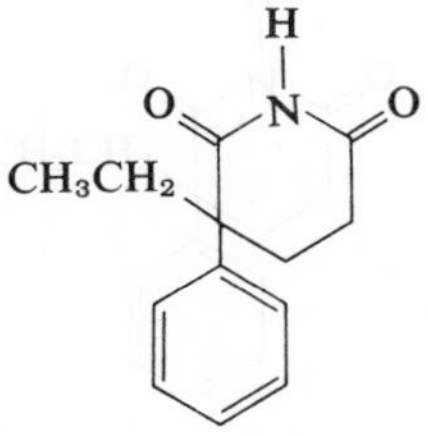

Synonym: 2-Ethyl-2-phenylglutarimide.
Pharmaceutical Preparations
Doriden[R] (USV)—Tablet: White, scored, containing 250 or 500 mg glutethimide. Capsule: Blue and white, containing 500 mg glutethimide.

General Comments: Glutethimide, a nonbarbiturate, is very similar to pheno-barbital in structure. It was introduced into medicine in Germany in 1954. This drug is a useful sedative and hypnotic, although its abuse has led to many cases of chronic and acute intoxication, resulting in a number of fatalities, dependence, and addiction.

Biochemistry: The enantiomorphs of glutethimide have entirely different metabolic routes. *d*-Glutethimide is metabolized by hydroxylation of the glutarimide ring to give "A." The *levo* isomer undergoes hydroxylation of the ethyl group to give "B" (Keberle *et al.*, 1963). Although glutethimide is

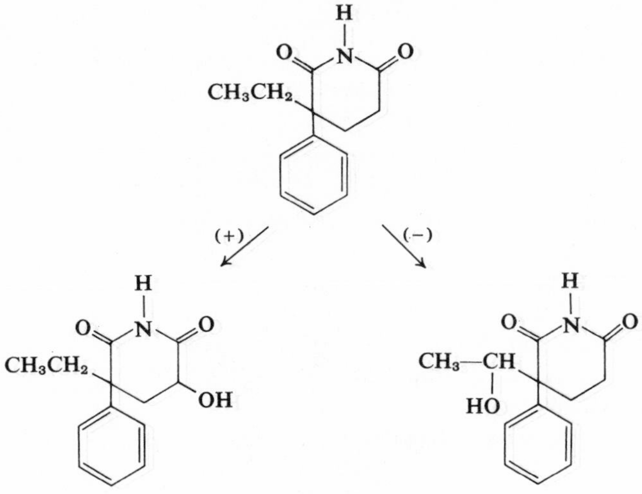

A   B

marketed as the racemic mixture, the hypnotic activity of the (+)-isomer is greater than that of the racemic mixture. This mixture, in turn, is more potent than the (−)-isomer.

The comparison of structural features of the barbiturates and glutethi-mide should be noted:

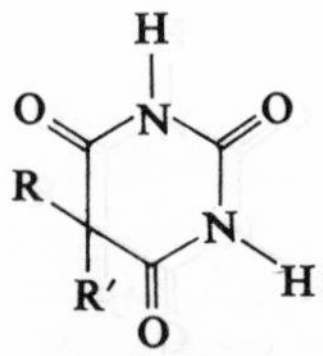

Barbiturate 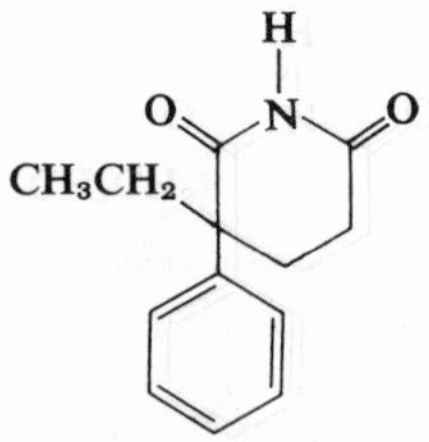   Glutethimide

It should be obvious from this comparison of glutethimide with barbiturates that glutethimide was produced in an effort to develop a less toxic drug with the sedative and hypnotic properties of barbiturates. Although glutethimide produces central nervous system depression similar to that produced by the barbiturates, the comparable side effects are greatly reduced.

Toxicology–Pharmacology: Glutethimide is a central depressant medication, with actions similar to those of the barbiturates. It may be slowly absorbed from the gastrointestinal tract due to its poor water solubility, resulting in an irregular period of activity. Its plasma half-life is reported to be about 11 hours (Curry *et al.*, 1971). It is entirely metabolized in man, the primary metabolite being 4-hydroxy-2-ethyl glutarimide. It has been found that this metabolite is about twice as potent as glutethimide in its central depressant properties, and may account for the prolonged coma in patients after overdose from glutethimide (Hansen, A. R., *et al.*, 1975).

Symptoms of acute intoxication are similar to those of acute barbiturate intoxication. Respiratory depression is not as severe, however. Hypotension is characteristic of glutethimide intoxication, and circulatory shock may represent a major therapeutic problem. Mydriasis and dryness of the mouth are also characteristic.

A dose of 5 g is enough to produce a severe intoxication, while the lethal dose is between 10 and 20 g.

A therapeutic dose of 250 mg yields peak blood levels of from 0.2 to 0.6 mg/dl (Widdop, 1970).

A dose of 2000 mg administered in two 1000-mg doses gave blood levels of 0.63–1.22 mg/dl in 2.0 hours (Parker *et al.*, 1970). Lethal blood levels are usually greater than 2.0 mg/dl.

▶ **GLYCOPYRROLATE**
Noncontrolled Substance

General Comments: Glycopyrrolate is 3-hydroxy-1,1-dimethyl-pyrrolidinium bromide α-cyclopentylmandelate and is a cholinergic blocking agent. It is encountered in phenobarbital preparations classified as Excepted Substances in a phenobarbital/glycopyrrolate ratio of 1/0.06.

▶ **HALOPERIDOL**
Dangerous Drug

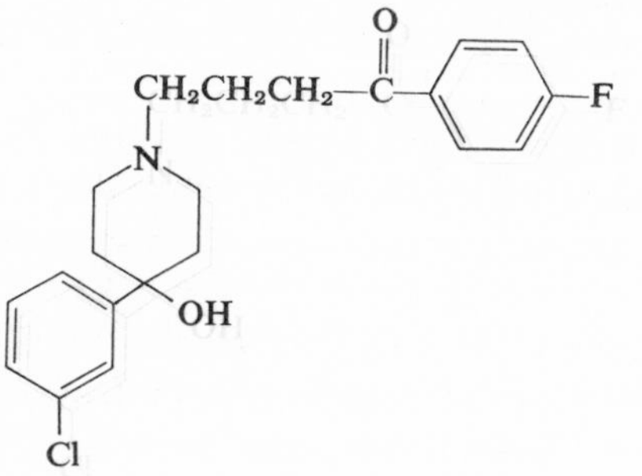

Synonym: 4-[4-(*p*-Chlorophenyl)-4-hydroxypiperidino]-4'-fluorobutyrophenone.

Pharmaceutical Preparations

Haldol[R] (McNeil)—Tablets, containing haloperidol, scored, labeled "McNeil": white, 0.5 mg; yellow, 1 mg; pink, 2 mg; green, 5 mg; aqua, 10 mg. Concentrate: each 1 ml containing 2 mg. Injection: each 1 ml containing 5 mg.

General Comments: Haloperidol is a butyrophenone derivative developed by Janssen Pharmaceutica (Belgium), which is pharmacologically similar to the phenothiazine tranquilizers. It has tranquilizing, antiemetic, hypotensive, and hypothermic actions. Since it is a tranquilizer, it is classified in this text as a Dangerous Drug.

Biochemistry: Haloperidol is an antipsychotic drug and was the prototype of the butyrophenone class. In this class, potent neuroleptic activity is associated with 4-tertiary amino-substituted derivatives. These derivatives have the following general structure:

$$ArCO(CH_2)_3NR$$

Ar = phenyl, substituted phenyl, or thienyl
NR = 4-substituted piperidino, tetrahydropyridino, or piperazino

The structural and chemical variations that influence antipsychotic potency are (Zirkle and Kaiser, 1970):

1. The nature and substitution of the aryl group
2. Replacement of the carbonyl group
3. Alterations in the propylene chain
4. Changes involving the basic amino group

Studies of the 4-piperidinobutyrophenone series, which includes halo-peridol, show the 4-aryl substituent to be advantageous for neuroleptic potency (Harper *et al.*, 1966).

Toxicology–Pharmacology: Haloperidol has antipsychotic effects similar to those of the phenothiazines. It induces feelings of tiredness, lowers the blood pressure, pulse rate, and body temperature, and is an antiemetic. It is useful for therapy in the manic phase of manic–depressive psychosis, and it is often effective in calming agitated, overactive, or hostile patients. It may also be used as a tranquilizer in presurgical medication.

It is a relatively long-acting drug. Peak plasma levels occur 2–6 hours after ingestion, and it may plateau for as long as 72 hours, being detectable for several weeks.

The major metabolic pathway seems to be *N*-dealkylation, which gives rise to β-(*p*-fluorobenzoyl)propionic acid, which is further metabolized to *p*-fluorophenylacetic acid.

Toxic effects include the potentiation of the depressant effects of barbiturates, analgesics, and other drugs having depressant effects on the central nervous system. Other untoward actions are similar to those of the phenothiazine tranquilizers (see **CHLORPROMAZINE**).

▶ **HARMINE**
Noncontrolled Substance

General Comments: Harmine and harmaline are two major alkaloids responsible for the hallucinogenic properties of the tropical vine *Banisteriopsis*. This genus is a tropical American vine numbering about 100 species.

There is a drink widely employed in northern South America for prophecy, divination, and, in general, as a magic hallucinogen. The drink has many indigenous names, but it is generally known as *ayahuasca, caapi*, or *yaje*.

Toxicology–Pharmacology: Harmine reportedly caused hallucinations in man when 25–75 mg was administered subcutaneously (Lewin, 1928). In animals, it acts as a central nervous system excitant. LSD-like effects were reported in mental patients given 150–200 mg intravenously, whereas oral administration produced the impression of a wavelike movement of the environment, as well as paresthesia and a lower sensitivity of the skin to contact and pain stimuli (Pennes and Hoch, 1957).

▶ **HEPTABARBITAL**
Schedule III

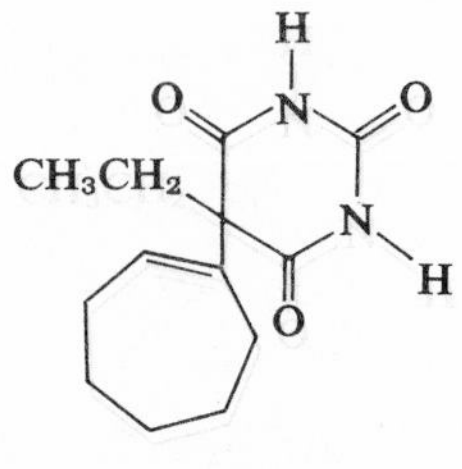

Synonyms: Heptabarbitone, 5-(1-cyclophepten-1-yl)-5-ethylbarbituric acid.
Pharmaceutical Preparations: Heptabarbital is not found in any pharmaceutical preparations sold in the United States.
General Comments: Heptabarbital is a short-acting barbiturate similar in action to secobarbital. It is listed under Schedule III as a "derivative of barbituric acid."
Biochemistry: Similar to that of cyclobarbital.
Toxicology–Pharmacology: Heptabarbital is a short-acting barbiturate used as a hypnotic and as a sedative for the treatment of hypertension, gastrointestinal disorders, anxiety neuroses, and other conditions in which mild sedation is indicated. The adult hypnotic dose is 200–400 mg.

Heptabarbital overdose is characteristic of hypnotic drug medication, with general depression of the central nervous system, and death from respiratory depression.

▶ **HEROIN**
Schedule I

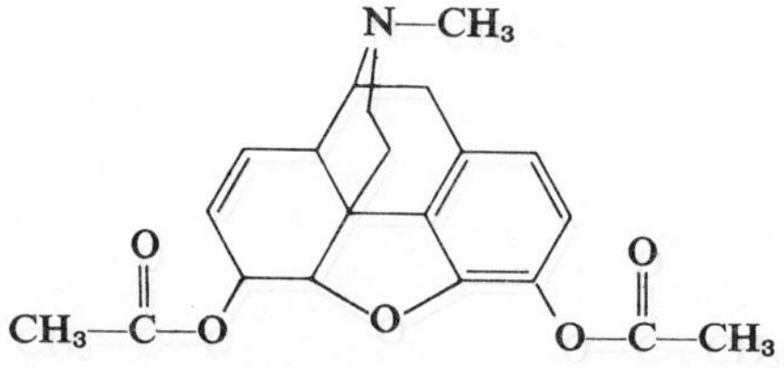

Synonyms: Diacetylmorphine, diamorphine, acetomorphine.
Pharmaceutical Preparations: Heroin is not found in any pharmaceutical preparations sold in the United States.
General Comments: Heroin is a semisynthetic narcotic analgesic that was first synthesized from morphine in 1874. Its use in medicine began in the early 1900s when the Bayer Company first started commercial production of a new pain remedy. It received widespread acceptance, and the medical profession

remained unaware for years of its potential for addiction. The Harrison Narcotic Act of 1914 established the first comprehensive control of heroin in the United States.

Pure heroin is a white powder with a bitter taste. Illicit heroin may vary in color from white to dark brown. The dark color may be due to impurities left from the manufacturing process or the presence of diluents such as food coloring, coca, or brown sugar.

Sugar, starch, powdered milk, procaine, methapyrilene, and quinine are among the diluents used.

Biochemistry: In 1898, the Bayer Company of Germany synthesized the diacetyl derivative of morphine in the hope of developing an analgesic to replace morphine without addictive properties. This derivative was named heroin, a term derived from the German *heroisch*, meaning large and powerful.

The acetylation of both the phenolic and alcoholic groups of morphine, however, yields a drug that is three times more analgetically potent and addictive than morphine. It has since been determined that O-acylation of the alcoholic hydroxyl enhances analgetic activity to a degree greater than the weakening effect normally associated with covering the phenolic hydroxyl. The increased activity thus probably arises from the greater susceptibility of the 3-acetyl group to hydrolysis producing 6-monoacetylmorphine. This latter metabolite of heroin is approximately four times as potent as morphine. Coupled with the potency of heroin, the resulting toxicity is greatly enhanced.

Heroin   6-Monoacetylmorphine

Toxicology–Pharmacology: Heroin is qualitatively equivalent to morphine in its narcotic actions, having the pharmacological characteristics of producing analgesia, euphoria, central nervous system and respiratory depression, and addiction. Due to the acetyl groups, the heroin molecule transverses the blood–brain barrier more readily than morphine, causing it to be two to three times more potent than morphine. It has been used therapeutically for the same purposes as morphine, as an analgetic for severe pain, and as a cough suppressant. Due to its pronounced addictive properties, it is no longer used therapeutically in the United States. It is of major significance as a drug of abuse in many parts of the world, however. Estimates of the number of heroin addicts in this country range up to 200,000.

Heroin must be administered by injection to retain most of its euphoric potency. Abusers usually inject it intravenously, but sometimes subcutaneously or intramuscularly. Due to the lack of control over the quality of street samples, the user does not know the potency of the drug he is using. If it is unusually potent, or adulterated with other drugs, he runs the risk of overdose. Overdose from heroin is characterized by torpor, rapidly progressing to stupor accompanied by irregular, slow, gasping respiration. Coma and respiratory arrest precede death. Death may occur within a few minutes of the injection, or after a comatose period of several hours. Treatment for narcotic overdose is specific and rapidly effective. Narcotic antagonists, such as nalline or naloxone, antagonize the respiratory and general depression of the narcotic drugs, bringing rapid recovery.

Death from heroin overdose is one of the most prevalent causes of drug overdose deaths in most major cities.

After death from heroin overdose, blood concentrations of free morphine may range from undetectable levels to greater than 0.10 mg/dl. The quantity found in the blood is dependent on the survival time after the injection. High concentrations are also found in the kidney, lung, and liver after intravenous administration. Since heroin is rapidly deacetylated in the blood and other body organs, no unchanged drug can be detected in the body.

Heroin users may be detected most readily by analysis of urine samples for morphine, and/or by challenge with a narcotic antagonist, which precipitates withdrawal symptoms. Morphine is excreted in the urine for several days after an injection of heroin.

▶ **HEXOBARBITAL**
Schedule III

Synonyms: Hexobarbitone, 5-cyclohex-1'-enyl-1,5-dimethylbarbituric-acid.
Pharmaceutical Preparations: Hexobarbital is not found in any pharmaceutical preparations sold in the United States.
General Comments: Hexobarbital is a short-acting barbiturate with actions similar to those of secobarbital. It is listed under Schedule III as a "derivative of barbituric acid."
Biochemistry: Hexobarbital is metabolized by oxidation of the cyclohexenyl ring, by N-demethylation, and, to a minor extent, by ring scission. Oxidation

to ketohexobarbital precedes demethylation. The hydroxylation of hexo-barbital to 3'-hydroxyhexobarbital is catalyzed by an $NADPH_2$-dependent microsomal enzyme system, whereas the oxidation reaction is effected by a soluble liver enzyme (Frey *et al.*, 1959, Toki *et al.*, 1963).

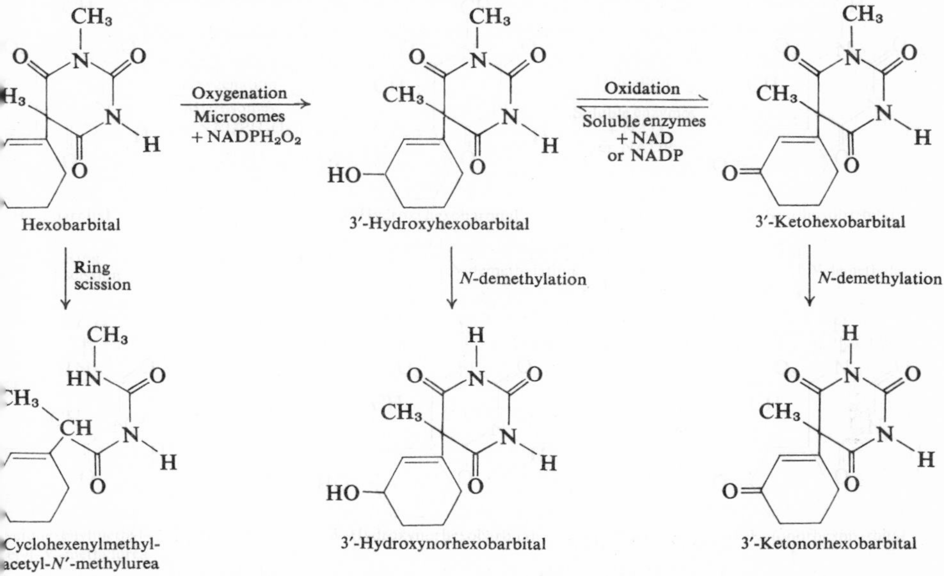

Hexobarbital → (Oxygenation Microsomes + $NADPH_2O_2$) → 3'-Hydroxyhexobarbital → (Oxidation Soluble enzymes + NAD or NADP) → 3'-Ketohexobarbital

Ring scission ↓ ; N-demethylation ↓ ; N-demethylation ↓

Cyclohexenylmethyl-acetyl-N'-methylurea ; 3'-Hydroxynorhexobarbital ; 3'-Ketonorhexobarbital

Toxicology–Pharmacology: Hexobarbital is classified as an ultra-short-acting barbiturate derivative. When injected intravenously, it causes unconscious-ness within 35–40 seconds, as does thiopental. It has a plasma half-life of about 5 hours (Brodie, 1952). Toxicity is characteristic of the barbiturate group, and could result in depression of the central nervous system, leading to respiratory arrest.

Therapeutic or lethal blood concentrations are not known.

▶ **HEXOCYCLIUM METHYLSULFATE**
Noncontrolled Substance
Encountered in Excepted Substances

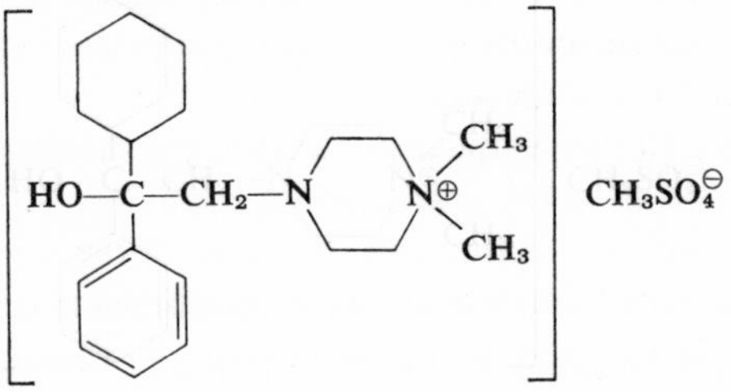

Pharmacology: Hexocyclium methylsulfate is a quaternary ammonium anticholinergic compound with autonomic blocking effects. It has atropine-like actions.

▶ **HOMATROPINE**
Noncontrolled Substance
Encountered in Excepted Substances

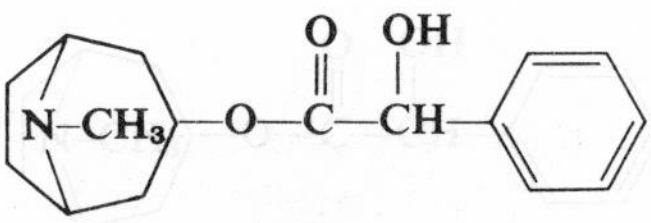

General Comments and Pharmaceutical Preparations: Homatropine is an ester of the cyclic base tropine with mandelic acid and may be prepared by esterification of these substances. The related substance atropine is an ester of tropine with *dl*-tropic acid. The following table indicates drugs and drug/homatropine ratios found in excepted preparations:

Drug	Drug/Homatropine Ratio
Amobarbital	1/0.15
Butabarbital	1/0.25
Pentobarbital	1/0.16
Phenobarbital	1/0.04

Toxicology–Pharmacology: Homatopine is a quaternary ammonium derivative of atropine, and as such has peripheral actions similar to those of atropine but lacks the central nervous system activity. It is used primarily to dilate the pupils of the eye for ophthalmological examinations. It is shorter acting than atropine and may be used as a 1 percent aqueous solution (as the hydrobromide) for dilating the pupils. Most of the effects disappear within 24 hours.

The methyl bromide salt of homatropine may be used as an antispasmodic and inhibitor of secretions in disorders of the gastrointestinal tract. It is considered to be less potent than atropine in antimuscarinic activity, and less toxic, but more potent in ganglionic blocking activities (Goodman and Gilman, 1970).

Side effects are similar to those of atropine: dryness of the mouth, disturbance of vision, postural hypotension, and impotence.

▶ **HYDROCODONE**
See **DIHYDROCODEINONE.**

▶ **HYDROMORPHINOL**
Schedule I

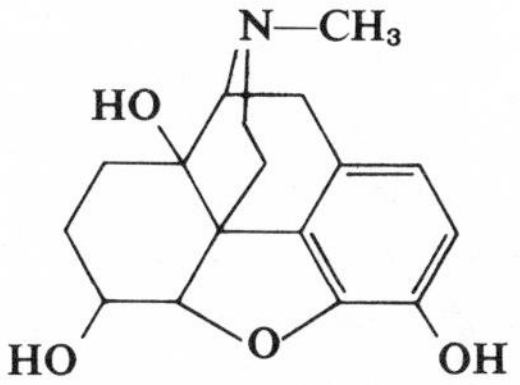

Synonym: 4,5-Epoxy-3,6,14-trihydroxy-*N*-methylmorphinan.
Pharmaceutical Preparations: Hydromorphinol is not found in any pharmaceutical preparations sold in the United States.
General Comment: Hydromorphinol is a narcotic analgesic that has no accepted medicinal value in the United States.
Biochemistry: The ketones are roughly three to five times as effective as their hydroxyl counterparts. However, their utility is limited because of higher dependence liability. Hydromorphinol has a higher physical-dependence potential than oxymorphone, which has accepted medicinal value in the United States.

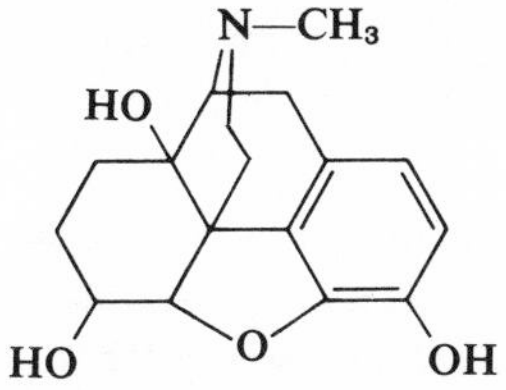

Hydromorphinol 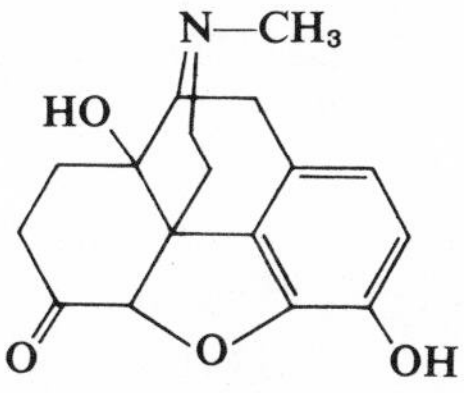   Oxymorphone

Toxicology–Pharmacology: Hydromorphinol is effective as an analgesic in an injectable dose of 1.0–1.5 mg, as compared with 10 mg for morphine. It is thus six to ten times more potent than morphine. It has a duration of action of 4–5 hours. It is an addictive drug similar to morphine and heroin. Overdose is characterized by depression of respiration and central nervous system depression. Narcotic antagonists such as nalline or naloxone are effective in the treatment of overdose with hydromorphinol.

▶ **HYDROMORPHONE**
Schedule II

Synonyms: Dihydromorphinone, dimorphone, novolaudon.
Pharmaceutical Preparations
Dilaudid^R (Knoll)—Ampules: each 1 ml containing 1, 2, 3, or 4 mg
    hydromorphone hydrochloride. Tablets: containing 1, 2, 3, or 4 mg
    hydromorphone hydrochloride. Suppositories: containing 3 mg hydro-
    morphone hydrochloride. Powder: for prescription compounding as
    hydromorphone sulfate.
Dilaudid^R Cough Syrup (Knoll)—Syrup: each 5 ml containing 1 mg hydro-
    morphone hydrochloride
General Comment: Hydromorphone is a semisynthetic narcotic analgesic
that has accepted medicinal value in the United States.
Biochemistry: Hydromorphone is obtained by hydrogenating morphine.
While hydromorphone and morphine have the same empirical formula,
hydromorphone has a ketone group in place of the hydroxyl in morphine,
and is also hydrogenated at a double bond of the morphine molecule.
    The actions of hydromorphone are very similar to those of morphine, the
most important effects being depression of the pain-perceiving mechanism and
of the respiratory center. The analgesic effect of hydromorphone is accepted
as being five times that of morphine. However, the duration of analgesia is
shorter.
    The habit-forming tendency of hydromorphone is considered to be about
the same as that of morphine. Being more active than morphine (but having a
shorter duration of action), it may be used in smaller but more frequent doses
by addicts. The manifestations of the withdrawal syndrome appear more
rapidly, reach greater intensity, and subside more quickly with hydromorphone than with morphine.
Toxicology–Pharmacology: Hydromorphone, or Dilaudid^R, is a commonly
used narcotic analgesic medication, about five times as potent as morphine in
its analgesic potency. It has a duration of action of 4–5 hours, and has an
addiction liability similar to that of morphine, so it may be used to relieve
pain without inducing sleep.
    Hydromorphone is probably less toxic than morphine or heroin, due to

its less severe depressant properties. However, as with the narcotic drugs, it can cause addiction, and death from overdose when used intravenously.

After a death from intravenous injection of hydromorphone a blood concentration of 0.017 mg/dl was reported (Walls, 1976).

▶ **6-HYDROXYDIMETHYLTRYPTAMINE**
Noncontrolled Substance

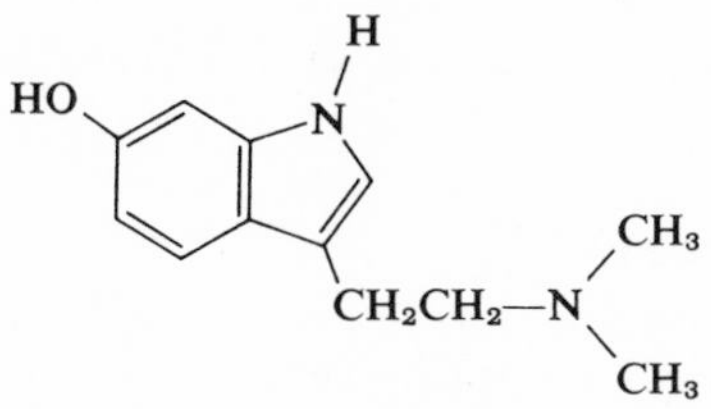

General Comments: 6-Hydroxydimethyltryptamine is an isomer of bufotenine (5-hydroxydimethyltryptamine). Their actions are similar.

▶ **7-HYDROXYDIMETHYLTRYPTAMINE**
Noncontrolled Substance

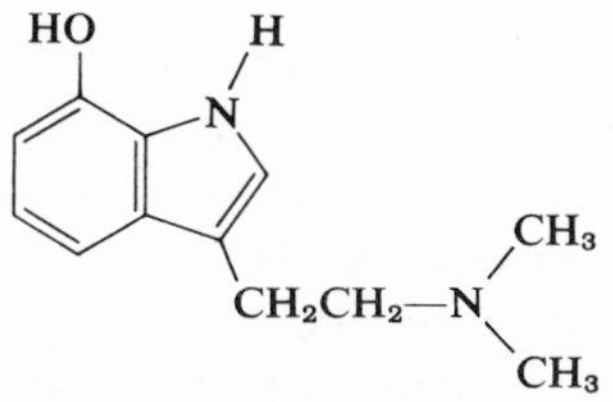

General Comments: 7-Hydroxydimethyltryptamine is an isomer of bufotenine (5-hydroxydimethyltryptamine). Their actions are similar.

▶ **HYDROXYPETHIDINE**
Schedule I

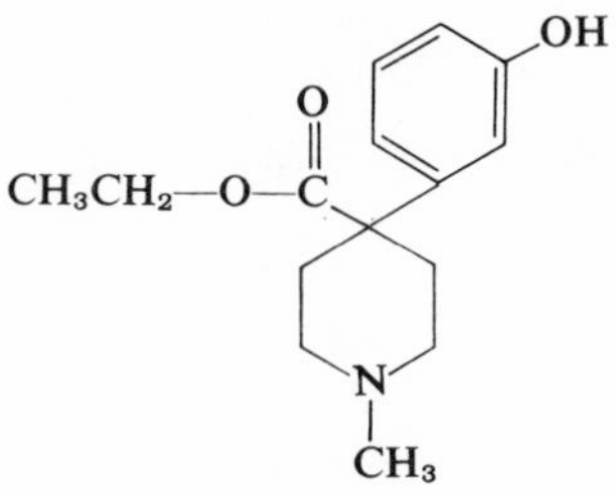

Synonym: Bemidone, oxypethidin, 4-(*m*-hydroxyphenyl)-1-methyl-iso-nipe-cotic acid ethyl ester.

Pharmaceutical Preparations: Hydroxypethidine is not found in any pharmaceutical preparations sold in the United States.

General Comment: Hydroxypethidine is a synthetic narcotic analgesic structurally similar to meperidine (pethidine) but with no accepted medicinal value in the United States.

Biochemistry: Similar to that of pethidine.

Toxicology–Pharmacology: Unknown. Probably similar to that of pethidine.

▶ **HYDROXYPHENAMATE**
Dangerous Drug

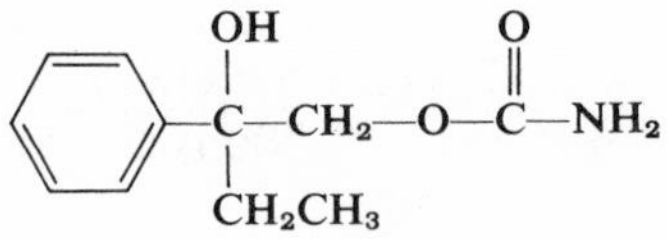

Synonyms: Carbamic acid β-ethyl-β-hydroxyphenethyl ester, 2-hydroxy-2-phenylbutyl carbamate.

Pharmaceutical Preparations: Hydroxyphenamate is not found in any pharmaceutical preparations sold in the United States.

General Comment: Hydroxyphenamate has pharmacological actions of tranquilizing drugs. It is therefore classified in this text as a Dangerous Drug.

Biochemistry: Similar to that of meprobamate.

Toxicology–Pharmacology: Unknown. Probably similar to that of meprobamate.

▶ **HYDROXYZINE**
Dangerous Drug

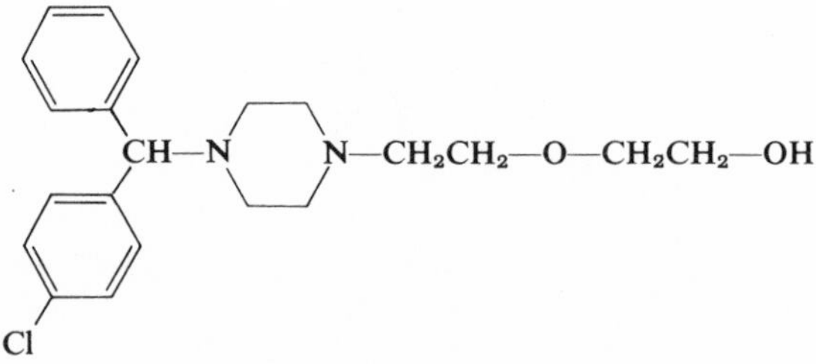

Synonyms: 2-[2-[4-(*p*-Chloro-α-phenylbenzyl)-1-piperazinyl]ethoxy]-ethanol; 1-(*p*-chlorodiphenylmethyl)-4-[2-(2-hydroxyethoxy)ethyl]piperazine.

Pharmaceutical Preparations

Atarax^R (Roerig)—Tablets, containing hydroxyzine hydrochloride: orange, 10 mg; green, 25 mg; yellow, 50 mg; red, 100 mg. Syrup: each 5 ml containing 10 mg hydroxyzine hydrochloride

Ataraxoid^R (Pfizer)—Tablets: green, labeled "321," containing 10 mg hydroxyzine hydrochloride and 5 mg prednisolone; blue, labeled "320," containing 10 mg hydroxyzine hydrochloride and 2.5 mg prednisolone

Cartrax^R (Roerig)—Tablets, containing 10 mg hydroxyzine hydrochloride, plus: yellow, 10 mg pentaerythritol tetranitrate; pink, 20 mg pentaerythritol tetranitrate

Enarax^R (Roerig)—Tablets: Scored, containing 25 mg hydroxyzine hydrochloride, plus: white, 5 mg oxyphencyclimine; black and white, 10 mg oxyphencyclimine

Vistarax^R (Pfizer)—Tablets, scored, containing 25 mg hydroxyzine hydrochloride, plus: white, labeled "180," 5 mg oxyphencyclimine; black and white, labeled "181," 10 mg oxyphencyclimine

Vistaril^R (Pfizer)—Capsules, containing hydroxyzine pamoate: two-tone green, labeled "541," 25 mg; green and white, labeled "542," 50 mg; green and gray, labeled "543," 100 mg. Suspension: each 5 ml containing 25 mg hydroxyzine pamoate. Vials, containing hydroxyzine hydrochloride: 25 mg/ml; 50 mg/ml

General Comment: Hydroxyzine is indicated primarily as a tranquilizer. It is therefore classified in this text as a Dangerous Drug.

Biochemistry: Hydroxyzine was first synthesized by chemists of the Union Chimique Belge, and used in France and Belgium prior to introduction into the United States. It is structurally related to some of the antihistamines, but has central nervous system (CNS) depressant, antispasmodic, antiemetic, and antifibrillatory actions, as well as antihistaminic actions.

A very large number of tertiary alkylamines containing one or more aromatic groups have mixed excitatory and depressant actions on the CNS. These compounds usually possess a wide spectrum of pharmacological activity, including antihistaminic, anticholinergic, and local anesthetic effects. In most cases, these drugs are employed for purposes other than the production of sleep, and the soporific property represents an undesirable side effect; however, occasionally such a drug is promoted as a sedative, "antianxiety," or hypnotic agent. This family of compounds comprises most of the antihistamines and centrally acting anticholinergic compounds as well as certain phenothiazine derivatives.

Generally, the depressant effects appear at low concentrations and the excitatory effects at high concentrations. In some cases, the excitatory effect is dominant even at low concentrations, and in other cases, the drug produces depression throughout the range of sublethal doses.

Unfortunately, while much is known about the peripheral effects of these drugs, there is a paucity of information regarding their mode of action on the CNS. They differ in several respects from the sedative–hypnotic drugs. For example, the soporific action usually cannot be intensified by simply increasing the dose.

Toxicology–Pharmacology: Hydroxyzine is structurally related to the antihistamines, but is used primarily as a tranquilizer. It has CNS depressant, antispasmodic, antihistaminic, antiemetic, and antifibrillatory actions. Its central depressant properties provide the basis for its use as a calming drug for the symptomatic treatment of emotional disorders characterized by anxiety, tension, and agitation. It may also be used to treat urticaria and other allergic dermatoses, motion sickness, and as pre- or postoperative sedation.

The toxicity of hydroxyzine is low, and death from overdose of this agent alone is unusual. It will potentiate the depressant actions of other depressant drug medications, however, and is often involved in mixed drug intoxications. High doses are characterized by drowsiness, dryness of the mouth, and, rarely, convulsions.

▶ **HYOSCINE**
Noncontrolled Substance
Encountered in Excepted Substances

General Comments: Hyoscyamus is the dried leaf of *Hyoscyamus niger* Linne (Fam. *Solanaceae*), which is an annual or biennial plant native to Europe but also grows in the northern and eastern parts of the United States. Hyoscyamus contains the alkaloids hyoscyamine and hyoscine (scopolamine). Scopolamine belongs to the class of cholinergic blocking drugs (parasympathetic). In general, it resembles atropine in its action on the autonomic nervous system, but its effects on the higher centers are different. Atropine is a stimulant on the central nervous system, whereas scopolamine is a depressant.

▶ **HYOSCYAMINE**
Noncontrolled Substance
Encountered in Excepted Substances

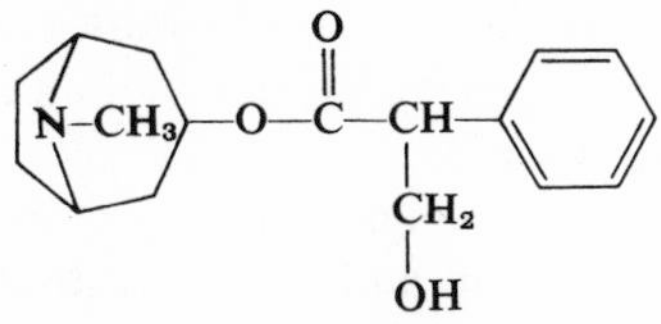

General Comments: Hyoscyamine has pharmacological actions qualitatively the same as those of its racemized form, atropine. Quantitatively, it is more potent than atropine. The following table shows the drugs and drug/hyoscyamine ratio found in excepted preparations:

Drug	Drug/Hyoscyamine Ratio
Butabarbital	1/0.008

Toxicology–Pharmacology: Hyoscyamine is the levorotary component of the racemic mixture known as atropine. Its actions are qualitatively similar to those of atropine in inducing an antagonism to the actions of the parasympathetic nervous system. Some of these inhibitory actions are to suppress the motility and secretions of the gut, dilate the pupils of the eye, and generally antagonize secretions of the salivary and other glands of the body. Hyoscyamine is used to relieve tremor in parkinsonism and to relieve pain of neuralgia, and it has a sedative effect that has been utilized to treat delirium tremens and mania.

Toxicity symptoms are similar to those of atropine.

▶ **IBOGAINE**
Schedule I

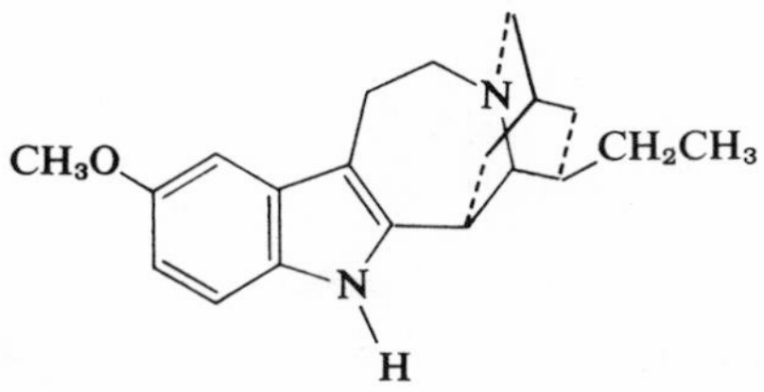

Synonyms: None found.
Pharmaceutical Preparations: Ibogaine is not found in any pharmaceutical preparations sold in the United States.

General Comments: Ibogaine is an alkaloid that has no accepted medical value in the United States. It is controlled under Schedule I hallucinogens.

Biochemistry: Ibogaine is an indole alkaloid from the root (1.27%), rootbark (2–6%), stems (1.95%), and leaves (0.35%) of the shrub *Tabernanthe iboga* Baill, *Apocynaceal*, found in Africa. The African natives use *iboga* extracts while stalking game to enable them to remain motionless for as long as 2 days while retaining mental alertness.

Little is known about the biological activity of ibogaine, even though its absolute sterochemistry is known and a total synthesis has been developed since 1966. It is known, however, that ibogaine is a cholinesterase inhibitor that causes hypertension and stimulation of appetite and digestion. In addition, it is a strong central stimulant and may cause hallucinations.

Toxicology–Pharmacology: Ibogaine has three main pharmacological actions. (1) It is a cholinesterase inhibitor, causing in man hypertension and stimulation of degestion and appetite. (2) It is a strong central stimulant, which is its most prominent effect, leading, in toxic doses, to convulsions, paralysis, and finally respiratory arrest. (3) It causes visual hallucinations, which are associated with severe anxiety and apprehension.

Locally, in certain areas of Africa, it has a reputation as a powerful stimulant and aphrodisiac, and warriors and hunters use the *Tabernanthe* plant constantly to keep awake during night watches. It is also employed as a hallucinogen in tribal ceremonies (Schultes and Hofman, 1973).

▶ **IBOMAL**
Schedule III

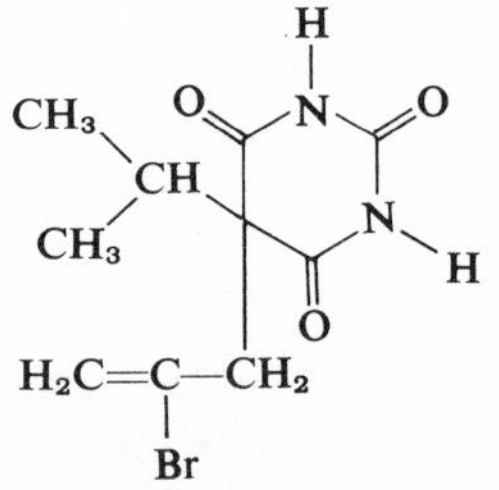

Synonym: 5-(2'-brom-allyl)-isopropyl barbituric acid.

Pharmaceutical Preparations: Ibomal is not found in any pharmaceutical preparations sold in the United States.

General Comments: Ibomal is an intermediate-acting barbiturate with actions similar to those of amobarbital. It is listed under Schedule III as a "derivative of barbituric acid."

Biochemistry: Ibomal, like butallylonal, has the keto derivative as its major metabolite:

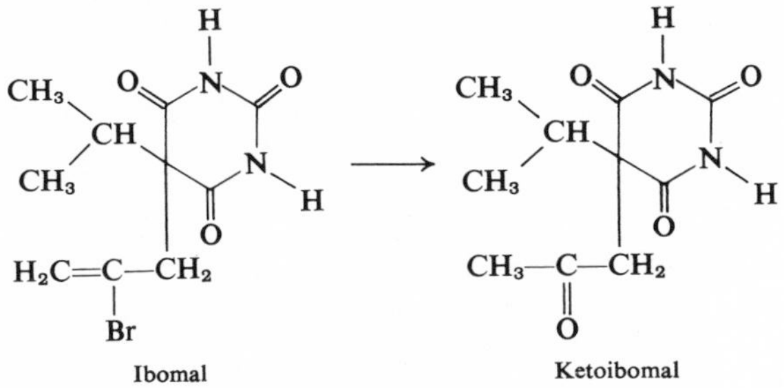

Ibomal   Ketoibomal

Toxicology–Pharmacology: Similar to that of butallylonal.

▶ **IMIPRAMINE**
Dangerous Drug

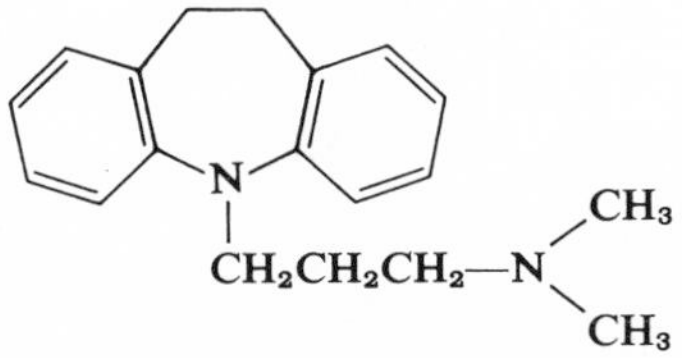

Synonym: 5-[3-(Dimethylamino)-propyl]-10,11-dihydro-2H-dibenz[b,f]-azepine.

Pharmaceutical Preparations
Imavate[R] (Robins)—Tablets
Imipramine[R] Hydrochloride (Phillips Roxane)—Tablets
Janimine[R] Filmtab (Abbott)—Tablets
Presamine[R] (USV)—Ampules and Tablets
SK-Pramine[R] (Smith Kline & French)—Tablets
Tofranil[R] (Geigy)—Ampules and Tablets
Tofranil-PM[R] (Geigy)—Capsules

General Comment: Imipramine is classified in this text as a Dangerous Drug because all pharmaceutical preparations containing imipramine require a prescription and thus bear the label "Caution: Federal law prohibits dispensing without a prescription."

Biochemistry: Imipramine is the prototype of the tricyclic antidepressants; however, the mode of action is unknown. It is not a stimulant like amphetamine, nor does it function as a monoamine oxidase inhibitor.

Tricyclic antidepressants potentiate the depressant effects of barbiturates on the central nervous system, increase the respiratory depression produced by narcotics, and potentiate the actions of meprobamate and of sympatho-mimetic drugs.

Imipramine is a member of a group of aminoalkyl derivatives of imino-benzyl synthesized by Hafliger and Schindler in 1951. In 1957, it was dis-covered that imipramine was relatively ineffective as an antipsychotic drug, but was a more specific drug in the treatment of depressive states. Following this discovery imipramine was introduced in Europe in 1958, then the United States in 1959, as an antidepressant drug (Kuhn, 1957).

The tricyclic antidepressants produce relatively little pharmacological effects at low doses. However, at higher doses, imipramine, like amitriptyline, may produce effects similar to those of the neuroleptic phenothiazines. Imipramine may also produce cholinergic blocking actions. These effects may be attributed in part to the secondary amino group in the side chain, since the imipramine derivatives without this group exhibit a decrease in potency of these central and peripheral effects.

The most significant biological properties of imipramine are related to its ability to alter the metabolism of biogenic amines and to prevent or reverse the biochemical effects of reserpine, thereby antagonizing the symp-toms such as sedation, ptosis, and hypothermia.

Imipramine forms a number of metabolites resulting from a combination of N-demethylation and aromatic ring hydroxylation reactions. The hydroxy derivatives resulting from the latter process form conjugates with glucuronic acid. In addition, hydroxylation of the ethylene bridge occurs. The two major metabolites are desipramine and 2-hydroxyimipramine:

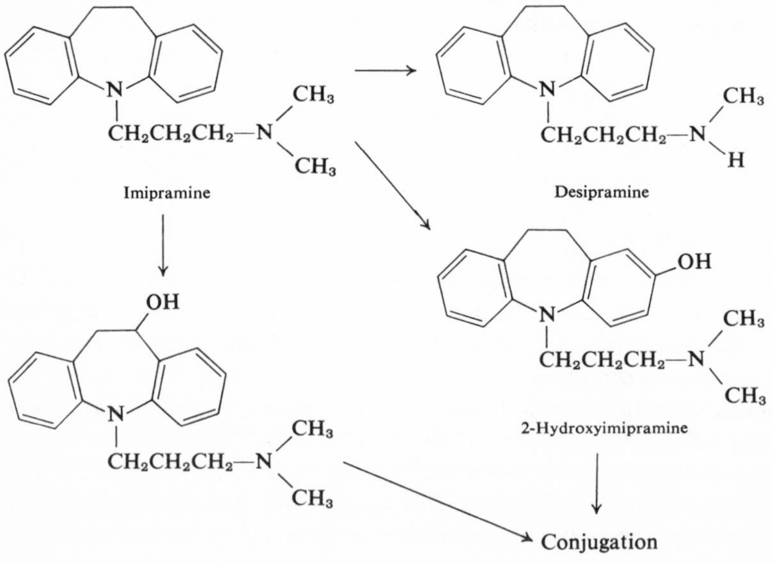

Toxicology–Pharmacology: Imipramine is one of a group of compounds known as tricyclic antidepressants. The mechanisms of their antidepressant action are unknown. They do not act as central stimulants, but have antihistaminic, anticholinergic, antispasmodic, and sympatholytic properties. Imipramine is effective in the treatment of endogenous depression showing the typical symptoms of mental and motor retardation, fatigue, hopelessness, and despair. It results in recovery in a high percentage of cases, although relief does not usually occur until after 1–4 weeks of therapy. It has also been effective in the treatment of enuresis in children.

Since long-term therapy is required for effectiveness, it is believed that the true actions are due to the major metabolite, desmethyl imipramine. It has been demonstrated that beneficial effects occur more rapidly when this compound is administered instead of imipramine.

Imipramine may result in severe toxic reactions when used in combination with monoamine oxidase inhibitors. Potentiation of the depressant effects of barbiturates or alcohol, or the respiratory depressant actions of narcotics, also occurs, and could lead to serious toxic reactions.

A single 100-mg dose of imipramine results in a therapeutic blood level of up to 0.004 mg/dl (Taylor and Egan, 1974), although 300 mg per day leads to blood concentrations of up to 0.060 mg/dl. After death from overdose, 0.20–1.00 mg/dl of imipramine may be found and often equivalent or higher concentrations of the major metabolite, desmethyl imipramine.

▶ **ISOMETHADONE**
Schedule II

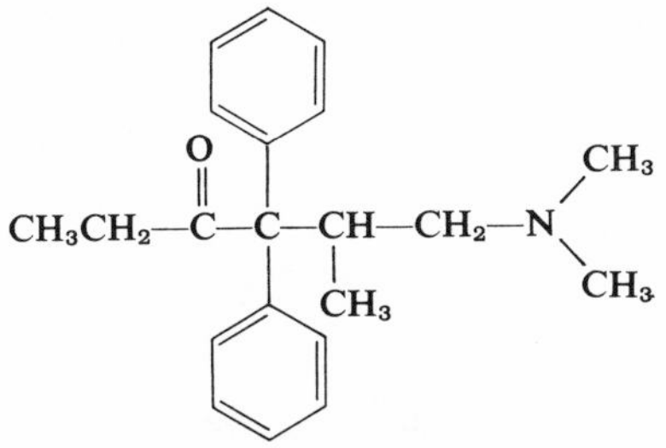

Synonyms: Isoamidone, isoadanone, 6-(dimethylamino)-5-methyl-4,4-diphenyl-3-hexanone.

Pharmaceutical Preparations: Isomethadone is not found in any pharmaceutical preparations sold in the United States.

General Comments: Isomethadone may be found in illicit preparations of methadone, as it is a synthetic by-product and difficult to separate from methadone. Pharmacologically, it is similar to methadone, but with a slightly higher toxicity.

Biochemistry: Methadone was first synthesized in 1948 by treating diphenyl-acetonitrile with 2-chloro-1-demethylaminopropane (Bockmühl and Ehrhart, 1948). This procedure resulted in the formation of, in addition to methadone, an isomer of methadone, isomethadone.

Most of the activity of (+)-isomethadone is from the *levo S*-isomer. It is interesting to note that the C-3 asymmetric center of the *levo S*-isomer of isomethadone has the same configuration as the C-3 asymmetric center of the more active (+)-isomer of propoxyphene:

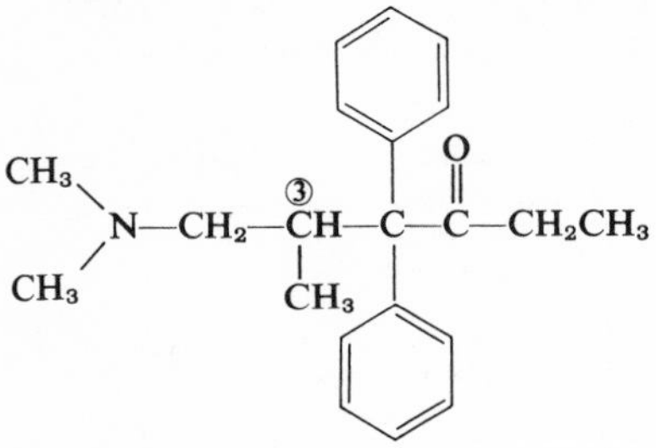

Isomethadone

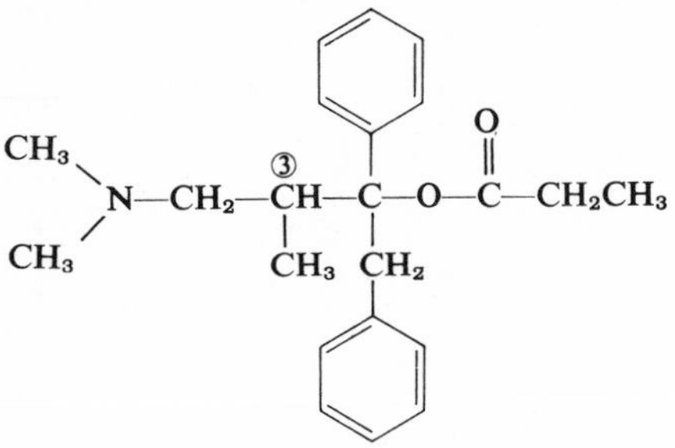

Propoxyphene

Toxicology–Pharmacology: See **METHADONE**.

▶ **ISOSORBIDE DINITRATE**
Noncontrolled Substance
Encountered in Excepted Substances

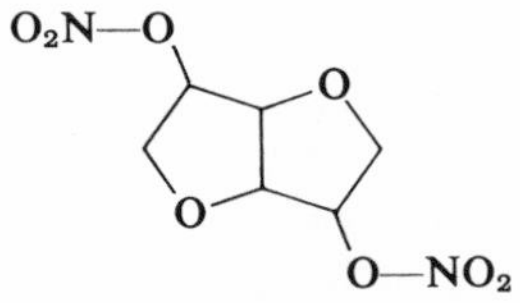

General Comments: Isosorbide dinitrate was first synthesized and studied pharmacologically in 1937. At that time, it appeared to offer little more advantage in the treatment of hypertension than any other organic nitrate. Later, it was discovered that it has useful coronary and peripheral vasodilating actions and that it will dilate constricted pulmonary vessels.

Isosorbide dinitrate is encountered in phenobarbital preparations classified as excepted preparations in a phenobarbital/isosorbide dinitrate ratio of 1/0.67.

▶ **KETOBEMIDONE**
Schedule I

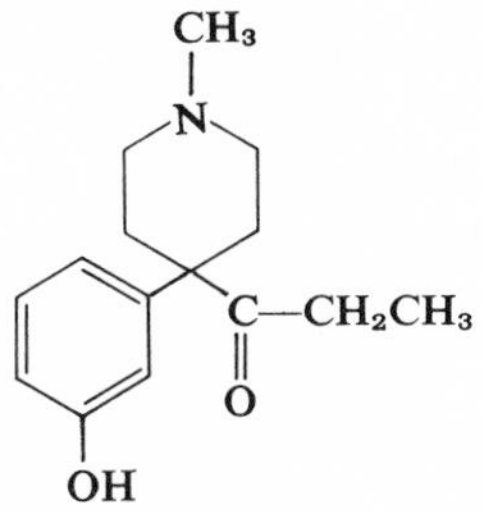

Synonyms: Cliradon, cymidon, Ketogan, ketogin, 1-[4-(*m*-hydroxyphenyl)-1-methyl-4-piperidyl]-1-propanone.

Pharmaceutical Preparations: Ketobemidone is not found in any pharmaceutical preparations sold in the United States.

General Comment: Ketobemidone is a synthetic bicyclic narcotic analgesic that has no accepted medicinal value in the United States.

Biochemistry: Ketobemidone is a derivative of meperidine (pethidine) in which the phenyl becomes *m*-hydroxyphenyl and the ester is changed to a ketone. Generally, when a substituent change at the C-4 position in meperidine occurs, the activity is diminished or has no improvement. However, in the case of ketobemidone, the opposite is true. Ketobemidone has twofold greater activity than meperidine and is equipotent with morphine (Avison and Morrison, 1950).

The shape and configuration of the group on nitrogen appear to play an important role in the activity of the molecule (Blair and Stephenson, 1960). In addition, other contributing factors are more rapid absorption and metabolism. However, complete data have not been obtained as yet.

Toxicology–Pharmacology: Ketobemidone is a narcotic analgesic that has been used as premedication for surgery. The duration of action and side effects are similar to those produced by equivalent doses of morphine. It has a weaker sedative action than morphine, however. Addictive or overdose properties are similar to those of morphine.

▶ **LACTOSE**
Noncontrolled Substance

General Comment: Lactose is a sugar commonly employed as a diluent in the formulation of capsules and tablets, especially those that are intended to dissolve completely.

▶ **LEVOMETHORPHAN**
Schedule II

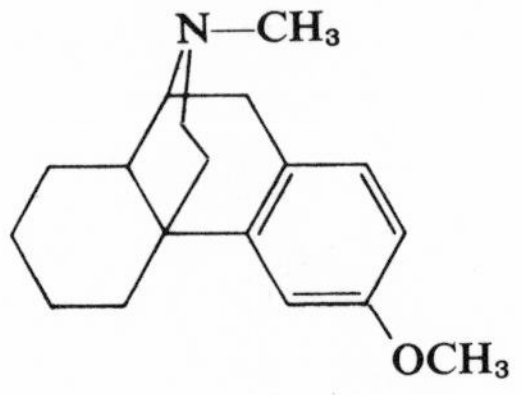

Synonym: *l*-3-Methoxy-*N*-methylmorphinan.
Pharmaceutical Preparations: Levomethorphan is not found in any pharmaceutical preparations frequently sold in the United States.
General Comment: Unlike the *dextro* isomer, dextromethorphan, which possesses antitussive properties, levomethorphan has narcotic analgesic actions that have accepted medicinal value in the United States.
Biochemistry: Levomethorphan is the methyl ether of levorphanol. Its stereochemical and physiological properties are similar to those of levorphanol.
Toxicology–Pharmacology: Similar to that of levorphanol.

▶ **LEVOMORAMIDE**
Schedule I

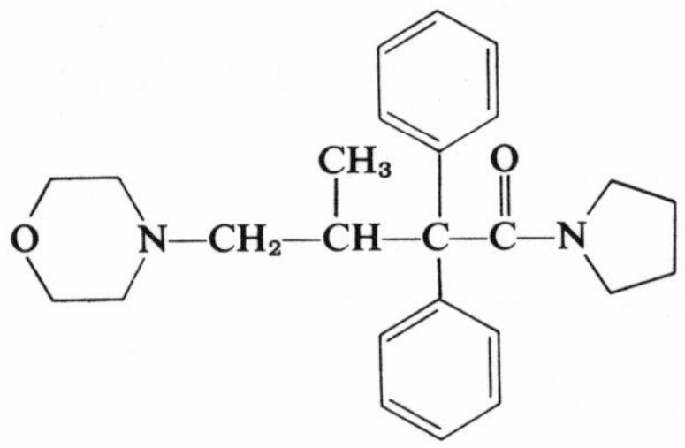

Synonyms: None found.
Pharmaceutical Preparations: Levomoramide is not found in any pharmaceutical preparations sold in the United States.
General Comments: The racemic racemoramide is known as the equal mixture of the two optical isomers. Both dextromoramide and levomoramide are separately listed as scheduled drugs without medical acceptance. An intermediate to these drugs is 4-cyano-2-dimethylamine-4,4-diphenylbutane, which is listed in Schedule II.
Biochemistry: Unknown.
Toxicology–Pharmacology: Unknown.

▶ **LEVOPHENACYLMORPHAN**
Schedule I

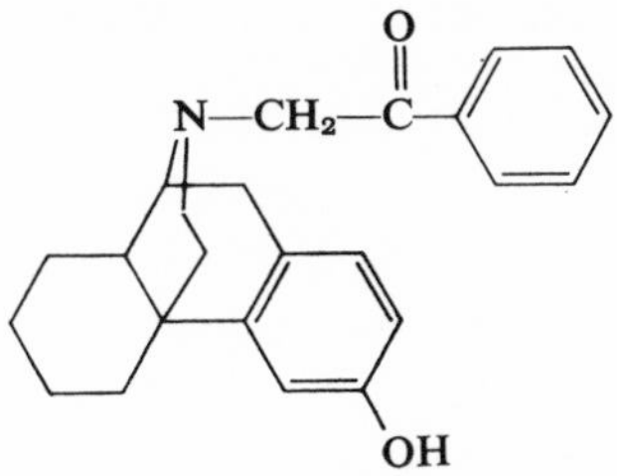

Synonym: *l*-3-Hydroxy-*N*-phenacylmorphinan.
Pharmaceutical Preparations: Levophenacylmorphan is not found in any pharmaceutical preparations sold in the United States.
General Comment: Levophenacylmorphan is a synthetic narcotic analgesic that has no accepted medicinal value in the United States.
Biochemistry: Unknown.
Toxicology–Pharmacology: Unknown.

▶ **LEVORPHANOL**
Schedule II

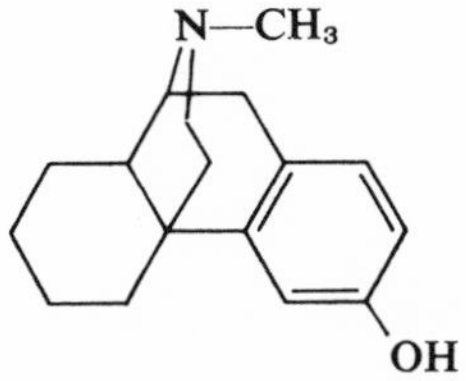

Synonym: 17-Methylmorphinan-3-ol.
Pharmaceutical Preparations: Levo-Dromoran^R (Roche)—Ampules: each 1 ml containing 2 mg levorphanol tartrate. Vials: 10 ml, each 1 ml containing 2 mg levorphanol tartrate. Tablets: containing 2 mg levorphanol tartrate.
General Comments: Levorphanol is a synthetic narcotic analgesic. It is the (−) isomer of the racemic compound, racemorphan, which is also listed as a Schedule II drug. The (+) isomer, dextrophan, once listed as a Schedule I drug, is no longer controlled.
Biochemistry: The synthesis of racemorphan has been developed along with its optical resolution (Schnider and Grussner, 1951). It was determined that practically all the analgetic activity and dependence liability of racemorphan were due to its *levo* enantiomorph, levorphanol. However, the toxicity of racemorphan has contributions from both the *levo* and *dextro* isomers.

Levorphanol is approximately four times as potent as morphine (Benson *et al.*, 1953).

Even though both racemorphan and levorphanol are clinically effective, only levorphanol is commercially available.

Toxicology–Pharmacology: Levorphanol is a narcotic–analgesic with qualitative actions similar to those of morphine. It is about five times as potent an analgesic as morphine, and is a more potent sedative. It may be administered orally in doses of 2–3 mg, which is equivalent to a 10-mg dose of morphine in effectiveness. It may be used to relieve severe pain in cancer, trauma, myocardial infarction, and other diseases, and is also used as preoperative medication and for postoperative pain.

It has an addiction liability similar to that of morphine.

Subcutaneous administration of 2–3 mg levorphanol tartrate produces a degree of analgesia similar to that obtained with 10–15 mg morphine. Maximal analgesia is developed in 60–90 minutes after subcutaneous injection, and in about 20 minutes after intravenous injection.

▶ **LIDOCAINE**
Noncontrolled Substance

General Comments: Lidocaine is a local anesthetic, but has use as an antiarrhythmic drug. It is encountered as a diluent in illicit preparations.

Toxicology–Pharmacology: Lidocaine is one of a group of compounds known as local anesthetics. It is effective in blocking sensations in areas where applied, and is effective when applied topically to the skin or mucous membranes as well as when injected. It is useful for infiltration and block anesthesia in general surgical and dental procedures. It is useful when applied locally as an ointment preparation to control itching, burning, and other unpleasant symptoms due to abrasions, hemorrhoids, eczema, and other conditions.

It also has antiarrhythmic activity when injected intravenously, and is used extensively for this purpose in emergency treatment of heart attack victims or other conditions causing cardiac arrhythmias.

Toxicity from lidocaine can result from unusually high doses, producing blood concentrations greater than 0.50 mg/dl. Toxicity reactions include dizziness, blurred vision, nausea, tremors, convulsions, and respiratory arrest.

Blood concentrations after a subcutaneous dose of 200 mg were 0.042

mg/dl after 30 minutes and 0.050 mg/dl at 2 hours (Schwartz *et al.*, 1974). Toxic effects (focal seizures, stuporous condition) have been reported at blood concentrations of 0.68–2.28 mg/dl (Gianelly *et al.*, 1967) and fatalities in two cases at 4.36 and 9.20 mg/dl (Borkwoski and Dluzniewaska, 1976).

▶ **LORAZEPAM**
Schedule IV

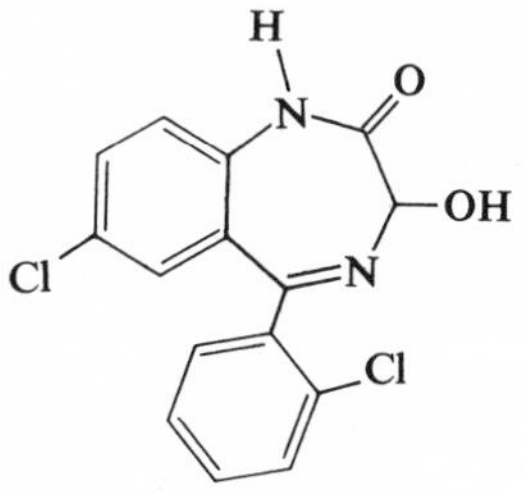

Synonym: *O*-Chlorooxazepam.

Pharmaceutical Preparations: Ativan[R] (Wyeth)—Tablets, white, scored, labeled "Wyeth": capsuled-shaped, containing 1.0 mg lorazepam; oval-shaped, containing 2.0 mg lorazepam

General Comment: Lorazepam was added to Schedule IV of the Controlled Substances Act in October, 1977.

Biochemistry: Lorazepam is the *O*-chloro derivative of oxazepam. The introduction of the chlorine in the *O* position of the phenyl ring causes a marked increase in pharmacological activity.

Toxicology–Pharmacology: Lorazepam is a potent antianxiety agent of the benzodiazepine group. Its clinical usefulness includes reduction of anxiety at low doses, sedation at higher doses, and reduction of frustration at low doses. As an antianxiety agent, it is two to four times more potent than diazepam. It also has marked sedative–hypnotic activity (Stein and Berger, 1971).

It is suggested for use as an antianxiety agent, in the treatment of sleep disorders, as preoperative medication, and as an adjunct to psychotherapy.

The usual dose for sleep induction is 2.5–5.0 mg; that for antianxiety is 1.5–3.0 mg per day (Collard, 1971). No toxic effects were observed in patients taking up to 22–25 mg per day for treatment of nervous tension and insomnia (Collard, 1971). It is more strongly antianxiety and tranquilizing than diazepam, but has fewer ataxic side effects (Schrappe, 1971).

Serum concentrations after a 2.5-mg dose reached 0.003 mg/dl at 2 hours, and after a 5 mg dose, the maximum concentration observed at 2 hours was 0.004 mg/dl (Knowles *et al.*, 1971).

▶ **LYSERGIC ACID**
Schedule III

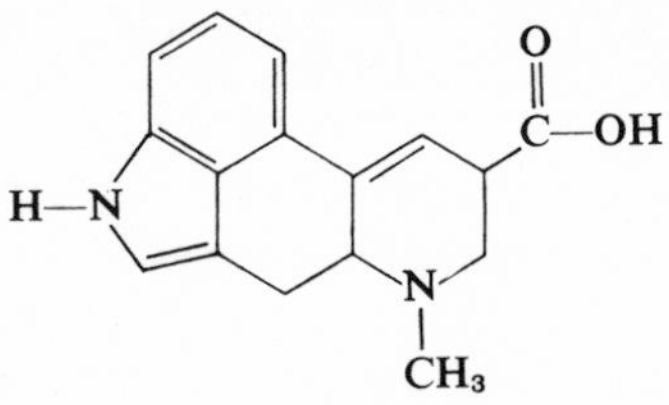

Synonyms: None found.

Pharmaceutical Preparations: Lysergic acid is not found in any pharmaceutical preparations sold in the United States.

General Comments: The listing of lysergic acid under Schedule III for depressants is pharmacologically improper. However, the reason for its inclusion is that it can serve as a precursor in the synthesis of lysergic acid diethylamide. Under Section 201 of the Controlled Substances Act, an immediate precursor may be placed in the same schedule as the controlled substance to which it is a precursor, or in any other schedule with a higher numerical designation. Since lysergic acid diethylamide is a Schedule I substance, lysergic acid could have legally been placed in Schedule I, II, III, IV, or V.

Biochemistry: Lysergic acid is one of the alkaloids found in dried sclerotium of *Claviceps purpurea* (Fries) Tulasne (Family *Hypocreaceae*), a parasitic fungus that develops on plants of rye, *Secale cereale* Linne (Family *Gramineae*). It may also be produced saprophytically in the fermentation of selected strains of *Claviceps paspali*, which is a fungus that grows on dead plant material.

The qualitative and quantitative composition of the alkaloid obtained from either source is influenced by a number of factors, but especially by the identity of the strain (chemical race) of organism involved.

Toxicology–Pharmacology: Lysergic acid possesses α-adrenergic blocking activity, and antagonizes the action of serotonin. It produces peripheral vasoconstriction and central vagal stimulation. It also possesses potent emetic properties as a result of stimulation of the chemoreceptor trigger zone.

▶ **LYSERGIC ACID AMIDE**
Schedule III

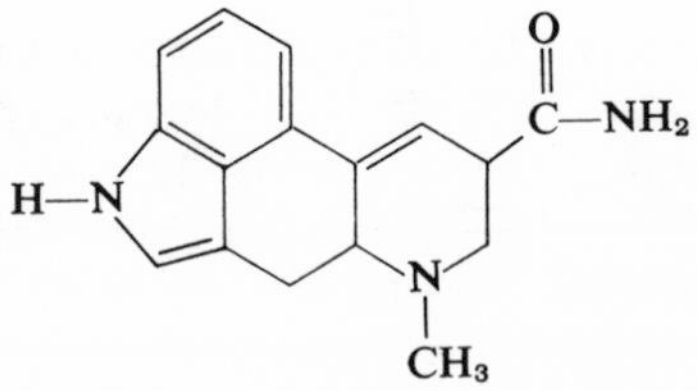

Synonyms: Lysergamide, ergine.

Pharmaceutical Preparations: Lysergic acid amide is not found in any pharmaceutical preparations sold in the United States.

General Comments: Like that of lysergic acid, the listing of lysergic acid amide under Schedule III for depressants is pharmacologically improper. Primarily, the reason for its inclusion is that it can serve as a precursor in the synthesis of lysergic acid diethylamide. Under Section 201 of the Controlled Substances Act, an immediate precursor may be placed in the same schedule as the controlled substance to which it is a precursor, or in any other schedule with a higher numerical designation. Since lysergic acid diethylamide is a Schedule I substance, lysergic acid amide could have legally been placed in Schedule I, II, III, IV, or V.

Biochemistry: Lysergic acid amide is also an ergot alkaloid (see **LYSERGIC ACID**). In addition, it has been found in the plants *Ipomoea violacea* L. and *Rivea corymbosa* L. (Mexican morning glories). Many horticultural varieties of morning glories are devoid of the psychotomimetic alkaloids. However, some, such as "Heavenly Blue" and "Pearly Gates," contain lysergic acid amide.

Lysergic acid amide is about 50–100 times less active than lysergic acid diethylamide (LSD).

Toxicology–Pharmacology: *d*-Lysergic acid amide is the main constituent of ololiuqui, the seeds of *Rivea corymbosa*. Ololiuqui is the small hallucinogenic seed used by the Aztecs or other Indians for purposes of divination. It is about 50–100 times less active as a hallucinogen than *d*-lysergic acid diethylamide. It has a much greater narcotic action than LSD, however. After ingestion of a 2.0-mg dose, Hofmann experienced tiredness, apathy, a feeling of mental emptiness and the unreality and complete meaninglessness of the outside world (Hofmann, 1963).

▶ **LYSERGIC ACID DIETHYLAMIDE**
Schedule I

Synonyms: LSD, LSD-25, lysergide, (+)-*N,N*-diethyl lysergamide.

Pharmaceutical Preparations: Lysergic acid diethylamide is not found in any pharmaceutical preparations sold in the United States.

General Comments: *d*-Lysergic acid diethylamide (LSD) was prepared by Hofmann for the first time in 1938 as part of a systematic chemical and pharmacological investigation of partially synthetic amides of lysergic acid. This work was conducted in the Sandoz Pharmaceutical-Chemical Research Laboratories in Basel with the intention of obtaining an analeptic drug. The basic reasoning behind this was the structural relationship of LSD to the well-known circulatory stimulant nikethamide:

Nikethamide

Limited pharmacological studies were carried out at this time. However, in 1943, Hofmann initiated the study again. During this work, an accidental observation led Hofmann to carry out a planned self-experiment with LSD. Thus, on April 16, 1943, the hallucinogenic properties of LSD were discovered (Hofmann, 1975).

Biochemistry: LSD is among several drugs with psychotropic actions which were investigated on the basis of electronic structures. Along with serotonin and chlorpromazine, LSD is a potent electron donor (Karreman *et al.*, 1959). Molecular orbital calculations utilizing HOMO were conducted on LSD and drugs in the amphetamine and tryptamine classes. It was determined that a close correlation existed between increasing HOMO energies and increase in hallucinogenic potencies (Snyder and Merril, 1965). In the tryptamine class, HOMO calculations indicated that methoxylation and disubstitution increased the energy of the HOMO.

Toxicology–Pharmacology: Although LSD is an alkaloid resembling ergonovine and its other ergot alkaloids, its significant effects are almost entirely on the central nervous system. Doses as low as 20–25 μg are capable of producing effects in some individuals. After ingestion of doses of from 25 to 250 μg, the individual experiences marked changes in mood. He may become quite emotional, and laugh or cry at slight provocation. Both euphoria and dysphoria occur. The most pronounced effects are the result of perceptual changes. They may be visual or tactile, and consist of either distortions or hallucinations. Intellectual processes are impaired, resulting in confusion and difficulty in thinking.

There are some sympathomimetic effects, consisting of mydriasis, hyperthermia, piloerection, and tachycardia. It also antagonizes the peripheral actions of LSD.

After overdose in four patients, symptoms consisting of psychosis, hyperexcitability, tachycardia, mydriasis, hyperthermia, and central nervous system and respiratory depression occurred. There were bleeding problems associated with platelet function impairment. Plasma levels of LSD were 2.1–26.0 ng/ml (Klock et al., 1975).

After intravenous administration of 2 μg/kg to normal subjects, plasma levels were 5.5 ng/ml at 1 hour, and 3.0 ng/ml at 4 hours. The plasma half-life was 175 minutes (Aghajanian and Bing, 1964).

▶ **MANNITOL HEXANITRATE**
Noncontrolled Substance
Encountered in Excepted Substances

$$O_2N-O-CH_2-\overset{\displaystyle \overset{H}{|}}{\underset{\displaystyle \underset{O_2N}{|}}{C}}-\overset{\displaystyle \overset{H}{|}}{\underset{\displaystyle \underset{O}{|}}{C}}-\overset{\displaystyle \overset{O}{|}}{\underset{\displaystyle \underset{H}{|}}{C}}-\overset{\displaystyle \overset{O}{|}}{\underset{\displaystyle \underset{H}{|}}{C}}-CH_2-O-NO_2$$

General Comments: Mannitol hexanitrate is a vasodilator similar to erythrityl tetranitrate. It is encountered in phenobarbital preparations classified as excepted preparations in a phenobarbital/mannitol hexanitrate ratio of 1/2.

▶ **MARIJUANA**
Schedule I
General Comments: Marijuana, as defined by Section 102 of the Controlled Substances Act, means the plant *Cannabis sativa* L., whether growing or not. It also includes every compound, manufacture, salt, derivative, mixture, or preparation of the plant, or its seeds. However, the law does not include:

1. The resin extracted from any part of such plant or any compound, manufacture, salt, derivative, mixture, or preparation of resin
2. The mature stalks of the plant
3. Fiber produced from the stalks
4. Oil or cake made from the seeds of the plant
5. Any other compound, manufacture, salt, derivative, mixture, or preparation of the mature stalks, fiber, oil, or cake
6. The sterilized seed of the plant, which is incapable of germination

Cannabis is probably the most widely diversified of all the psychoactive, drug-producing plants. It is diversified in its growth, scientific terminology, and common terminology.

In North America, *Cannabis* is commonly known as marijuana or marihuana. In India, it is known as bhang, ganja, and charas. The common name in Algeria and Morocco is kif, while in South America the names dagga, machona, and liamba are heard. Other names heard around the world are kabak in Turkey, takrouri in Tunisia, and djoma in Africa. The American drug culture has extended *Cannabis* terminology to muggles, reefer, joints, weed, Texas tea, tea, gage, loco-weed, sticks, grass, boo, jive, rope, gates, goof-butts, mooters, Mary Jane, pot, and possibly others that these authors are unaware of.

The possibility that the genus *Cannabis* comprises more than one species has been a matter for considerable controversy over a long period of time. The literature on the botany of *Cannabis* is complicated and confusing because of numerous specific and varietal names, most of which have never been properly published or described according to the rules of botanical nomenclature. Thus, the genus has been considered to be monotypic, and most taxonomists have, in the past, agreed that *Cannabis sativa* L. included all variants. The following are some of the specific epithets that have so far been proposed in the literature (Schultes *et al.*, 1974):

Cannabis americana Houghton et Hamilton [*Am. J. Pharm.* **80**(1908):17], nomen nudum

Cannabis erratica Sievers ex Pallas [*Neue Nord. Beytr.* **7**(1796):174], nomen nudum

Cannabis foetens Gilibert [*Exercit. Phytol.* **2**(1792):450], nomen illegitimum

Cannabis generalis E. H. L. Krause [*Strud. Fl. Deutschland*, Ed. 2, **4**(1905): 199]

Cannabis gigantea Crevost [*Bull. Econ. Indochine N.S.* **20**(1917):613]

Cannabis indica Lamarck [*Encycl.* **1**(1783):695]

X Cannabis intersita Sojak [*Novit. Bot. Del. Sem. Hort. Bot. Univ. Carol Prage* (1690):20]

Cannabis lupulus Scopoli [*Pl. Carniol.* Ed. 2, **2**(1772):263]

Cannabis macrosperma Stokes [*Bot. Mat. Med.* **4**(1812):539]

Cannabis pedemontana Camp [*J. N. Y. Bot. Gard.* **36**(1936):114], nomen nudum in synon

Cannabis ruderalis Janischewsky [*Uchen. Zap. Gas. Saratov. Univ.* **2**, Pt. 2 (1924):14]

Cannabis sativa Linnaeus [*Sp. Pl.* (1753):1027]

A study of these names indicates that three were originally described by Linnaeus, Lamarck, and Janischewsky, and were separately named *Cannabis sativa*, *Cannabis indica*, and *Cannabis ruderalis*, respectively. These three species have been taxonomically classified, properly described, and type specimens recorded and critically compared (Schultes *et al.*, 1974). The following quotation from this article describes the distinguishing characters of these three species and proposes a taxonomic key to identify them:

> While we recognize our present incomplete knowledge of characters, we offer the following key to distinguish the several species discussed above:
>
> 1) Plants usually tall (up to 5 to 18 feet), laxly branched, Akenes smooth, usually lacking marbled pattern on outer coat, firmly attached to stalk and without definite articulation.
>
> *C. sativa*
>
> 1a) Plants usually small (4 feet or less), not laxly branched, Akenes usually strongly marbled on outer coat with a definite abscission layer, dropping off at maturity.
>
> 2) Plants very densely branched, more or less conical, usually 4 feet tall or less. Abscission layer a simple articulation at base of Akene.
>
> *C. indica*
>
> 2a) Plants not branched or very sparsely so, usually 1 to 2 feet at maturity. Abscission layer forms a fleshy caruncle-like growth at base of Akene.
>
> *C. ruderalis*

The "distinctions which have been made between the taxa known as *C. sativa*, *C. indica* and *C. ruderalis* relate to characteristics of the fruit" (Stearn, 1974). When Linnaeus classified *C. sativa* in 1753 and gave India as the country of origin, the actual botanical data and description were based on plants grown in Northern Europe in 1737. To study the plant, botanists are faced with complexities regarding the variability of present-day cultivated vs. truly wild *Cannabis* (noting that there can be no wild hemp except in areas where it is native). A complete clarification of the botany of *Cannabis* will require field studies, where the plant is native or has not been subjected to cultivation (Schultes *et al.*, 1974).

In 1972, the study of meiosis and pollen fertility in hybrids representing combinations of 38 different populations of *Cannabis* was reported (Small, E., 1972). It was determined that these populations shared the same chromosome end-arrangement, and there was no reduction in pollen fertility of first-generation hybrids. This indicated that sterility barriers were not developed. The results of these interfertility studies do not preclude the possibility that sterility barriers may exist, however. It is known that "acceptable" species exist in certain genera in which few or no sterility barriers are present (Raven, 1974). Recognition of species mainly or totally on the presence of sterility barriers is a point of view accepted by some taxonomists. To other taxonomists, definable morphological differences are necessary.

The term "species" is a unit of classification for both plants and animals. It is characterized by a population of similar specimens alike in their structural and functional characteristics, which breed only with each other (sometimes with fertile offspring), have a common ancestry, and, in nature, maintain structural characters through countless generations. From a practical standpoint, two types of data may be utilized for the purpose of defining species: (1) internal separation, which is of a genetic–physiological nature expressed through incompatibility and intersterility, and through weakness of the hybrid offspring; and (2) external separation, which considers criteria of flower, fruit, seed, anatomical, and vegetative characters, resulting from environmental and ecological geographic factors.

The anatomy of *C. sativa* and *C. indica* from type locations has been examined (Anderson, 1974). Very substantial differences between the wood characteristics of these plants were found. These findings substantiate Lamarck's description of *C. indica* in 1783 and Linnaeus's description of *C. sativa* in 1753. The anatomy of the wood is widely recognized as the most conservative character of plants that cannot be an intraspecific response to environmental factors.

The fact remains that this genus has not yet been proved unequivocally to be monotypic of polytypic. However, several court rulings defining "marijuana" have been made, stating that *Cannabis sativa* L. refers to all forms of *Cannabis* plant material, on the basis of legislative intent. Cases cited include:

1. United States vs. Gaines, 489 F. 2d 690 (5th Cir., 1974)
2. United States vs. Honeyman *et al.* (Crim. No. 71-1035-RHS, N.D. Cal, Sept. 13, 1972)
3. United States vs. Honneus, 16 Cr. L. 2338 (First Circ., Dec. 24, 1974)
4. United States vs. Lewallen, 16 Cr. L. 2404 (U.S.D.C.W. Wisc., Jan. 19, 1974)
5. United States vs. Moore, 330 F. Supp. 684 (E.D. Pa., 1970), Affd. 446F. 2d 448 (3rd Cir., 1971), Cert. Dis. 406 U.S. 909 (1972)
6. United States vs. Rothberg, 351 F. Supp. 1115 (E.D.N.Y., 1972) Affd. 480 F. 2d 534 (2d Cir., 1973)
7. United States vs. Walton, 43 L.W. 2333 (D.C. Cir., Jan 28, 1975)

In U.S. vs. Gaines, 489 F. 2d 690 (5th Circ., 1974), it was stated:

> Gaines further argues that it was error for the trial court to refuse to instruct the jury as to the statutory definition of marihuana. We disagree and affirm.
> Noting that the Federal statutory definition of marijuana refers only to *Cannabis sativa* L., Gaines calls our attention to the fact that while the Government's expert chemist agreed that there are three species of marihuana; i.e. *Cannabis sativa* L., *Cannabis indica* and *Cannabis ruderalis*, the chemist was unable to differentiate between the three. Building upon the premise that *Cannabis sativa* L. is the only species of marihuana expressly prohibited by statute, Gaines argues that the court's refusal to give the jury an instruction containing the statutory definition of marihuana deprived the

jury of considering whether the Government's expert was sufficiently trained and whether he sufficiently tested the substance to prove beyond a reasonable doubt that, in fact, the substance examined was *Cannabis sativa* L. and not *Cannabis indica.*

The Third Circuit recently considered the issue raised by Gaines and concluded that *Cannabis indica* is included within the statutory definition of marihuana. U.S. v. Moore, 3 Cir. 1974, 446 F. 2d 448. Similarly, the Second Circuit, while recognizing the possibility that there may be some botanical opinion that *Cannabis* is polytypic, found that "there is no question but that the lawmakers, the general public and overwhelming scientific opinion considered that there was only one species of marihuana...Whether this is scientifically exact or not, the statute provided at the time of the offense a sufficient description of what was intended to be prohibited to give notice to all of the illegality of appellants' actions" (U.S. v. Rothberg. 2 Cir. 1973, 480 F. 2d 534, 536).

We are in full agreement with what has been said by our sister Circuits, and thus find no error in the District Court's refusal to instruct the jury with respect to the statutory definition of marihuana.

In U.S. vs. Walton, 16 Cr. L 2415 (1/23/75), the U.S. Court of Appeals for the D.C. Circuit rejected an argument stating the Government had failed to meet its burden of proof under 21 U.S.C. Sec. 802(15) in that the marijuana was not shown to be *Cannabis sativa* L. The court rejected this contention, stating:

> We think the fact that 21 U.S.C. Sec. 802(15) defines marijuana as *Cannabis sativa* L. is not sufficient to support the contention that Congress meant to outlaw the distribution of only one species.

In Walton, it was stated:

> Thus, Walton's argument is that Congress meant to outlaw the euphoric effects of the *sativa* L. species but not the euphoric effect of other species. This result seems manifestly unreasonable and furthermore could raise the most serious equal protection problems if it were adopted, i.e. an individual convicted for distribution of *sativa* L. could state with more than a little justification that no legitimate legislative purpose permits the government to jail persons who obtain a THC "high" from *sativa* L. but to not prosecute persons who obtain the exact same "high" from another species. Moreover, Walton's expert concedes that at present there is no reliable biochemical or spectrographic method for distinguishing between the various species of marihuana. Thus, unless the Government has access to the growing plant, an unlikely situation, it cannot at present prove that a given defendant possesses one kind of marihuana or another. It may be that the government has the capacity to develop a method but since Congress did not have the benefit of any such method when it enacted the statute in issue here, one must certainly pause to consider why Congress would enact a law the violations of which could not (be) proven on the basis of present knowledge. Even if Congress did have such a method it is apparently conceded that only citizens with expert botanical knowledge could distinguish between the various species of marihuana. This suggests a serious due process

question: could the Government prosecute an individual for possession of *sativa* L. when there are no means whereby the average citizen can distinguish between *sativa* L. and other species to thus conform his conduct to the requirements of the law? It presses us to extremes to hold that Congress would enact a law the violations of which are not detectable to the group of citizens to whom the law is addressed.

In Walton, it was further noted that every Federal Appeals Court that had considered this question had reached a similar conclusion, and the following cases were cited:

1. U.S. vs. Honneus, 16 Cr. L. 2338 (1st Cir. 12/24/74)
2. U.S. vs. Kinsey, #74-2014 (2d Cir. 10/31/74)
3. U.S. vs. Gaines, 489 F. 2d 690 (5th Cir. 1974)
4. U.S. vs. Rothberg, 480 F. 2d 534, 13 Cr. L. 2314 (2d Cir.), cert. den. 414 U.S. 856 (1973), aff'g, 351 F. Supp 1115 E.D.N.Y. 19 (1972)
5. U.S. vs. Moore, 446 F. 2d 448 (3d Cir 1971). aff'g. 330 F. Supp. 684 (E.D. Pa. 1970) See also St. vs. Romero, 74 N.M. 642, 397 P. 2d 26
6. People vs. Savage, 64 Cal. App. 2d 314, 148 P. 2d 654
7. Martinez vs. People, 160 Colo. 333, 417 P. 2d 485
8. St. vs. Alley, 263 A. 2d 66 (Me. 1970)
9. St. vs. Allison, 466 S.W. 2d 712 (Mo. 1971)
10. St. vs. Economy, 61 Nev. 394, 130 P. 2d 264

In Walton, it was recognized that the definition of marijuana set forth in 21 U.S.C. Sec. 802(15) was carried forward from the Marijuana Tax Act of 1937 without comment. It was further noted in Walton that there was no suggestion until the late 1960s that there was a possibility that marijuana had a polytypic status. Walton recognized that such issue was still very much in doubt (Lowry, 1976).

Biochemistry: The primary pharmacologically active constituents of *Cannabis* are the isomers of tetrahydrocannabinol. The pure steroisomer, $(-)\Delta'$-3,4-*trans*-tetrahydrocannabinol, and the $(-)\Delta^{1,6}$-isomer have been isolated and identified from *Cannabis* resin (Gaoni and Mechoulam, 1964).

(−) Δ'-3,4-*trans*-Tetrahydrocannabinol

The resin contains additional isomers that differ from each other in the location of the unsaturation of the monomethyl-substituted ring. In addition, isomers are present that differ in the steric arrangement at C-1, C-3, and C-4.

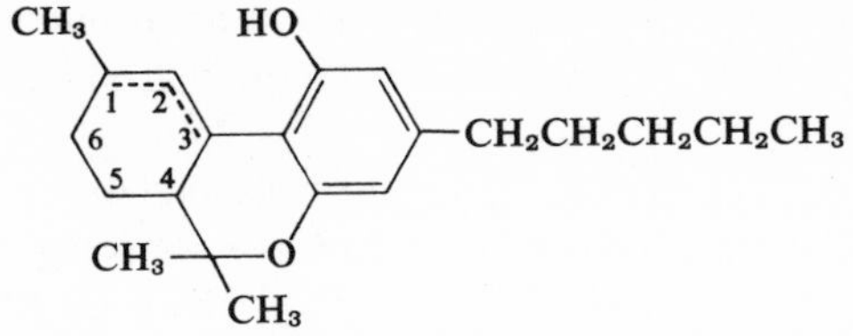

Numerous psychopharmacologically inactive compounds related to tetrahydrocannabinol have been isolated and identified from *Cannabis*. Among these compounds are cannabidiol, cannabidiolic acid, cannabigerol, and cannabinol:

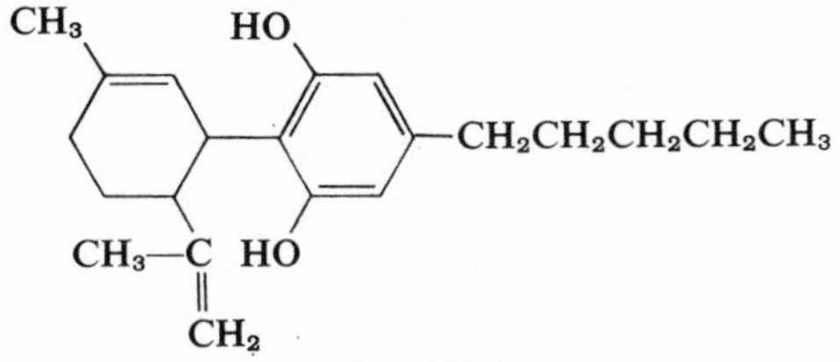

Cannabidiol

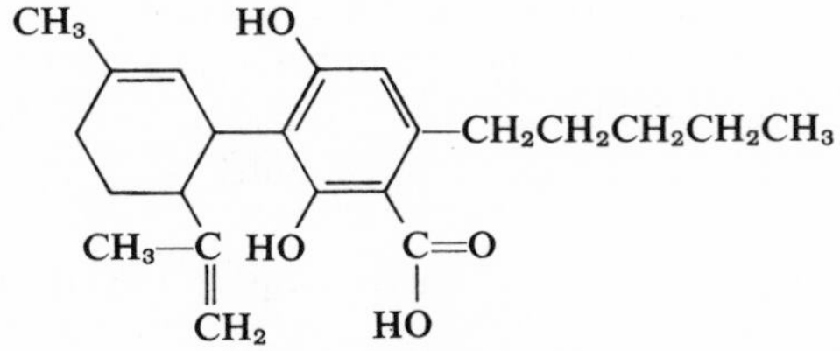

Cannabidiolic acid

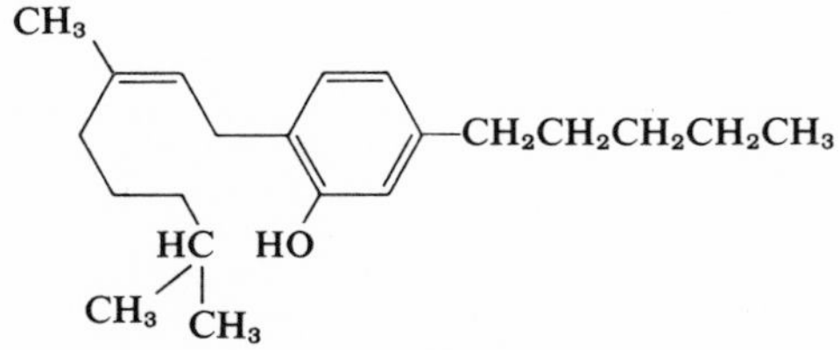

Cannabigerol

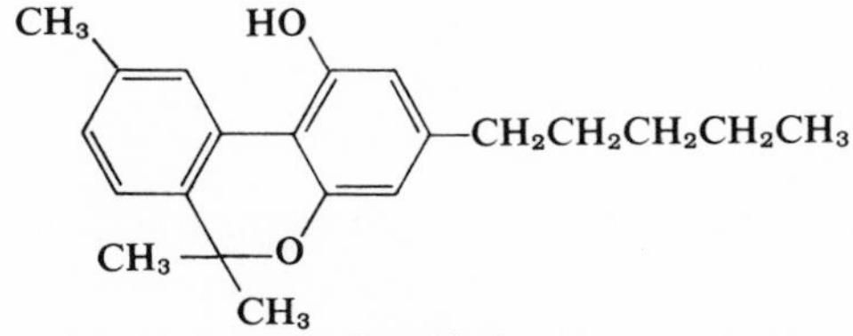

Cannabinol

When cannabidiol is heated in the presence of an acid catalyst, it is converted into a mixture of tetrahydrocannabinols that are pharmacologically active. It has been proposed that a similar conversion may occur in the plant or during the process of smoking the plant material (Adams *et al.*, 1940).

Saturation of the double bond in the unsaturated ring causes activity to decrease. In addition, shortening of the alkyl chain on the aromatic ring decreases activity, whereas branching of the chain increases activity.

Toxicology–Pharmacology: The plant of the genus *Cannabis* (marijuana) has been used by mankind for over 2000 years as a medicinal preparation or as a mild intoxicant. It is usually taken by smoking, but may also be ingested as a tea, an alcoholic extract, or in foods. The primary active component of the plant is Δ^9-tetrahydrocannabinol (THC), although some of the other related cannabinoids may add to or modify the activity when combined with the effect of THC.

The only physiological changes effected by THC are an increase in pulse rate and conjunctival vascular congestion. Dryness of the mouth and throat, and occasional dizziness or nausea, have also been noted. A marked increase in appetite and hunger is characteristic, although no explanation for this effect has been found. Subjectively, the most common reaction is the development of a dreamy state of altered consciousness, in which ideas seem disconnected, uncontrollable, and free-flowing. Space and time perception may be distorted, so that minutes seem like hours, and near objects appear far distant. Alterations of mood occur, the most characteristic being a feeling of well-being (euphoria), excitement, and laughter and hilarity to minimal stimuli.

Although some degree of tolerance develops to the effects after repeated use, no physical dependence, withdrawal symptoms, or craving occurs.

▶ **MAZINDOL**
Schedule III

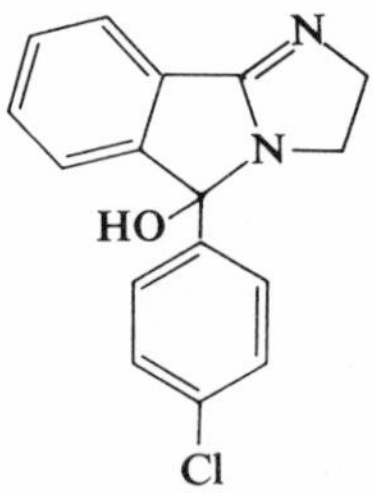

Synonym: 5-*p*-Chlorophenyl-5-hydroxy-2,3-dihydro-3*H*-imidazo-(2,1a)-iso-indole.

Pharmaceutical Preparations: Sanorex[R] (Sandoz)—Tabelts: labeled "78," on one side and "71" on the other, containing 1 mg mazindol; scored, labeled "78-66," containing 2 mg mazindol

General Comment: Mazindol is an isoindole that has pharmacological activity similar to that of the prototype drugs used in obesity, the amphetamines, and therefore has similar abuse potential.

Biochemistry: Imidazoline derivatives have been investigated following the observation that tolazoline is a potent adrenolytic and vasodilator (Chess and Yonkman, 1946):

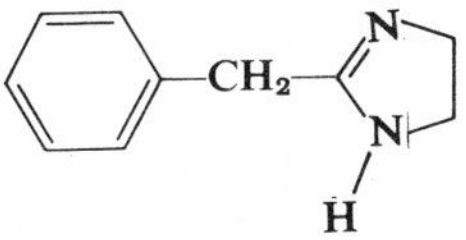

Tolazoline

From a series of 2-aminomethyl-2-imidazolines, an anorexiant sympathomimetic drug with relatively weak cardiovascular actions was developed. This drug, mazindol, causes mild stimulation in some people and mild depression in others. The mechanism of anorexiant action is unknown, but it has been postulated that lowering of brain 5-hydroxytryptamine and elevation of dopamine may be involved.

Toxicology–Pharmacology: Mazindol, an imidazoisoindole, is primarily an anorectic agent. Its pharmacological activity is in many ways similar to that of the prototype drugs used in obesity, the amphetamines. As with the amphetamines and other stimulants, drug dependence can occur, and consequently this drug is subject to abuse.

Adverse reactions may include overstimulation of the nervous system, restlessness, dizziness, insomnia, headache, weakness, dryness of the mouth, nausea, and other gastrointestinal disturbances. No data are available on overdose with mazindol.

▶ **MEBUTAMATE**
Schedule IV

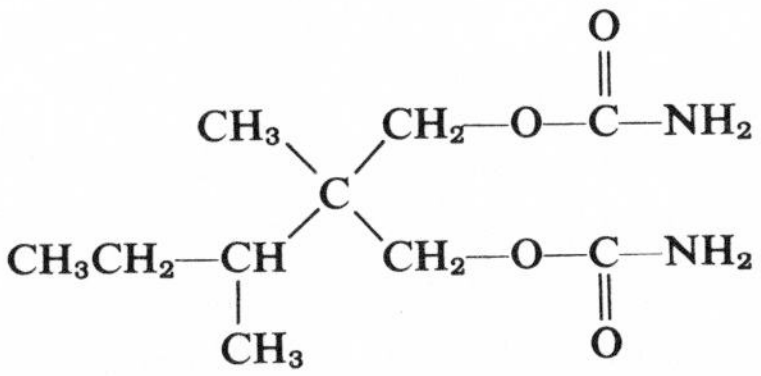

Synonym: 2-sec-Butyl-2-methyl-1,3-propanediol dicarbamate.

Pharmaceutical Preparations: Mebutamate is not found in frequently distributed pharmaceutical preparations sold in the United States.

General Comment: Mebutamate, a congener of meprobamate, is a sedative indicated for treatment of early, mild, or labile hypertension.

Biochemistry: Mebutamate is a bis-carbamate analogue of meprobamate. It

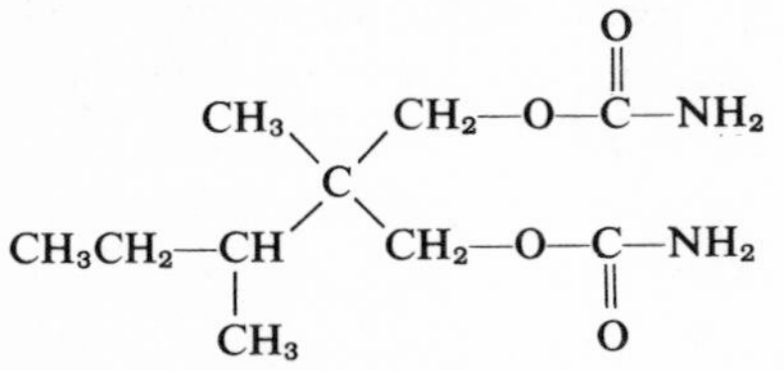

Mebutamate 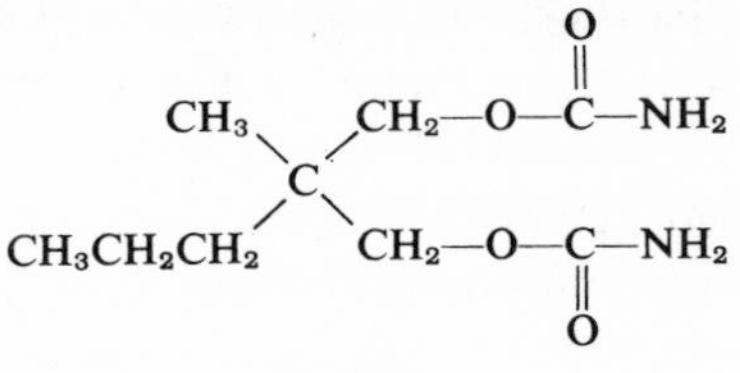   Meprobamate

has been investigated as a central relaxant and is specifically indicated for hypertension (Berger *et al.*, 1961). Although clinical studies with dogs indicate mebutamate's antihypertensive efficacy, supportive data in man are lacking.

Toxicology–Pharmacology: Mebutamate is a congener of meprobamate, and has some sedative and tranquilizing effects similar to those of meprobamate. It has antihypertensive action in the treatment of early or mild hypertension through an action on the vasomotor control centers in the brainstem. Its primary therapeutic usefulness is in the treatment of hypertension.

After a 300-mg dose of mebutamate, a blood concentration of 0.67 mg/dl was obtained after 1 hour. After 3 hours, the concentration was 0.48 mg/dl (Douglas *et al.*, 1962). Lethal concentrations are not known, but may be presumed to be in excess of 5.00 mg/dl due to its similarity to meprobamate.

▶ **MECLOQUALONE**
Schedule I

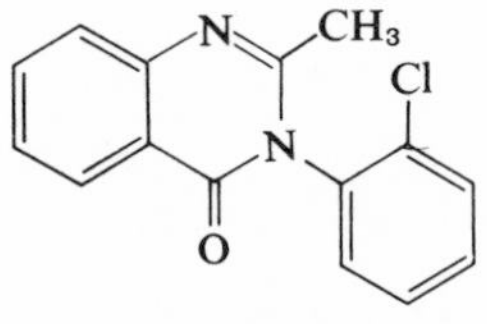

Synonym: 2-Methyl-3(2′-chlorophenyl)-4(3*H*)-quinazolinone.

Pharmaceutical Preparations: Mecloqualone is not found in any pharmaceutical preparations sold in the United States.

General Comments: Mecloqualone is a nonbarbiturate hypnotic of the quinazolinone series to which methaqualone also belongs. Mecloqualone is not accepted for medicinal use in the United States.

Biochemistry: Mecloqualone is a quinazolinone hypnotic and a derivative of methaqualone. The derivatization comes about by the replacement of the methyl group in the o-tolyl moiety by chlorine. The resulting structural modification substantially increases activity. The hypnotic activity of the o-chloro derivative is higher than that of the m- or p-chloro compounds. However, the o-chloro derivative is the least toxic (Boissier *et al.*, 1967).

Toxicology–Pharmacology: Not known. Probably similar to that of methaqualone.

▶ **MEPHENTERMINE**
Noncontrolled Substance

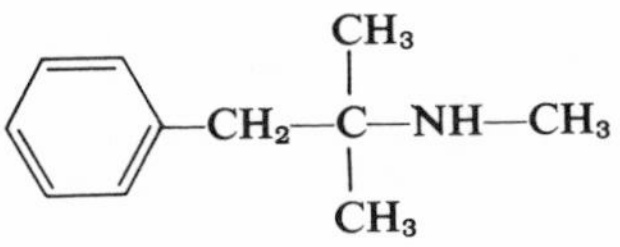

General Comments: Mephentermine is a sympathomimetic amine with characteristic activity useful for treatment of hypotensive conditions. It is also therapeutically useful as a nasal decongestant. Mephentermine closely resembles ephedrine, both qualitatively and quantitatively.

Toxicology–Pharmacology: Mephentermine is a sympathomimetic amine with pressor activity, used for the treatment of hypotensive conditions. As a sympathomimetic agent, it is also a bronchodilator, and may be used as a decongestant. It is effective in treatment of shock, hypotension following surgery, and hypotension resulting from heart disease. It is usually administered intramuscularly or intravenously. Adverse side effects include headache, anxiety, weakness, dizziness, tremor, palpitation, and some central stimulation.

▶ **MEPHOBARBITAL**
Schedule IV

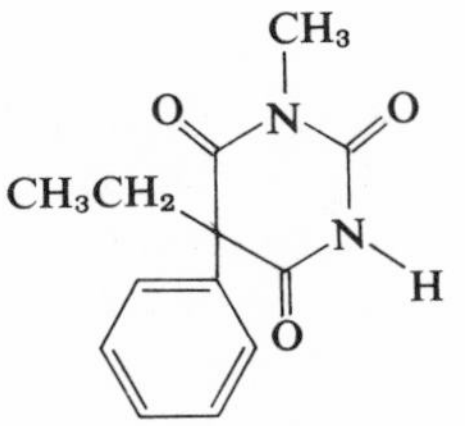

Synonym: 5-Ethyl-1-methyl-5-phenylbarbituric acid.

Pharmaceutical Preparations

Mebaral[R] (Winthrop)—Tablets: 32, 50, 100, and 200 mg mephobarbital
Mebroin[R] (Winthrop)—Tablets, scored: containing 250 mg mephobarbital
Also see Chapter 6.

General Comment: Mephobarbital is a long-acting barbiturate with less sedative action than phenobarbital.

Biochemistry: Mephobarbital is a derivative of phenobarbital having a methyl group at the 3 position of the barbiturate ring. The N-dealkylation and the oxygenation of C^5-substituents are competing reactions in the metabolism of mephobarbital. In this competition, demethylation occurs more rapidly, and mephobarbital is metabolized to phenobarbital:

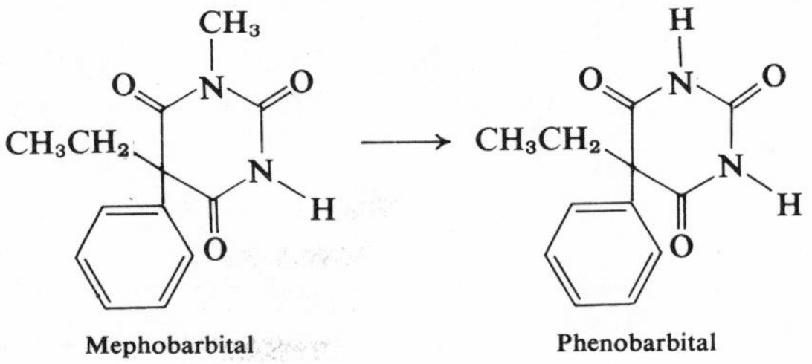

Mephobarbital   Phenobarbital

Toxicology–Pharmacology: Mephobarbital is a long-acting barbiturate, similar in actions to phenobarbital. It is a less potent sedative than phenobarbital, and is used primarily as an anticonvulsant in petit mal and grand mal epilepsy. It is also used as a general sedative, due to the slow release of phenobarbital as demethylation of the parent compound occurs.

Doses of 400–600 mg per day may be used in epilepsy, while a sedative dose for adults is 32–100 mg, three times a day.

A 600-mg oral dose, taken daily for five days, gave a plasma level of 1.50 mg/dl, 12 hours after the last dose. The phenobarbital concentration was 3.2 mg/dl, 60 hours after the last dose (Butler and Woddall, 1958).

▶ **MEPROBAMATE**
Schedule IV

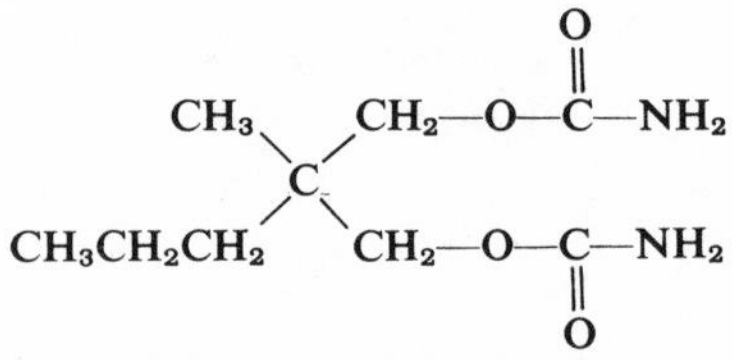

Synonym: 2-Methyl-2-n-propyl-1,3-propanediol.

Pharmaceutical Preparations

Deprol[R] (Wallace)—Tablets: light pink, scored, containing 400 mg meprobamate and 1 mg benactyzine

Equanil[R] (Wyeth)—Tablets: white, scored, containing 200 or 400 mg meprobamate; yellow, coated, containing 400 mg meprobamate. Capsules: red
and clear, labeled "WYETH-44," containing 400 mg meprobamate.

Meprospan[R] (Wallace)—Capsules: blue-top, containing 400 mg meprobamate; yellow-top, containing 200 mg meprobamate

Meprotabs[R] (Wallace)—Tablets: white, coated, containing 400 mg meprobamate

Miltown[R] (Wallace)—Tablets: white, scored, containing 400 mg meprobamate; white, coated, containing 200 mg meprobamate

Qidbamate[R] (Mallinckrodt)—Tablets: containing 400 mg meprobamate

Sk-Bamate[R] (Smith Kline & French)—Tablets: white, containing 200 or 400
mg meprobamate

Also see Chapter 6.

General Comments: None.

Biochemistry: Meprobamate was introduced in 1955 as a treatment for
anxiety. Basically, the metabolism of meprobamate leads to inactivation. In
addition to the unchanged drug, the glucuronide conjugate and a hydroxyl
derivative are found as metabolites.

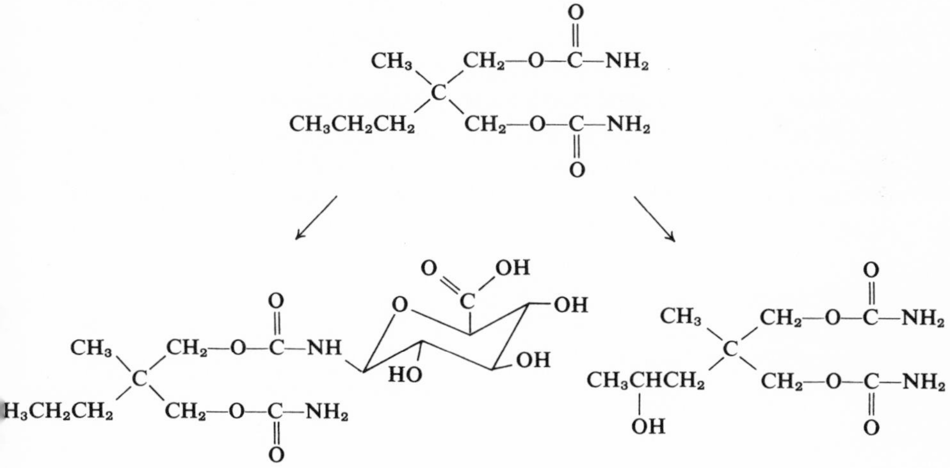

Meprobamate was synthesized in 1951 along with several mono- and
dicarbamate derivatives of propanediol. In 1954, it was determined that
meprobamate was the most potent anticonvulsant in the series. Following

this, it was determined that meprobamate was an effective muscle relaxant that had a duration of action eight times longer than that of mephenesin, an antianxiety agent in use prior to meprobamate (Ludwig and Piech, 1951; Berger, 1954).

Toxicology–Pharmacology: Meprobamate is widely used for its tranquilizing and muscle-relaxant properties. It exerts a "taming" effect on animals and protects mice from death from convulsions induced by convulsant drugs or induced by electroshock. Monkeys given a dose of meprobamate lose their fear, hostility, and aggressiveness and become tame.

Meprobamate is used in humans to provide relief in anxiety and tension states, in the treatment of musculoskeletal disorders, and sometimes as an anticonvulsant in mild forms of epilepsy.

Some physical and psychological dependence has been observed after prolonged usage. Sudden withdrawal of the drug after prolonged and excessive use may be followed by recurrence of preexisting symptoms, such as anxiety, anorexia, or insomnia, or by withdrawal reactions, such as vomiting, ataxia, tremors, muscle twitching, confusion, hallucinations, and, in rare instances, epileptic-type seizures. Due to its tranquilizing actions, meprobamate has synergistic actions when combined with alcohol or other depressant medications. Therapeutic dosage may be up to 2.40 g per day, although therapeutic effects are usually achieved with 300–400 mg three or four times a day. After a single 400-mg dose, a blood concentration of 0.50 mg/dl was observed, while after a 1200-mg dose, a blood concentration of 2.00 mg/dl was obtained.

Fatal overdose does not usually occur with blood concentrations of less than 10.0 mg/dl, although nonfatal poisonings have been described with concentrations ranging from 1.1 to 10.2 mg/dl (Maes et al., 1969). Tolerance to meprobamate is illustrated by a report of two motor-vehicle drivers found to have concentrations of 9.0 and 9.6 mg/dl of meprobamate in their blood (Graves and Schwartz, 1974).

▶ **MEPRODINE**
Schedule I

Synonym: 3-Ethyl-1-methyl-4-phenyl-4-propionyloxypiperidine.
Pharmaceutical Preparations: Meprodine is not found in any pharmaceutical preparations sold in the United States.
Biochemistry: Similar to that of prodine.
Toxicology–Pharmacology: Both α- and β-meprodine are listed in most texts as narcotic analgesics. It is the homologue of prodine with an ethyl group in place of the piperidine methyl group. The toxicity is similar to that of prodine.

▶ **MESCALINE**
Schedule I

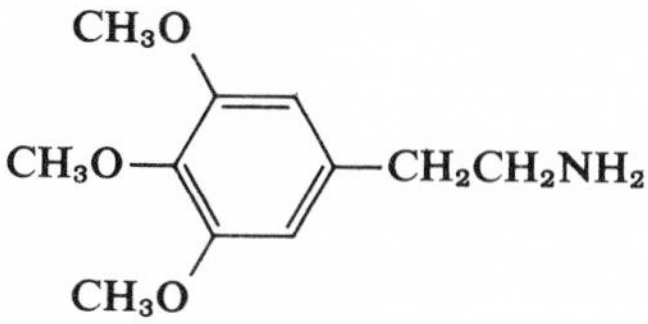

$$CH_3O$$

$$CH_3O- -CH_2CH_2NH_2$$

$$CH_3O$$

Synonym: 3,4,5-Trimethoxyphenethylamine.
Pharmaceutical Preparations: Mescaline is not found in any pharmaceutical preparations sold in the United States.
General Comments: Mescaline is the primary active hallucinogen of the peyote cactus. It can also be produced synthetically. A dose of 350–500 mg mescaline produces illusions and hallucinations lasting from 5 to 12 hours.
Biochemistry: A large number of psychotomimetic drugs from botanical sources have originated in Central America and Mexico. In these areas, the drugs have been used therapeutically and in religious ceremonies dating back to ancient Indian civilizations of 1000 years B.C.

The three major drugs from Mexican plants are mescaline, psilocybin, and the alkaloids of ololiuqui. Mescaline is the principal alkaloid from *Lophophora williamsii* (Lem.) Coulter. This plant is a cactus that grows in the deserts of northern Mexico and the Southwestern United States and is more commonly referred to as peyote.

Mescaline is readily absorbed and is concentrated in the kidney, liver, and spleen. Surprisingly, it does not reach a high concentration in the brain. About 60–90 percent is excreted unchanged in the urine. In addition to the unchanged drug, about 25 percent is changed during metabolism to an inactive metabolite, 3,4,5-trimethoxyphenylacetic acid. The metabolic scheme is shown below:

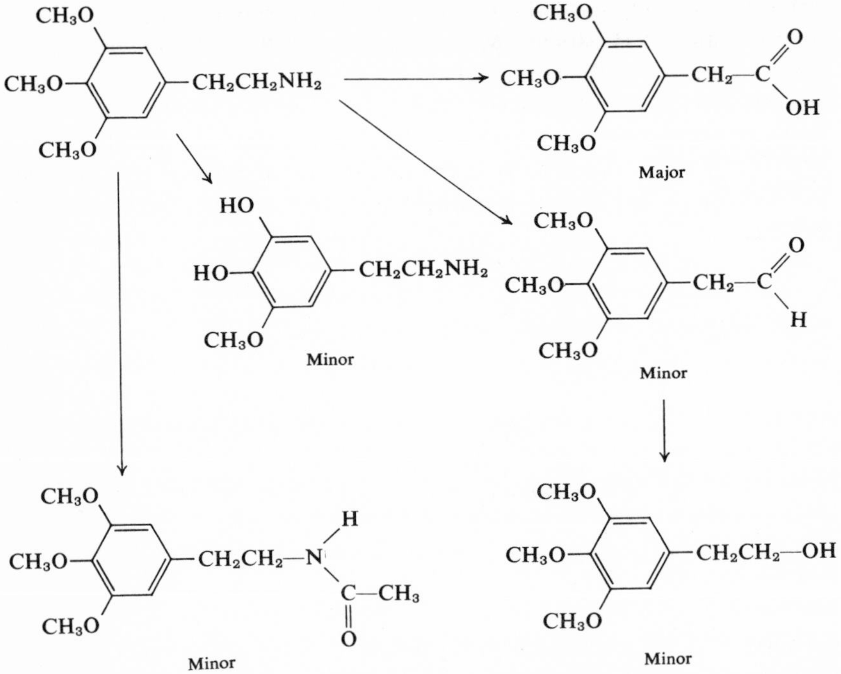

CH₃O—, CH₃O—, CH₃O— (ring) —CH₂CH₂NH₂ → CH₃O—, CH₃O—, CH₃O— (ring) —CH₂—C(=O)OH   **Major**

HO—, HO—, CH₃O— (ring) —CH₂CH₂NH₂   **Minor**

CH₃O—, CH₃O—, CH₃O— (ring) —CH₂—C(=O)H   **Minor**

CH₃O—, CH₃O—, CH₃O— (ring) —CH₂CH₂—N(H)—C(=O)—CH₃   **Minor**

CH₃O—, CH₃O—, CH₃O— (ring) —CH₂CH₂—OH   **Minor**

It has been shown that branching of the ethylamine chain by a methyl group increases psychotropic potency. An example of such a branching is 3,4,5-trimethoxyamphetamine.

Toxicology–Pharmacology: Mescaline is a hallucinogenic drug, inducing gradual changes in spatial and temporal consciousness. Time is experienced as emptiness or timelessness. It induces visual hallucinations, often consisting in brightly colored lights and geometric designs. In addition, the usual oral dose of 5 mg/kg causes, in humans, anxiety, sympathomimetic effects, hyperreflexia of the limbs, and static tremors. Mescaline has been used as an experimental tool for the investigation of schizophrenia and other psychotic states.

Mescaline does not induce addiction, and there has been no demonstration of abstinence symptoms when the drug is withdrawn.

When ingested as the crude peyote buttons, 2–20 buttons are required for the hallucinogenic properties (Fischer, 1958). No data are available on blood concentrations after use of mescaline. Toxic effects are usually limited to results of gastrointestinal irritation, nausea and vomiting being common effects, and psychological disturbances.

Mescaline is metabolized to 3,4,5-trimethoxy phenylacetic acid and 3,4-dihydroxy-5-methoxy phenylacetic acid, which is excreted as a glutamine conjugate. Human subjects given mescaline orally excreted 81.9 percent of the administered dose in the urine during the first 12 hours (Charalampous *et al.*, 1964).

▶ **METAZOCINE**
Schedule II

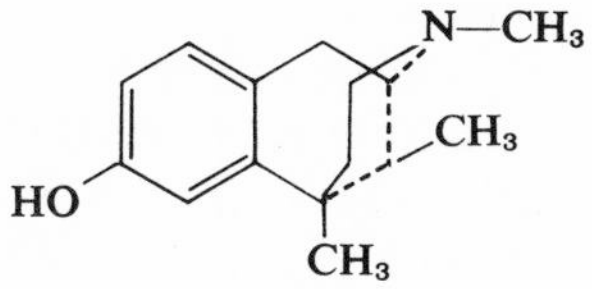

Synonym: 1,2,3,4,5,6-Hexahydro-8-hydroxy-3,11-trimethyl-2,6-methano-3-benzazocine.

Pharmaceutical Preparations: Metazocine is not frequently found in pharmaceutical preparations sold in the United States.

General Comment: Metazocine is a synthetic narcotic analgesic in the benzomorphinan series.

Biochemistry: Metazocine is a synthetic narcotic analgetic in the 6,7-benzomorphan class. Both the *dextro* and *levo* isomers are potent analgetics, but the *dextro* isomer is more toxic. It is similar to other 5,9-dialkylbenzomorphans with respect to lack of the property to suppress the morphine abstinence syndrome. It is comparable to morphine in the relief of postoperative pain, however.

Toxicology–Pharmacology: Unknown.

▶ **METHADOL**
Schedule I

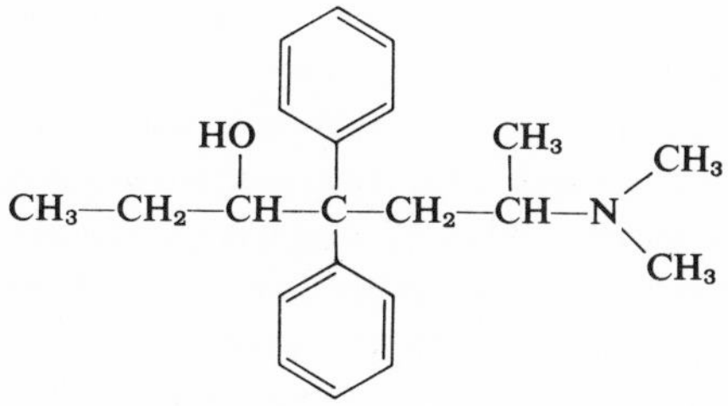

Synonym: (α,β)-6-Dimethylamino-4,4-diphenylheptan-3-ol.

Pharmaceutical Preparations: Methadol is not found in any pharmaceutical preparations sold in the United States.

General Comments: Methadol is structurally similar to methadone, and is thus a narcotic analgesic. However, it has not been accepted for medicinal use in the United States. It is controlled as separate substances under Federal law, specifically listing its isomers, α-methadol and β-methadol.

Biochemistry: Methadol is produced by the reduction of methadone. This reduction forms a second asymmetric center in the molecule, thus producing four isomers. For example, $R(-)$-methadone produces α$(+)$-methadol and β$(-)$-methadol, while $S(+)$-methadone produces α$(-)$- methadol and β$(+)$-methadol. It has been determined that the α$(-)$ isomer is the most potent methadol isomer. This may seem strange, as it is formed from the least potent methadone isomer, $S(+)$-methadone. From this information, it would seem that the C-3 rather than the C-6 configuration is of prime importance (Veath *et al.*, 1964). The next most potent isomer is β$(-)$-methadol.

Toxicology–Pharmacology: Similar to that of methadone.

▶ **METHADONE**
Schedule II

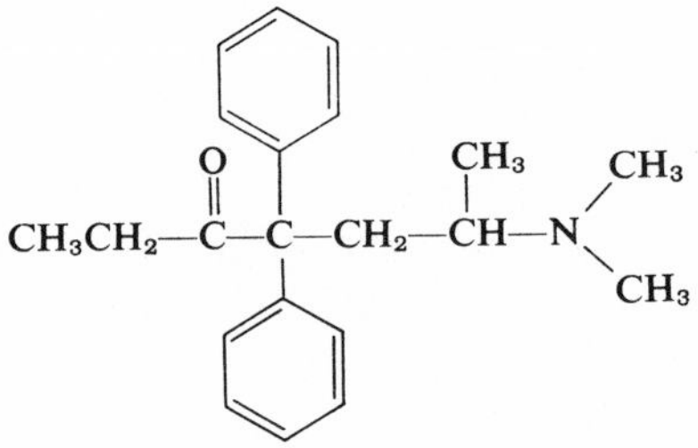

Synonyms: Amidon, amidone, phenadon, phenadone, $(+)$-6-dimethylamino-4,4-diphenylheptan-3-one.

Pharmaceutical Preparations: Dolophine^R (Lilly)—Ampules: each 1 ml containing 10 mg methadone hydrochloride. Tablets: containing 5 or 10 mg methadone hydrochloride.

General Comments: Under the Federal methadone regulations, methadone has not, until recently, been available from community pharmacies for use as an analgesic without specific approval of each pharmacy by FDA. This restriction was intended to prevent widespread availability of the drug outside of hospitals and formal methadone treatment programs. A suit by the American Pharmaceutical Association (APhA), upheld in the U.S. Court of Appeals for the District of Columbia Circuit, eliminated this restriction, and methadone is now available in community pharmacies for prescription as an analgesic, subject only to the restrictions of Schedule II of the Controlled Substances Act.

The closed distribution system that governs use of methadone for maintenance and detoxification of narcotic addicts will continue in effect under the regulations promulgated under the Narcotic Addict Treatment Act of 1974. These regulations require registration with the Drug Enforcement Administration (DEA) for all maintenance and detoxification treatment, except (1) when such treatment is provided for hospitalized patients as an incidental adjunct to medical or surgical treatment of conditions other than addiction or (2) when a narcotic drug is administered for up to 3 days on an emergency basis to treat withdrawal symptoms while arrangements are being made to refer a patient to a treatment and rehabilitation program.

Methadone is currently the only narcotic drug approved for detoxification and maintenance treatment of narcotic addiction. In the future, the Department of Health, Education and Welfare will be preparing revised regulations under the Narcotic Addict Treatment Act of 1974 that will apply to the use of methadone or any other narcotic drug for maintenance or detoxification (Schmidt *et al.*, 1976).

Biochemistry: Methadone is a potent synthetic narcotic analgesic. The two major urinary excretion products are the unchanged methadone and the demethylated, cyclized pyrrolidine:

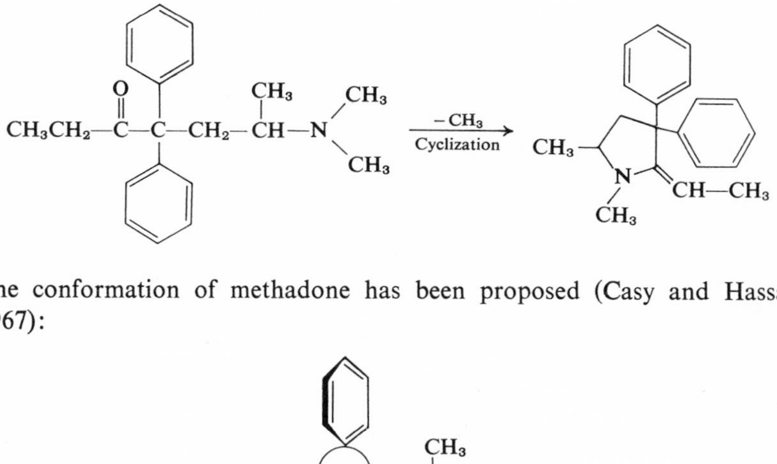

The conformation of methadone has been proposed (Casy and Hassan, 1967):

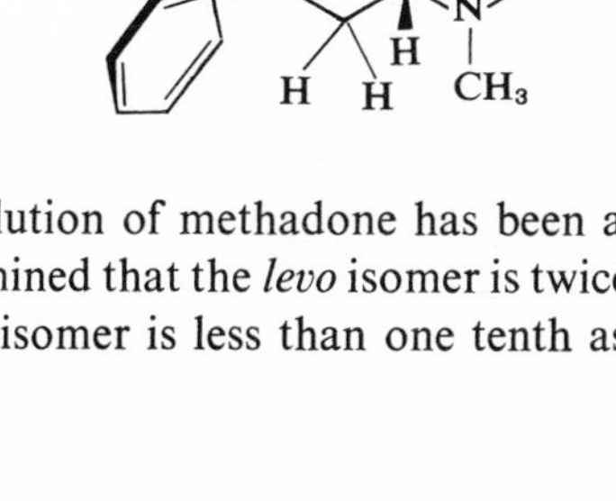

The optical resolution of methadone has been accomplished, and from this it has been determined that the *levo* isomer is twice as potent as morphine. However, the *dextro* isomer is less than one tenth as effective as morphine.

Basically, however, the racemic mixture is equivalent in its pharmacological actions to the *levo* isomer.

Toxicology–Pharmacology: The pharmacological effects of methadone are qualitatively the same as those of morphine. It is therefore a narcotic drug having the classic properties of inducing analgesia, sleep, tolerance, and addiction. The distinctive properties of methadone are its efficacy when taken by the oral route and its extended duration of action. Like other narcotic drugs, it causes sedation and respiratory depression. It also has significant antitussive effects. It is not especially effective for rapid relief of pain after a single dose, but is excellent for use in chronic severe pain.

Methadone has mild euphoric actions in nondependent patients, but its effect is more pronounced in dependent patients. Its addictive property is less than that of heroin or morphine, but it produces cross-tolerance to heroin and other opiates. In heroin addicts, tolerance to methadone can be established and maintained with a constant daily oral dose, so that it becomes possible to block the action of heroin and eliminate the hunger for narcotic drugs.

The most significant use of methadone today is not for its analgetic properties, but for its ability to suppress the craving for heroin in heroin addicts. In the numerous "methadone maintenance" programs now operating, methadone is given orally in doses of 20–130 mg to addicts, suppressing withdrawal symptoms, and permitting rehabilitation treatment. Methadone does not induce the euphoria of heroin, and effectively suppresses the craving for the latter drug.

Plasma levels of methadone after a single oral dose of 15 mg were maximal at 4 hours with 0.0075 mg/dl (Inturresi and Verebely, 1972). In methadone maintenance patients taking daily oral dosages of 100–120 mg, maximum blood concentrations of 0.083 mg/dl were observed at 2 hours after dosing. At 24 hours, the concentrations were 0.046 mg/dl (Inturresi and Verebely, 1972).

Due to the long-acting nature of the drug, the overdose victim often lies unconscious for long periods of time, during which time much of the drug is metabolized. In deaths, the blood concentrations may vary from less than 0.01 to 0.30 mg/dl (Garriott *et al.*, 1973; Robinson and Williams, 1971).

▶ **METHAMPHETAMINE**
Schedule II

$$CH_2CH-NH-CH_3$$
$$\overset{\displaystyle CH_3}{|}$$

Synonyms: Methylamphetamine, deoxyephedrine, desoxyephedrine, phenyl-methylaminopropane, N,α-dimethylphenethylamine.

Pharmaceutical Preparations

Desoxyn[R] (Abbott)—Tablets: containing 2.5 or 5 mg methamphetamine hydrochloride

Fetamin[R] (Mission)—Tablet: containing 5 mg methamphetamine hydrochloride

Obetrol[R] (Obetrol)—See **AMPHETAMINE**

The following pharmaceutical preparation, Phelantin[R], appears to be controlled under the Federal Controlled Substances Act as a Schedule III preparation. However, no specific explanation for control can be determined.

 Phelantin[R] Kapseals (Parke-Davis)—Capsule: containing 2.5 mg methamphetamine hydrochloride, 30 mg phenobarbital, and 100 mg phenytoin

General Comments: None.

Biochemistry: See Toxicology–Pharmacology below and **AMPHETAMINE.**

Toxicology–Pharmacology: The pharmacological actions of methamphetamine are similar to those of amphetamine, but it exhibits a different ratio between central and peripheral actions. Small doses of methamphetamine have prominent central stimulant actions with significant peripheral actions. Larger doses produce rises in blood pressure due to cardiac stimulation.

Moderate doses of methamphetamine produce an elevation of mood, a sense of increased energy and alertness, and decreased appetite. The latter property accounts for the extensive use of amphetamines to aid in combating obesity. Tolerance and some psychological dependence occur as the result of chronic use of amphetamine, and oral and intravenous abuse has been common. Methamphetamine has been available from illicit sources in the crystalline form and is commonly known as "crystal." This is soluble in aqueous solution and may be injected intravenously. In serious abuse, methamphetamine is injected intravenously (mainlining) in large doses in the range 500–1000 mg, and at intervals as short as 2 hours. This may lead to use of as much as 1500 mg in a single day, and abuse may be as long as 6 or 7 days.

Following intravenous injection, the user experiences a sudden, generalized, overwhelming, pleasureful feeling called a "flash" or a "rush." He has intense fascination with all his thoughts and activities, which extends even to the paranoid fear and anger that almost inevitably follow. Sexual interest is enhanced in most people. Appetite for food is completely suppressed. During a period of chronic use of the drug, a weight loss of 20–30 pounds may occur. Solid food seems impossible to swallow during this period. Abscesses, nonhealing ulcers, and brittle fingernails develop, probably secondary to the malnourished state.

At the start of a "run" with methamphetamine, the activity of the user is purposeful, but after some hours it becomes less so, at times is compulsive, and ultimately becomes grossly disorganized. Paranoid reactions develop sooner or later. After initial experimentation, a pattern of use of the drug is to inject it every 2 hours around the clock for 3–6 days, during which the subject remains awake continuously; rarely, the "run" continues 12 days. The user is then so exhausted, disorganized, tense, or paranoid that he ceases using the drug and goes to sleep, although sometimes a barbiturate is needed to induce sleep. After a "run" of 3 or 4 days, the subject sleeps 12–18 hours, but after a longer "run" he may be semicomatose for 4 or 5 days. On waking, the subject is famished and his paranoid state is largely dissipated, but he may express lethargy and depression. Prolonged psychoses or brain damage may result from such use. Crimes of violence may be committed by users.

After a 10-mg oral dose of methamphetamine, a blood concentration of 0.003 mg/dl was observed in 1 hour (Lebish *et al.*, 1970). After death from intravenous overdose, blood concentrations of methamphetamine may vary from 0.01 to 0.56 mg/dl (Cravey and Reed, 1970; Patterson and Peat, 1976).

Methamphetamine is excreted in the urine as the unchanged drug, and its major metabolite, amphetamine. Approximately 6% of the dose is excreted as amphetamine in 24 hours, and 11% in 48 hours. About 61% of the dose is excreted as unchanged drug in 24 hours, and 68% in 48 hours (Rowland and Beckett, 1966).

▶ **METHAPYRILENE**
Noncontrolled Substance

General Comment: Methapyrilene is an antihistaminic drug that is encountered in abused drug samples due to its common use as an adulterant for heroin. **Toxicology–Pharmacology:** Methapyrilene is in the class of antihistaminic drugs. Its primary usefulness is to counteract histaminic responses in the body, due to allergic manifestations of hay fever, rhinitis, allergic cough, chronic urticaria, and other conditions. In addition to this property, methapyrilene, as many other antihistaminics, has some central depressant actions. It often induces drowsiness, even when used in therapeutic doses. As a result of this property, it is also often used in over-the-counter sedative proportions used to treat insomnia. It is thus readily available to the public. In addition, methapyrilene is one of the commonest substances used to "cut" illicit heroin samples in some parts of the United States. It may then be detected (as a metabolite) in urine samples of drug abusers.

Methapyrilene is rapidly metabolized in the body after oral administration, and is seldomly detected in blood samples after therapeutic usage. It is more commonly detected as a metabolite in urine. Although few deaths from overdose have been reported, massive overdose results in central nervous system depression, and possible convulsions. In a death from methapyrilene and alcohol, a blood level of 0.44 mg/dl was recorded, with a blood alcohol of 90 mg/dl (Fatteh, 1972).

▶ **METHAQUALONE**
Schedule II

Synonym: 2-Methyl-3-O-tolyl-4-($3H$)-quinazolinone.
Pharmaceutical Preparations
Quaalude[R] (Rorer)—Tablets: white, scored, containing 150 or 300 mg methaqualone
Sopor[R] (Arnar-Stone)—Tablets, scored yellow, 150 mg methaqualone; orange, 300 mg methaqualone
General Comments: None.
Biochemistry: Methaqualone is a quinazolinone derivative. It was evaluated as a hypnotic in 1955 and finally produced commercially in 1965.

It has been determined in rats that methaqualone acts on the respiratory chain prior to the point of electron transfer from NADH to cytochrome b (Seth and Parmar, 1965).
Toxicology–Pharmacology: Methaqualone has hypnotic effects similar to those of the barbiturates. It has anticonvulsant properties in experimentally induced convulsions in animals, and it has antitussive properties comparable to those of codeine. When taken orally in doses of 150–200 mg, it induces sleep, usually within 10–20 minutes.

Methaqualone is prescribed extensively as a nighttime sedative–hypnotic. It has become one of the most popular street drugs in many cities of the United States, and has to some extent replaced the barbiturates in this respect (Pascarelli, 1973). As a result, it is often encountered in confiscated drug samples, in blood samples from motor-vehicle drivers, and in autopsy samples analyzed in medical examiners' offices (Garriott and Latman, 1976).

After a 300-mg oral dose, the average plasma concentration was 0.30

mg/dl in 2 hours. At 4 hours, the concentration had fallen to 0.19 mg/dl, and at 8 hours, to 0.06 mg/dl. The plasma half-life was 2.6 hours (Morris *et al.*, 1972). After one 400-mg dose, a maximum plasma concentration of 0.54 mg/dl was observed at 2 hours, in one subject, while a range of 0.10–0.40 mg/dl occurred in the remaining group at 2 hours (Waggoner *et al.*, 1973).

▶ **METHARBITAL**
Schedule III

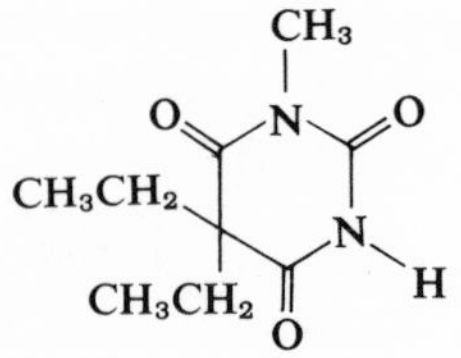

Synonym: 5,5-Diethyl-1-methylbarbituric acid.
Pharmaceutical Preparations: Gemonil[R] (Abbott)—Tablets: containing 100 mg metharbital.
General Comments: Metharbital is a long-acting barbiturate that has anti-epileptic action similar to that of phenobarbital but is less potent. It appears to be less depressant and hypnotic than phenobarbital. Its listing in Schedule III is improper and should be under Schedule IV.
Biochemistry: Metharbital is the N-1 methyl derivative of barbital. Like barbital, it is a long-acting barbiturate. However, it is demethylated at a much less rapid rate as compared with mephobarbital. The oxidation of the C-5 substituent appears to lead to competition metabolically with demethylation:

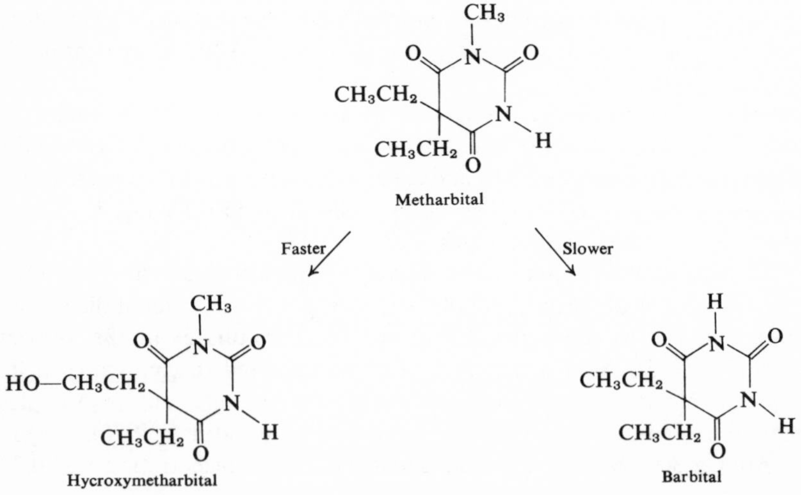

Metharbital

Faster / Slower

Hycroxymetharbital

Barbital

Toxicology–Pharmacology: Metharbital is a long-acting barbiturate, differing from barbital only in having a methyl substituent at a nitrogen atom. It is used primarily for its anticonvulsant potential, and is recommended for control of grand mal, petit mal, myoclonic, and mixed types of seizures. It has generally low toxicity, although dizziness and drowsiness may occur as adverse side effects. It is metabolized in the liver by demethylation to barbital.

Metharbital is usually effective in doses of 100–300 mg per day, although some patients may require up to 600–800 mg per day. After administration of 300 mg metharbital per day, no parent drug was detected in the plasma 8 hours after dosage (Butler, 1958). It may be presumed to be similar to barbital in toxicity and in lethal blood concentrations.

▶ **METHENAMINE**
Noncontrolled Substance

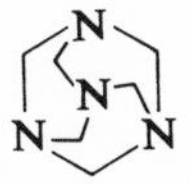

General Comment: Methenamine is a urinary antibacterial that has been encountered in cases of drug abuse because of its similarity to amphetamines in name only.

Toxicology–Pharmacology: Methenamine has mildly irritant and antiseptic properties. It is used primarily as a urinary antiseptic, although, today, much more effective agents are available. At acid pH, methenamine is converted to formaldehyde. It is this product that probably has the antiseptic actions.

In large doses, methenamine induces violent inflammation of the urinary tract, resulting in albuminuria, hematuria, and tenesmus. It has no known systemic or other toxic actions.

▶ **METHOCARBAMOL**
Dangerous Drug

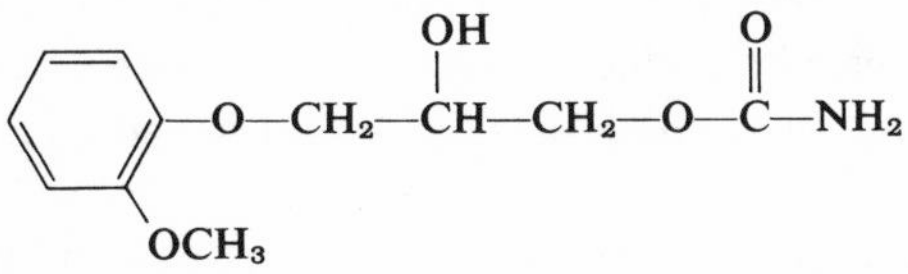

Synonym: 3-(*O*-Methoxyphenoxy)-1,2-propanediol-1-carbamate.

Pharmaceutical Preparations

Robaxin[R] (Robins)—Injection: each 1 ml containing 100 mg methocarbamol.
  Tablets: white, scored, containing 500 mg methocarbamol; white,
  scored, capsule-shaped, containing 750 mg methocarbamol.

Robaxisal[R] (Robins)—Tablets: Pink and white laminated, containing 400 mg
  methocarbamol and 325 mg aspirin

General Comments: Methocarbamol is a skeletal muscle relaxant. It is listed
in this text as a Dangerous Drug because all pharmaceutical preparations
containing methocarbamol require a prescription and bear the legend "Caution: Federal law prohibits dispensing without a prescription."

Biochemistry: Methocarbamol is a muscle relaxant with actions and chemistry similar to those of mephenesin, its prototype.

Toxicology–Pharmacology: Methocarbamol is a centrally acting muscle
relaxant. It produces little sedation in doses that are effective for muscle-relaxant activity. It may be given intramuscularly or intravenously to relieve
severe pain from muscle spasm. In fracture and accident cases, it relieves
spasm and muscle soreness.

  Adverse effects may include lightheadedness, dizziness, drowsiness,
nausea, allergic manifestations, blurred vision, and fever. Severe toxicity
reactions are rare, however.

  The usual adult dosage is 1.5–2 g four times a day.

▶ **METHOHEXITAL**
Schedule IV

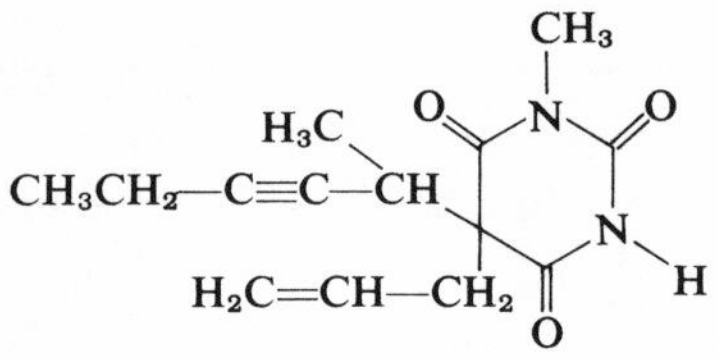

Synonyms: Methohexitone, 1-methyl-5-allyl-5-(1-methyl-2-pentynyl) barbituric acid.

Pharmaceutical Preparations: Brevital[R] (Lilly)—Injection.

General Comments: Methohexital is improperly listed in Schedule IV with
phenobarbital and barbital, which are long-acting barbiturates. Even though
it is not available for abuse, methohexital should be more appropriately listed
in Schedule III.

Biochemistry: In the metabolic competition of N-demethylation and oxidation, it is the (ω-1) oxidation of the 5-methylpentynyl substituent that supersedes. The metabolite hydroxymethohexital has been found as the major metabolite, while the *N*-demethylated product may be found in less than 1% of the initial dose:

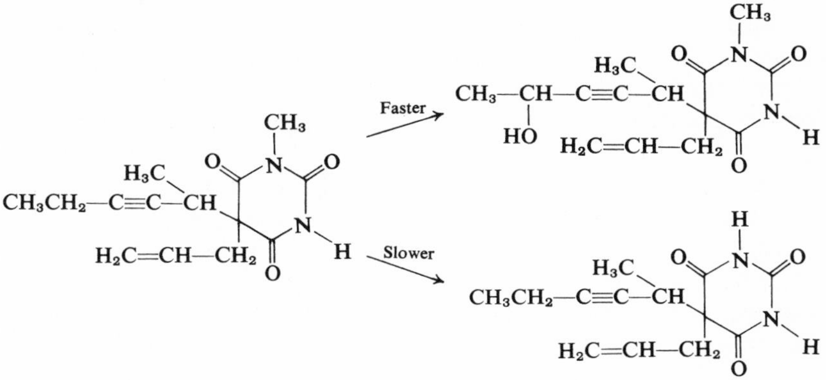

Toxicology–Pharmacology: Methohexital is classified pharmacologically as an ultra-short-acting barbiturate. It is used for the rapid induction of anesthesia, as an intravenous anesthetic for short surgical procedures, or as an agent for inducing a hypnotic state.

It is rapidly metabolized by the liver, and excreted primarily as hydroxymethohexital (Welles *et al.*, 1963).

Methohexital has a plasma half-life of only about 3.5 hours (Brodie, 1952). After a 525-mg oral dose, an average blood concentration of 0.17 mg/dl was observed in 30 minutes. After 1 hour, a blood concentration of 0.14 mg/dl was seen (Bush *et al.*, 1966).

▶ **METHOTRIMEPRAZINE**
Dangerous Drug

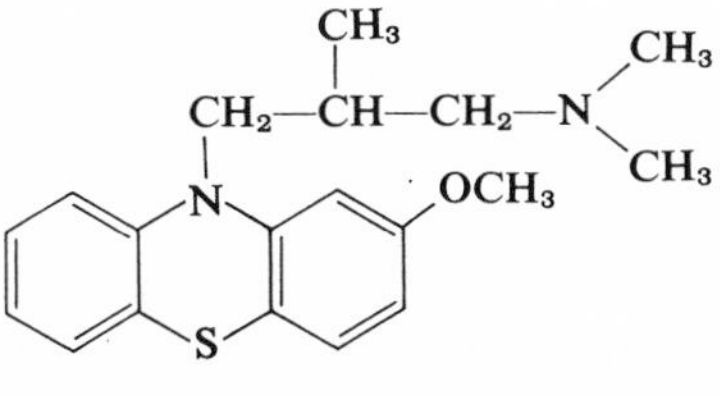

Synonym: (−)-10-[3-(Dimethylamino)-2-methylpropyl]-2-methoxyphenothiazine.
Pharmaceutical Preparations: Levoprome[R] (Lederle)—Ampules: each 1 ml containing 20 mg methotrimeprazine.
General Comments: Methotrimeprazine is a phenothiazine tranquilizer and is

therefore classified in this text as a Dangerous Drug. It is also a potent non-narcotic analgesic and sedative used in nonambulatory patients by intra-muscular injection.

Biochemistry: In a study with methotrimeprazine in mice, a loss of coordin-ated motor ability was observed to vary directly with the concentration of un-metabolized drug in the brain. This primarily suggests that methotrimepra-zine, not a metabolite, is responsible for the pharmacological action (Afifi and Way, 1967).

Toxicology–Pharmacology: Methotrimeprazine is a 2-methoxy derivative of trimeprazine, a phenothiazine tranquilizer. It acts as a nonnarcotic analgesic and sedative. It is used for the relief of pain of various types, and for sedation. The analgesic effect is comparable in man to that of morphine and pethidine, 15–20 mg methotrimeprazine being equivalent to 10 mg morphine or 75 mg pethidine hydrochloride.

Habituation, dependence, or addiction with large doses has not been observed, and respiratory depression with usual therapeutic doses is not usually observed.

Methotrimeprazine exerts additive effects with central nervous system depressant drugs, and should be used with caution when other depressants are in use.

About 17 percent of a dose of trimeprazine is excreted unchanged in the urine, and about 10 percent as sulfoxide conjugates. Fourteen percent of the dose appeared unchanged in the feces (Allgen *et al.*, 1963).

▶ **METHOXAMINE**
Dangerous Drug

Synonym: α-(1-Aminoethyl)-2,5-dimethoxygenzyl alcohol.
Pharmaceutical Preparations: Vasoxyl[R] (Burroughs Wellcome)—Injection.
General Comments: Methoxamine is a sympathomimetic amine used for its vasopressor effect. It is listed in this text as a Dangerous Drug because phar-maceutical preparations of methoxamine require a prescription and bear the legend "Caution: Federal law prohibits dispensing without a prescription."
Biochemistry: Similar to that of phenylpropanolamine.
Toxicology–Pharmacology: Methoxamine is a sympathomimetic agent, hav-ing almost exclusively properties of α-receptor stimulation. The effect is

therefore an increase in blood pressure due entirely to vasoconstriction. It has no stimulant action on the heart and causes little or no stimulation of the central nervous system.

When given intravenously or intramuscularly, it causes a rise in systolic and diastolic blood pressure that persists for 60–90 minutes; a reflex slowing of the heart rate is experienced.

It is used during surgical procedures to maintain blood pressure or restore it to normal levels, and may be used in preoperative medication in hypotensive patients. It may also be used as an adjunct in the treatment of hypotension associated with hemorrhage, trauma, or surgery, but is not a substitute for blood or plasma when these are required.

The bradycardia produced by methoxamine may also be of value in treatment of paroxysmal supraventricular tachycardia, and it may be used for this purpose.

High dosage may cause high blood pressure, and excessive bradycardia, headache, urinary urgency, vomiting, and pilomotor erection. It may precipitate a hypertensive crisis if used in combination with monoamine oxidase inhibitors.

▶ **4-METHOXYAMPHETAMINE**
Schedule I

$$CH_3O\text{—}\text{—}CH_2\text{—}\underset{\underset{NH_2}{|}}{CH}\text{—}CH_3$$

Synonyms: 4-Methoxy-α-methylphenethylamine, *p*-methoxyamphetamine, PMA.

Pharmaceutical Preparations: 4-Methoxyamphetamine is not found in any pharmaceutical preparations sold in the United States.

General Comments: 4-Methoxyamphetamine is a psychotomimetic amphetamine that has no accepted medicinal value in the United States. It produces many of the effects of amphetamines, but has the added capability of producing hallucinations.

Biochemistry: Behavioral studies in rats involving the trimethoxy-, dimethoxy-, and monomethoxyamphetamines, LSD, and mescaline showed 4-methoxyamphetamine to be the most potent hallucinogen, with the exception of LSD. The severe and prolonged disruption of behavior produced by 4-methoxyamphetamine suggests that it might cause an irreversible inhibition of an enzyme, possibly catechol *O*-methyltransferase.

Toxicology–Pharmacology: 4-Methoxyamphetamine is a hallucinogenic derivative of amphetamine. It has been responsible for overdose reactions in deaths in areas when it has been available. In one report of eight fatalities, blood concentrations of 4-methoxyamphetamine ranged from 0.03 to 0.19 mg/dl (Robinson *et al.*, 1973), and in three additional ones, 0.28–0.43 mg/dl was found (Barnhill *et al.*, 1974).

It is apparently excreted as metabolized products, as none could be detected in urine of subjects taking doses up to 629 mg.

▶ **5-METHOXYDIMETHYLTRYPTAMINE**
Noncontrolled Substance

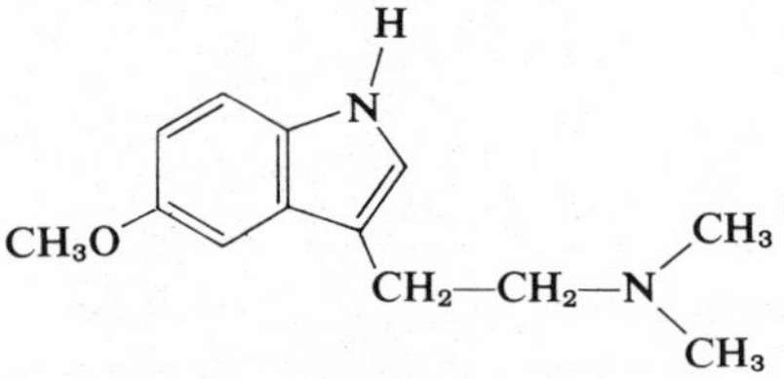

General Comments: 5-Methoxydimethyltryptamine is the *O*-methyl derivative of bufotenine. It is also found in South American snuff powders. The introduction of the *O*-methyl group causes an increase in hallucinogenic properties. Thus, 5-methoxydimethyltryptamine has more pronounced hallucinogenic activity than bufotenine (Fabig and Hawkins, 1956).

▶ **5-METHOXY-3,4-METHYLENEDIOXYAMPHETAMINE**
Schedule I

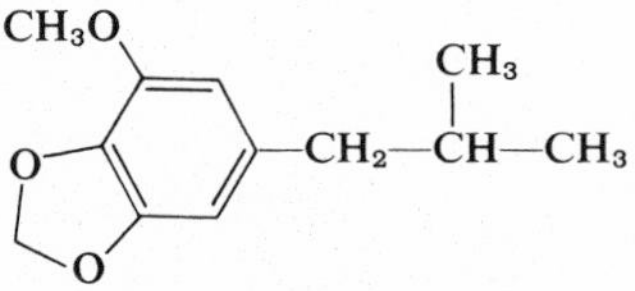

Synonyms: 3,4-Methylenedioxy-5-methoxyamphetamine, MMDA.
Pharmaceutical Preparations: 5-Methoxy-3,4-methylenedioxyamphetamine is not found in any pharmaceutical preparations sold in the United States.
General Comments: 5-Methoxy-3,4-methylenedioxyamphetamine is a psychotomimetic amphetamine that has no accepted medicinal value in the United States. Chemically and pharmacologically, it is related to the amphetamines as well as mescaline. In addition to central nervous system stimulating properties, it is capable of producing a false sense of well-being and hallucinations.

Produced illicitly, it may be encountered in powder, tablet, or liquid form. It is usually taken orally, but may be "snorted" though the nose (like cocaine) or injected intravenously.

Biochemistry: Similar to that of mescaline.

Toxicology–Pharmacology: 5-Methoxy-3,4-methylenedioxyamphetamine (MMDA) acts as a hallucinogenic agent in man. It has a behavioral and toxicological pattern similar to that of trimethoxyamphetamine. It exerts the hallucinogenic effect in humans at a dose of about 1.0 mg/kg, and effects a "hypnogogic dementia" at less than 2.0 mg/kg. Its potency is greater than that of trimethoxyamphetamine and about three times greater than that of mescaline (Shulgin, 1964).

▶ **METHOXYPHENAMINE**
Noncontrolled Substance

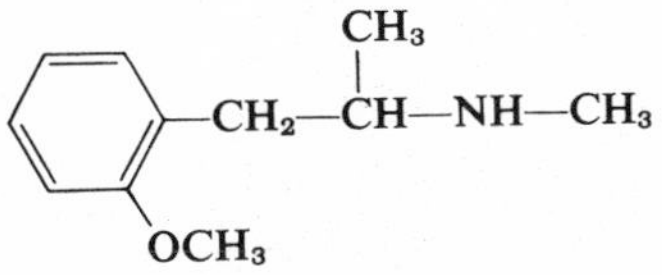

General Comments: Methoxyphenamine is a sympathomimetic amine with predominant actions of bronchodilation and inhibition of smooth muscle. Its pressor activity is considerably less than that of ephedrine. It is encountered in cases of drug abuse because of the similarity of its name to amphetamines.

Toxicology–Pharmacology: Methoxyphenamine is an orally active sympathomimetic amine. Its predominant actions are bronchial dilation and inhibition of smooth muscle. It does not have stimulant actions on the central nervous system. It is used primarily as a bronchodilator in the treatment of bronchial asthma, and in treatment of allergic rhinitis, acute urticaria, and gastrointestinal allergy.

▶ **p-METHOXYPHENETHYLAMINE**
Noncontrolled Substance

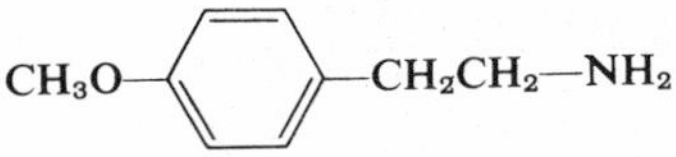

General Comments: p-Methoxyphenethylamine is a sympathomimetic amine with actions comparable to those of ephedrine. It is encountered in cases of drug abuse because of the similarity of its name to amphetamines.

▶ **METHOXYPROMAZINE**
Dangerous Drug

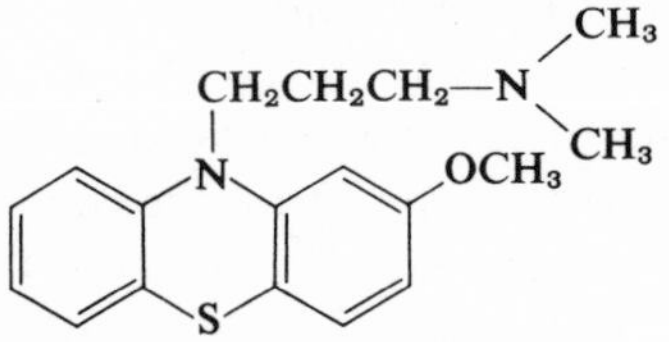

Synonyms: Methopromazine, 10-(3-dimethylaminopropyl)-2-methoxypheno-thiazine.
Pharmaceutical Preparations: Methoxypromazine is not found in any pharmaceutical preparations sold in the United States.
General Comment: Methoxypromazine is a phenothiazine tranquilizer. Because it is classified pharmacologically as a tranquilizer, it is listed in this text as a Dangerous Drug by definition.
Biochemistry: Similar to that of promazine.
Toxicology–Pharmacology: Similar to that of promazine.

▶ **5-METHOXYTRYPTAMINE**
Noncontrolled Substance

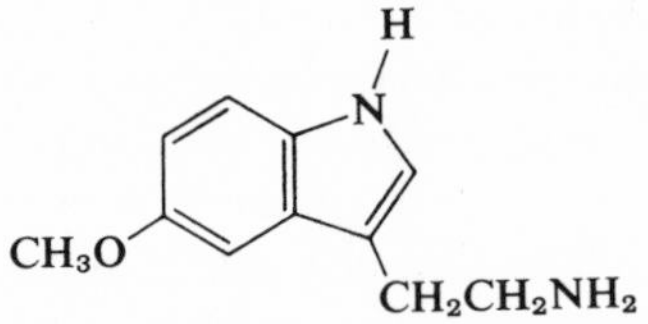

General Comments: 5-Methoxytryptamine was proposed as a potentiator for hypnotics and sedatives. It has been claimed to be more active than serotonin. It is the *O*-methyl derivative of 5-hydroxytryptamine, which is serotonin:

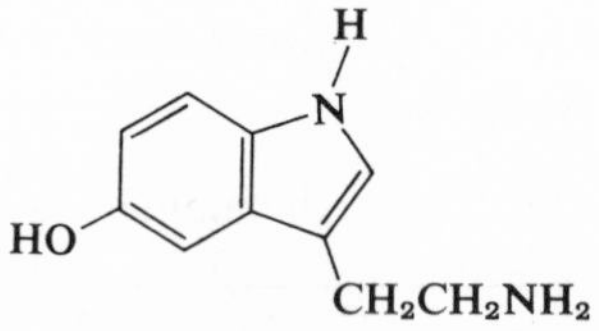

Serotonin

▶ **METHSCOPOLAMINE**
Noncontrolled Substance

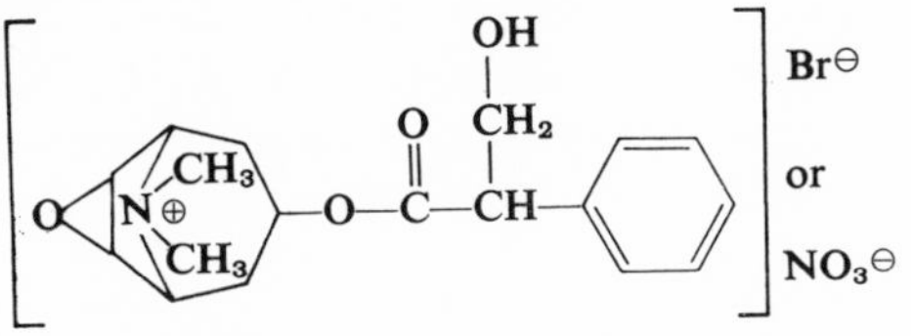

General Comment: Methscopolamine is the quaternary salt of scopolamine formed with either methylbromide or methylnitrate.

Toxicology–Pharmacology: Methscopolamine is an anticholinergic drug that has the effect of decreasing the acidity and volume of gastric secretion. It does not have any effects on the central nervous system. It is used as an adjunct in the therapy and treatment of peptic ulcer and gastric disorders associated with spasm, hyperactivity, and hypermotility.

As with other anticholinergic medications, dryness of the mouth usually occurs, and occasional side effects are blurring of vision, dizziness, drowsiness, and constipation.

▶ **METHYLDESORPHINE**
Schedule I

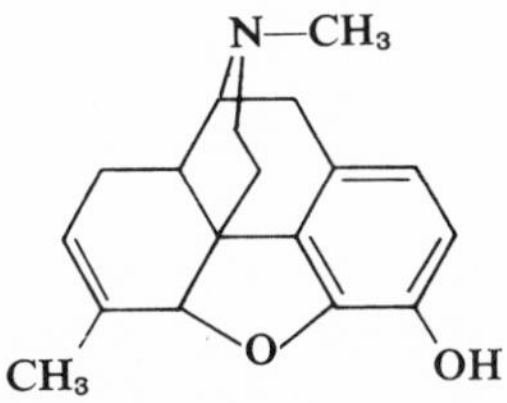

Synonym: 6,7-Dehydro-4,5-epoxy-3-hydroxy-N,6-dimethylmorphinan.

Pharmaceutical Preparations: Methyldesorphine is not found in any pharmaceutical preparations sold in the United States.

General Comments: Methyldesorphine is a synthetic narcotic analgesic chemically derived from morphine. It has no accepted medicinal value in the United States.

Biochemistry: See **METHYLDIHYDROMORPHINE.**

Toxicology–Pharmacology: See **METHYLDIHYDROMORPHINE.**

▶ **METHYLDIHYDROMORPHINE**
Schedule I

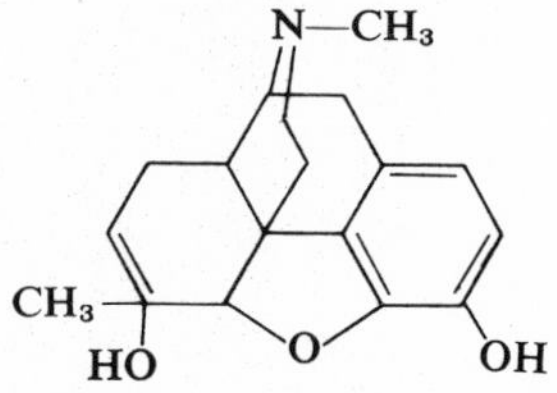

Synonyms: Methydromorphine, 4,5-epoxy-3,6-dihydroxy-N,6-dimethylmorphinan.

Pharmaceutical Preparations: Methyldihydromorphine is not found in any pharmaceutical preparations sold in the United States.

General Comments: Methyldihydromorphine is a synthetic narcotic analgesic chemically related to morphine. It has no accepted medicinal value in the United States.

Biochemistry: The alcoholic hydroxyl group in morphine has been modified in several ways with varying effects on analgetic activity. The product formed from the dehydration of 6-methyldihydromorphine has a great improvement of analgetic activity. This product, 6-methyl-Δ^6-desoxymorphine, is nearly ten times as active as morphine with a short duration of action. However, it has a high dependence potential (Small, L. F., and Rapoport, 1947; Isbell and Fraser, 1950).

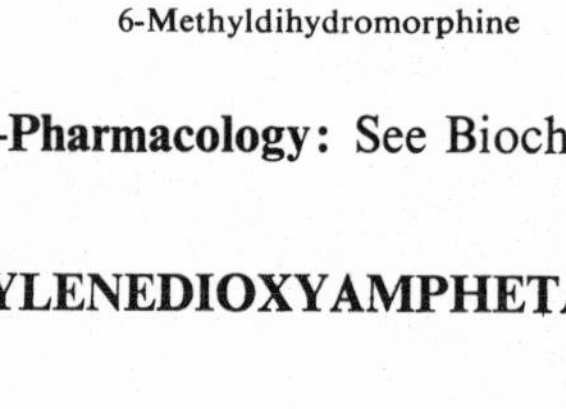

6-Methyldihydromorphine 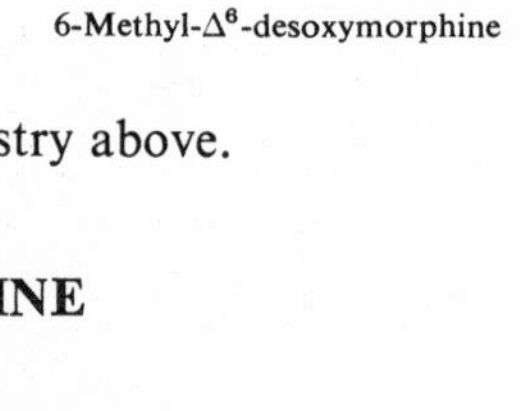   6-Methyl-Δ^6-desoxymorphine

Toxicology–Pharmacology: See Biochemistry above.

▶ **3,4-METHYLENEDIOXYAMPHETAMINE**
Schedule I

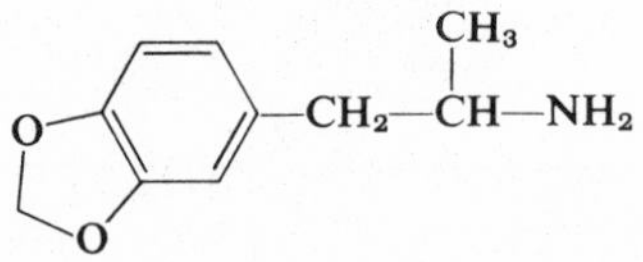

Synonyms: MDA, 3,4-methylenedioxy-α-methylphenethylamine.

Pharmaceutical Preparations: 3,4-Methylenedioxyamphetamine is not found in any pharmaceutical preparations sold in the United States.

General Comments: 3,4-Methylenedioxyamphetamine is a psychotomimetic amphetamine possessing the stimulatory properties of the amphetamines in addition to hallucinogenic properties similar to that of mescaline. It is controlled as a hallucinogen under Schedule I. Sold in the illicit market as MDA, it is encountered in powder, tablet or liquid form. It may be taken orally, "snorted" (like cocaine), or injected intravenously. The "trip" from this drug is reported to be devoid of the visual and auditory distortions that are characteristic of the experience with LSD.

The medical hazards from abuse of 3,4-methylenedioxyamphetamine are similar to those with methamphetamine.

Biochemistry: Similar to that of 3-methoxy-4,5-methylenedioxyamphetamine.

Toxicology–Pharmacology: 3,4-Methylenedioxyamphetamine (MDA) is a substituted amphetamine, having primarily central stimulant and euphoranti effect in humans. The effective dose is between 120 and 150 mg. Onset of effects occurs from 30 to 60 minutes after ingestion and may persist for about 8 hours. In general, MDA engenders a sense of physical well-being, with heightened tactile sensations. True hallucinations, perceptual distortions, closed-eye imagery, common with hallucinogens such as LSD, mescaline, and psilocybin, are usually absent with MDA. An intensification of feelings with increased perception of self-insight and aesthetic enjoyment are usually experienced. Adverse aftereffects may consist of marked physical exhaustion and anxiety, lasting up to 2 days (Ratcliffe, 1974).

The physical effects are characteristic of central nervous system sympathomimetic agents. The pupils of the eyes are dilated, and the systolic and diastolic blood pressures are increased.

The fatal dose of MDA is, as yet, unknown. In one fatality involving oral ingestion of homemade capsules containing 30 mg MDA, a blood concentration of 0.5 mg/dl was reported. Methamphetamine was also detected in the urine (Finkle, 1969a).

▶ **METHYLERGOMETRINE**
Noncontrolled Substance

General Comments: Methylergometrine is a semisynthetic homologue of ergonovine, an ergot alkaloid, prepared from lysergic acid. It is medically accepted as an oxytocic and is prepared pharmaceutically by Sandoz and sold under the trade name Methergine^R.

Toxicology–Pharmacology: Similar to that of ergonovine.

▶ **2-METHYL-3-MORPHOLINE-1,1-DIPHENYLPROPANE CARBOXYLIC ACID**
Schedule II

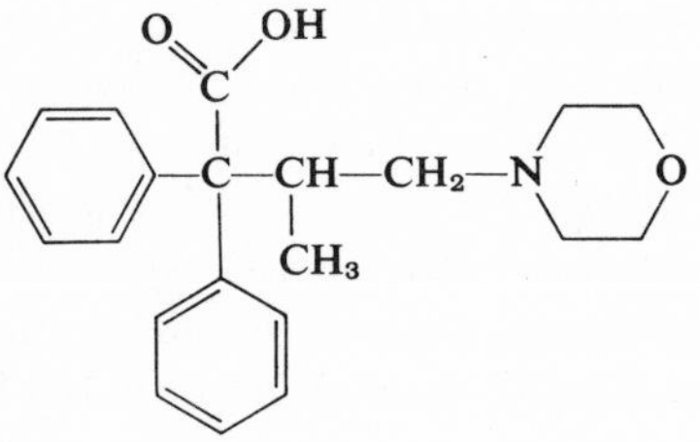

Synonyms: None found.

Pharmaceutical Preparations: 2-Methyl-3-morpholine-1,1-diphenylpropane carboxylic acid is not found in any pharmaceutical preparations sold in the United States.

General Comments: 2-Methyl-3-morpholine-1,1-diphenylpropane carboxylic acid is listed as a Schedule II controlled substance because it is an immediate precursor in the synthesis of moramide. Under Section 201 of the Controlled Substances Act, an immediate precursor may be placed in the same schedule as the controlled substance to which it is a precursor, or in any other schedule with a higher numerical designation. Since moramide is a Schedule I substance, this substance could have legally been placed in Schedule I, II, III, IV, or V.

Biochemistry: Unknown.

Toxicology–Pharmacology: Unknown.

▶ **METHYLPHENIDATE**
Schedule II

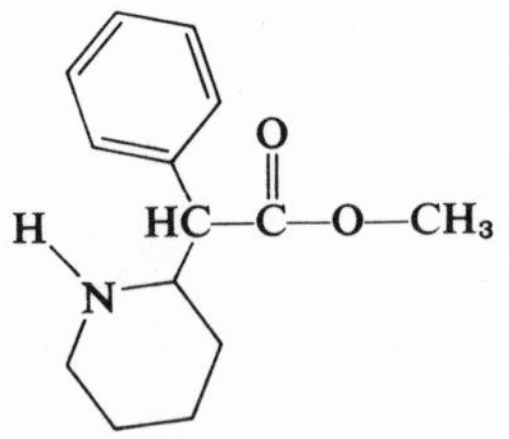

Synonym: α-Phenyl-2-piperidinacetate.

Pharmaceutical Preparations: Ritalin[R] (Ciba)—Tablets, scored, containing methylphenidate hydrochloride: peach, 20 mg; pale green, 10 mg; pale yellow, 5 mg

General Comments: None.

Biochemistry: Methylphenidate may inhibit the metabolism of coumarin anticoagulants, anticonvulsants, and tricyclic antidepressants.

Toxicology–Pharmacology: Methylphenidate is a mild central nervous system (CNS) stimulant, more potent than caffeine but less effective than amphetamine in increasing motor and mental activities. It has little effect on blood pressure or respiration. It has been used in various types of depression, in the treatment of overdosage from depressant drugs, and as a general stimulant. It may also be useful in treatment of narcolepsy, and in treatment of hyperkinetic children, which is an important current application for this drug.

Chronic use of methylphenidate leads to tolerance and psychological dependence. Overdosage results in overstimulation of the CNS, and excessive sympathomimetic effects, including agitation, tremors, hyperreflexia, muscle twitching, hallucinations, confusion, and convulsions.

After a 20-mg dose of methylphenidate, plasma levels of 0.0010–0.0028 mg/dl were observed in 1 hour, and levels of 0.0013–0.0058 mg/dl were found at 3 hours after dosing (Milberg et al., 1975). Death from overdosage of methylphenidate alone is rare, and toxic levels have not been reported.

▶ **1-METHYL-4-PHENYLPIPERIDINE-4-CARBOXYLIC ACID**
Schedule II

Synonyms: None found.

Pharmaceutical Preparations: 1-Methyl-4-phenylpiperidine-4-carboxylic acid is not found in pharmaceutical preparations sold in the United States.

General Comments: 1-Methyl-4-phenylpiperidine-4-carboxylic acid is listed as a Schedule II controlled substance because it is an immediate precursor in the synthesis of pethidine (meperidine). Under Section 201 of the Controlled Substances Act, an immediate precursor may be placed in the same schedule as the controlled substance to which it is a precursor, or in any other schedule

with a higher numerical designation. Since pethidine is a Schedule II substance, this substance could have legally been placed in Schedule II, III, IV, or V.
Biochemistry: Unknown.
Toxicology–Pharmacology: Unknown.

▶ *N*-METHYL-3-PIPERIDYLBENZILATE
Schedule I

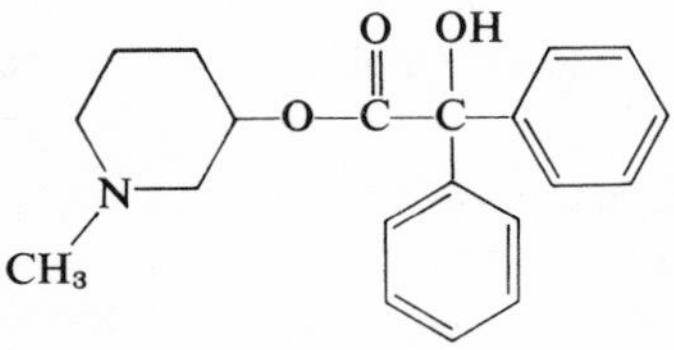

Synonyms: JB-336, LBJ.
Pharmaceutical Preparations: *N*-methyl-3-piperidylbenzilate is not found in any pharmaceutical preparations sold in the United States.
General Comments: None.
Biochemistry: *N*-methyl-3-piperidylbenzilate was synthesized in 1958 along with a series of similar compounds having the following general structure:

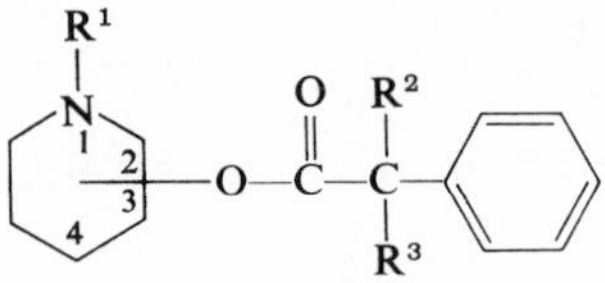

The compounds were designed using the piperidine ring of atropine while modifying the tropic acid side chain with substituted glycobolic acids (Abood *et al.*, 1958). Of this series of compounds, it was found that maximum hallucinogenic activity was exhibited when R^1 was either a methyl or an ethyl group while R^2 was a hydroxyl group. Major variations in central nervous system (CNS) activity were observed with different substituents at R^3. The potency decreased in the order cycloalkyl > phenyl > unsaturated alkyl > alkyl. Within the cycloalkyl group, cyclopentyl exhibited the greatest potency.
Toxicology–Pharmacology: *N*-methyl-3-piperidylbenzilate was synthesized in 1958 and studied because of its potent anticholinergic and CNS activity. It exhibits powerful psychotomimetic and antidepressant activity. In doses of above 1 mg, like its counterpart *N*-ethyl-3-piperidylbenzilate, it produces long-lasting hallucinogenic effects.
    This drug appeared on the illicit market in 1967 identified by its street name LBJ.

▶ **METHYLTESTOSTERONE**
Dangerous Drug

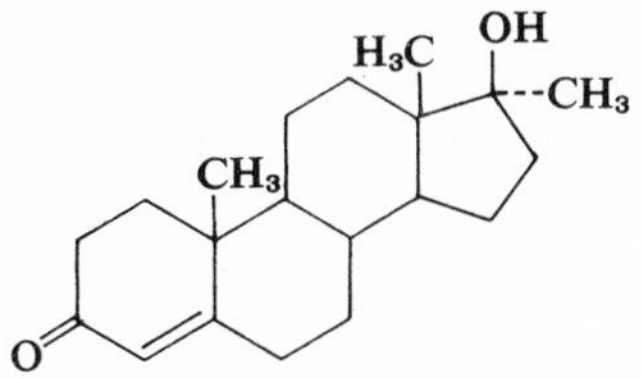

Synonyms: 17β-Hydroxy-17-methylandrost-4-en-3-one, 17α-methyltestosterone.

Pharmaceutical Preparations
Android^R (Brown)—Tablets
Estratest^R (Reid-Provident)—Tablets
Gevrine^R (Lederle)—Capsules
Gynetone^R (Schering)—Tablets
Metandron^R (Ciba)—Buccal Tablets and Tablets
Oreton^R (Schering)—Buccal Tablets and Tablets
Os-Cal Mone^R (Marion)—Tablets
Premarin^R with Methyltestosterone (Ayerst)—Tablets
Testand-B^R (Geriatric)—Tablets
Test-Estrin^R (Marlym)—Capsules and Vaginal Inserts
Testred^R (ICN)—Capsules
Tylosterone^R (Lilly)—Tablets
Virilon^R (Star)—Capsules

General Comments: Methyltestosterone does not occur naturally. It is synthesized from cholesterol. The actions and uses of methyltestosterone are similar to those of testosterone, a male sex hormone. It may be encountered in cases of drug abuse when persons attempt to use this drug as an aphrodisiac.

Methyltestosterone is classified in this text as a Dangerous Drug because all preparations containing this drug require a prescription and thus bear the label "Caution: Federal law prohibits dispensing without a prescription."

Biochemistry: The metabolitic products of methyltestosterone have been identified as 17α-methyl-5α-androstane-3α,17β-diol, 17α-methyl-5β-androstane-3α,17β-diol, and 17α-methyl-5α-androstane-3β,17β-diol (Segaloff *et al.*, 1965).

Toxicology–Pharmacology: Methyltestosterone is a synthetic derivative of cholesterol. It has actions similar to those of testosterone, but is three to five times less effective than testosterone. The androgenic hormones (such as testosterone) maintain the secondary sexual characteristics and are necessary for development of sexual organs in the male. Methyltestosterone may be used in the treatment of hypoganadism in the young male, and in various testicular developmental abnormalities in which inadequate testosterone is secreted. It may also be used for suppressing certain breast cancers, and in certain gynecological conditions. Other circumstances in which methyltestosterone may be effective are to restore sexual function in impotence, and for anabolic functions. In the latter circumstances, male hormones increase protein synthesis in the body, aiding in weight gain and muscular development.

Untoward effects may include jaundice from intrahepatic biliary obstruction, and priapism.

▶ **α-METHYLTRYPTAMINE**
Noncontrolled Substance

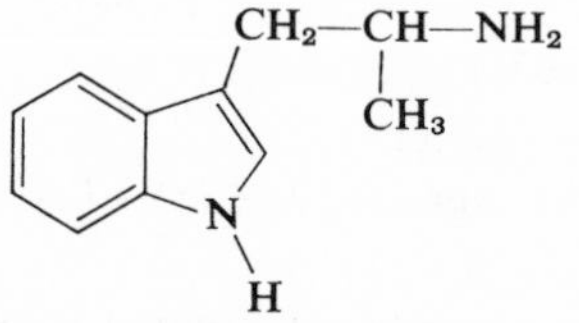

General Comment: α-Methyltryptamine is a synthetic indole alkaloid similar chemically and pharmacologically to bufotenine, but with little or no hallucinogenic activity.
Toxicology–Pharmacology: Unknown.

▶ **N-METHYLTRYPTAMINE**
Noncontrolled Substance

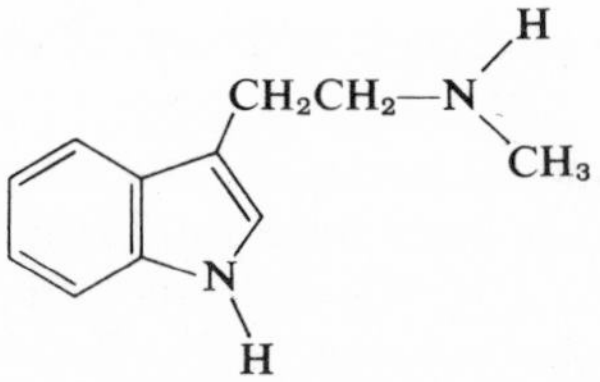

General Comments: N-Methyltryptamine is a naturally occurring indole

alkaloid found in the South American legume *Anadenanthera peregrina*. It is chemically and pharmacologically similar to bufotenine.
Toxicology–Pharmacology: Similar to that of bufotenine.

▶ **METHYPRYLON**
Schedule III

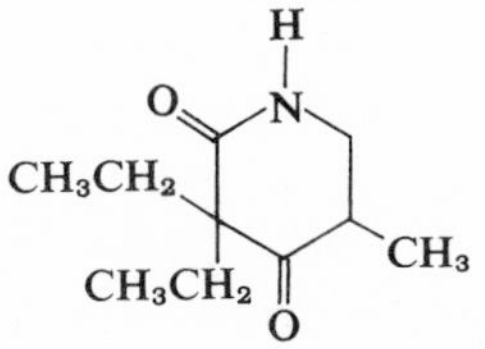

Synonym: 3,3-Diethyl-5-methyl-2,4-piperidinedione.
Pharmaceutical Preparations
Noludar[R] (Roche)—Tablets: scored, containing 200 mg methyprylon
Noludar[R]-300 (Roche)—Capsules: amethyst and white, containing 300 mg methyprylon
General Comments: None.
Biochemistry: See Toxicology–Pharmacology below.
Toxicology–Pharmacology: Methyprylon is a nonbarbiturate hypnotic–sedative drug, having central depressant actions similar to those of secobarbital and pentobarbital in onset and duration of effects. It is used primarily as a nighttime hypnotic, producing an average duration of sleep of 7 hours. The usual sleep-inducing dosage is 200 or 300 mg.

Habituation, tolerance, and addiction have been reported with chronic use, and the abstinence syndrome is similar to those with many central depressants, including insomnia, confusion, hallucinations, and generalized convulsions.

After overdosage, coma and depression of the cardiac and respiratory systems are conspicuous manifestations.

After oral administration of 650 mg methyprylon to adults, plasma concentrations of 0.57 mg/dl was observed in 1 hour. In 2 hours, the concentration was 1.02 mg/dl, and at 3 hours, 0.79 mg/dl (Randall *et al.*, 1956).

After overdosage, levels above 3.00 mg/dl were associated with coma. The patients had pupillary constriction, lateral nystagmus, and some had seizures (Bailey and Jatlow, 1973). The half-life of methyprylon is about 4 hours.

Methyprylon is almost completely metabolized, above 0.3 percent being excreted unchanged in the urine. Other metabolites included 5-carboxypyrithyldione, 6-oxo-methyprylon, and methypyritheldione (Bösche *et al.*, 1969).

▶ **METHYSERGIDE**
Noncontrolled Substance

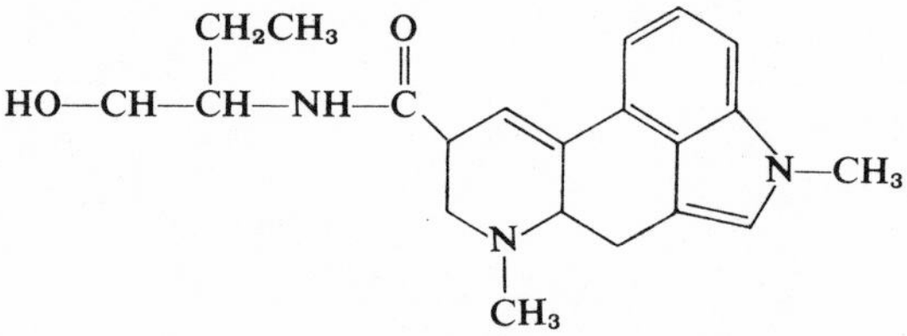

$$
\begin{array}{c}
\text{CH}_2\text{CH}_3 \quad \text{O} \\
| \quad\quad || \\
\text{HO—CH—CH—NH—C}
\end{array}
$$

General Comments: Methysergide is chemically and pharmacologically re-lated to methylergometrine. It is used as a prophylactic agent in the manage-ment of all forms of migraine headache. It may be encountered in cases of drug abuse because of the similarity of its name to lysergic acid diethylamide.
Toxicology–Pharmacology: Methysergide is similar in structure to ergono-vine and other ergot alkaloids. It does not, however, have oxytocic properties, and is not effective in the acute phase of migraine headache, as are the other ergot alkaloids. It is of primary effectiveness in the prophylactic treatment of migraine headache. It must be given for a day or two for its prophylactic effect to develop.

Untoward effects in patients taking methysergide include fibrosis in peritoneal, pleuropulmonary, cardiac, and other tissue, vasoconstriction in arteries, nausea, vomiting, and diarrhea, and edema. These toxic side effects may necessitate withdrawal from the drug in up to 30 percent of patients. The usual dosage of methysergide is 4–8 mg daily.

▶ **METOPON**
Schedule II

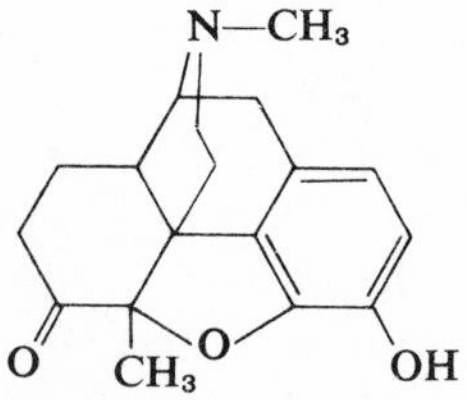

Synonyms: Dihydromethylmorphinone, methyldihydromorphinone, 4,5-epoxy-3-hydroxy-N,5-dimethyl-6-oxomorphinan.
Pharmaceutical Preparations: Metopon is not frequently found in pharma-ceutical preparations sold in the United States.
General Comments: None.

Biochemistry: Metopon may be produced synthetically in a four-step reaction process from dihydrothebaine:

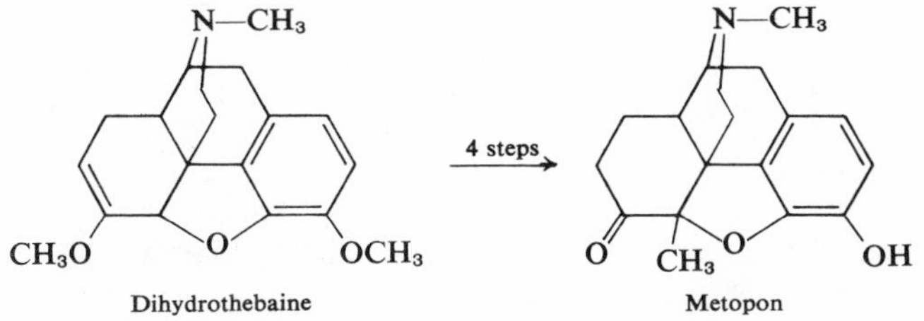

Dihydrothebaine   Metopon

Generally, the introduction of new substituents into the aromatic or alicylic rings of the morphine molecule causes a decrease in analgetic activity. Metopon is an exception to this rule. It is effective orally and is about three times as potent as morphine (Gates and Shepard, 1962).

The low yields obtained in the synthesis of metopon probably account for the lack of commercial production for medicinal use.

Toxicology–Pharmacology: Metopon is a synthetic narcotic analgesic. It is approximately three times as effective as morphine in analgesic potency. It has a duration of action of around 4–5 hours.

Like other synthetic narcotic agents, metopon has central depressant and euphoriant actions, and induces tolerance and addiction when used repeatedly.

Therapeutic doses of metopon induce relief from pain and euphoria. Higher doses or overdose results in central and respiratory depression. The estimated minimum lethal dose of metopon is 100 mg.

▶ **MORAMIDE**
Schedule I

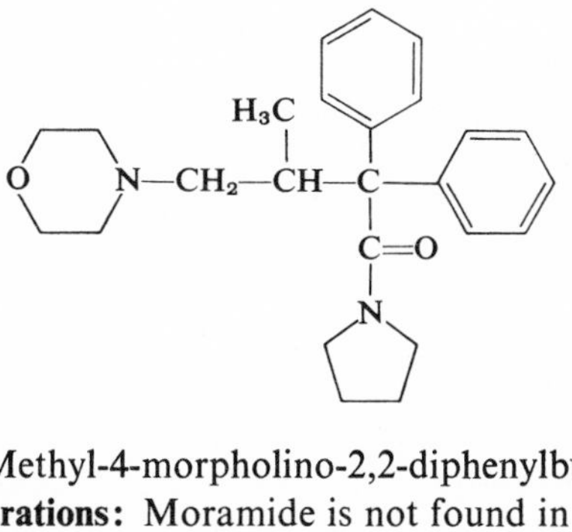

Synonym: ($\pm$)-1-(3-Methyl-4-morpholino-2,2-diphenylbutyryl)-pyrrolidine.
Pharmaceutical Preparations: Moramide is not found in any pharmaceutical preparations sold in the United States.

General Comments: See **DEXTROMORAMIDE** and **LEVOMORAMIDE.**
Biochemistry: See **DEXTROMORAMIDE** and **LEVOMORAMIDE.**
Toxicology–Pharmacology: The *dextro* isomer of moramide is a synthetic
narcotic analgesic, with an analgesic potency about twice that of morphine.
A dose of 5–7.5 mg provides relief from pain for 4–5 hours. It retains most of
its analgetic potency when given orally and may exhibit cumulative effect on
repeated dosage.

Like other narcotics, dextromoramide may induce tolerance and addiction if taken repeatedly. Addicted individuals may take up to 400 mg daily.
The estimated lethal dose is 500 mg.

▶ **MORPHERIDINE**
Schedule I

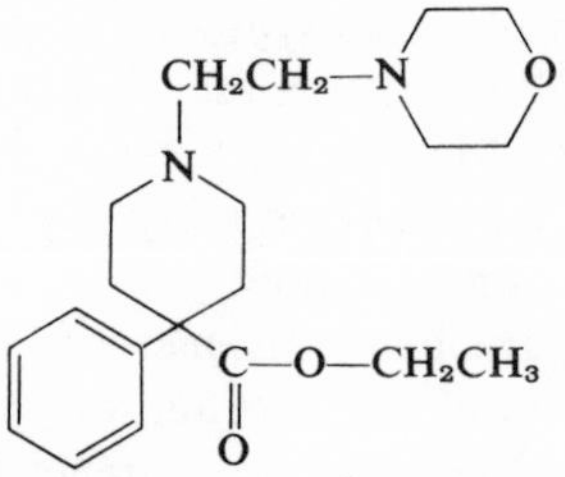

Synonyms: Morpholinoethylnorpethidine, ethyl-1-(2-morpholinoethyl)-4-
phenylpiperidine-4-carboxylate.
Pharmaceutical Preparations: Morpheridine is not found in any pharmaceu-
tical preparations sold in the United States.
General Comment: Morpheridine is a synthetic narcotic analgesic that has no
accepted medicinal value in the United States.
Biochemistry: Unknown.
Toxicology–Pharmacology: Unknown.

▶ **MORPHINE**

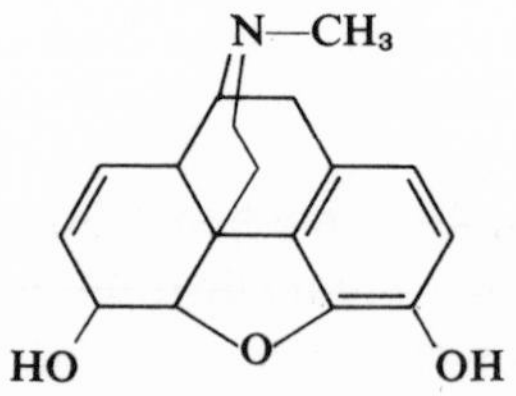

Schedule II

or

Schedule III for any material, compound, mixture, or preparation (or any salts thereof) containing not more than 50 mg morphine per 100 ml or per 100 g with one or more active nonnarcotic ingredients or recognized therapeutic amounts

Synonyms: Morphia, morphina, 7,8-dehydro-4,5-epoxy-3,6-dihydroxy-*N*-methylmorphinan.

Pharmaceutical Preparations: Morphine Sulfate[R] (Vitrine)—Tablets and Injection.

General Comment: Formerly, morphine base, morphine hydrochloride, and morphine sulfate were official. However, at present, only the sulfate is recognized, although the *U.S. Pharmacopeia* permits the use of "a suitable salt of morphine" in preparing morphine injection.

Biochemistry: Morphine occurs naturally as the *levo* enantiomer. It has five asymmetric centers at positions 5, 6, 9, 13, and 14:

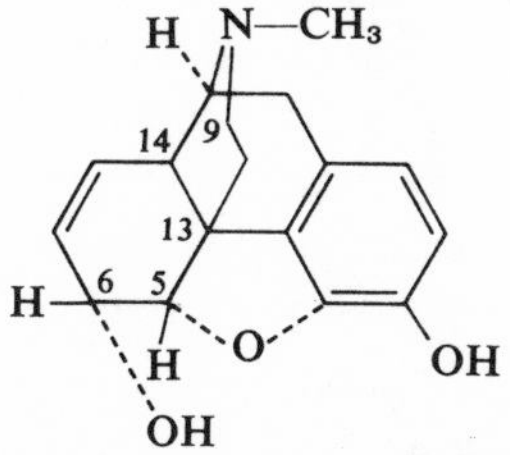

The absolute configuration of morphine has been determined and confirmed by optical rotatory studies (Bentley and Cardwell, 1955):

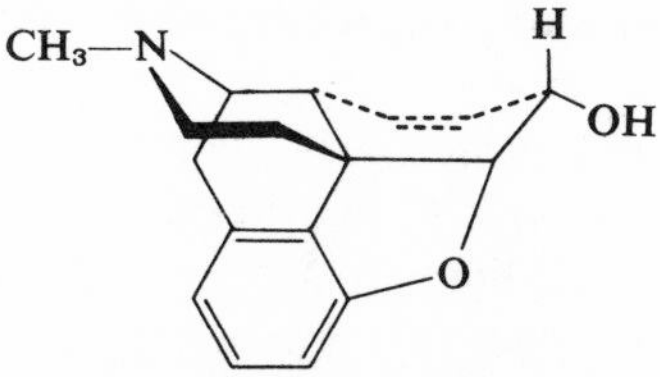

The *dextro* enantiomer of morphine has been synthetically prepared and determined to have no analgetic properties (Goto *et al.*, 1957).

The analgetic potency of morphine may be markedly increased by substitution of a 2-arylethyl group on the nitrogen (May and Sargent, 1965). It may be decreased by replacement of the *N*-methyl with ethyl, propyl, or butyl. However, *N*-amyl and *N*-hexyl derivatives will restore the analgetic activity equivalent to the *N*-methyl (Joshi *et al.*, 1965).

Toxicology–Pharmacology: Morphine is the prototype of narcotic analgesic drugs. It is the principal alkaloid of opium, and was isolated from the plant in 1803 by Derosne. Opium itself had been in use as a medicinal or sedative for some 3500 years. Morphine continues to be one of the most important drugs in common clinical use (Eddy and Mary, 1973). Although more than 150 derivatives of morphine have been synthesized and tested, and thousands of synthetic narcotics have been made and tested, many of them much more potent than morphine itself, morphine continues to be one of the most useful and effective analgesics available.

The classic pharmacological properties of morphine, and of subsequent narcotic analgesics, are: analgesia, sedation (sleep), euphoria, and, with continued use, tolerance and addiction. After an average dose of morphine administered intramuscularly, the patient characteristically experiences a pleasant drowsiness characterized by muscular relaxation, freedom from anxiety, a rapid flow of ideas, shortening of the sense of time, disappearance of fears, doubts, and inhibitions, lessened physical activity, dimness of vision, and lethargy. Pain and hunger are abolished, respiration is slowed, and the pupils are small. Sleep usually ensues, and dreams may be experienced.

Morphine relieves pain by increasing the threshold for the perception of pain and by altering the psychic response so the patient is better able to tolerate pain. It is effective against pain arising in the viscera as well as in the muscles, joints, and elsewhere, and is more effective against dull continuous pain than against sharp and intermittent pain. The maximum analgesic action appears in 60–90 minutes after subcutaneous injection of 10 mg morphine; after intravenous administration, it begins within 20 minutes.

Morphine is a respiratory depressant, producing an abnormal sensibility of the respiratory center to carbon dioxide. This is of little significance with therapeutic doses but is a serious toxic reaction after overdose. In the gastrointestinal tract, morphine antagonizes peristalsis, inducing constipation after chronic use.

Plasma concentrations of morphine range up to 0.01 mg/dl up to 2 hours after intravenous injection with 10-mg doses. It clears rapidly from plasma, however, with an initial half-life of 1.9–3.1 hours; a second, prolonged half-life of 10–44 hours was observed. Detectable blood concentrations were present for 48 hours (Vesell and Passananti, 1971). In patients receiving regular injections of morphine for pain, however, concentrations of 0.04 mg/dl or higher may be observed.

After death from overdose with morphine sulfate, a blood concentration of 0.265 mg/dl was detected (Garriott, 1977). Morphine becomes concentrated in the bile after metabolism to morphine glucuronide, and may be present there in very large concentrations. Up to 22.0 mg/dl have been found in bile.

Morphine is much more commonly detected on toxicological investigations as the main metabolite of heroin. After injection of heroin, morphine is detected in the blood or tissues. In blood, fatalities from heroin overdose had concentrations of morphine averaging 0.042 mg/dl (Baselt *et al.*, 1975b).

The depressant effects of morphine may be potentiated and prolonged by alcohol and other central nervous system depressants (analgesics, antihistamines, barbiturates, narcotics, phenothiazines, sedative–hypnotics).

▶ **MORPHINE METHYLBROMIDE**
Schedule I

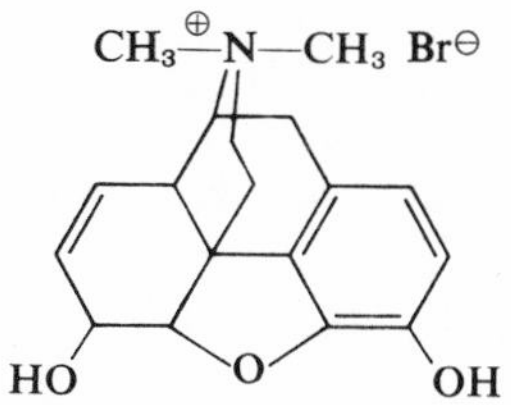

$$CH_3 \overset{\oplus}{-} N - CH_3 \ Br^{\ominus}$$

Synonym: Morphosan.
Pharmaceutical Preparations: Morphine methylbromide is not found in any pharmaceutical preparations sold in the United States.
General Comments: See **MORPHINE.**
Biochemistry: See **MORPHINE.**
Toxicology–Pharmacology: Morphine methylbromide is a quarternary homologue of morphine formed by interaction of morphine with methylbromide. It is a narcotic analgesic that has no accepted medicinal value in the United States. Pharmacology and toxicology are similar to those of morphine.

▶ **MORPHINE METHYLSULFONATE**
Schedule I

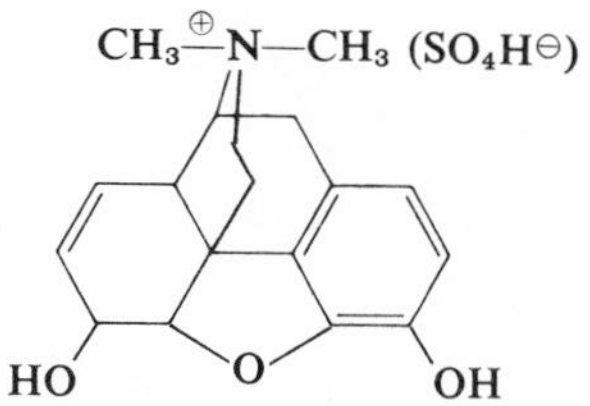

$$CH_3 \overset{\oplus}{-} N - CH_3 \ (SO_4 H^{\ominus})$$

Synonyms: None found.
Pharmaceutical Preparations: Morphine methylsulfonate is not found in any pharmaceutical preparations sold in the United States.
General Comments: See **MORPHINE.**

Biochemistry: See **MORPHINE.**

Toxicology–Pharmacology: Morphine methylsulfonate is a quarternary homologue of morphine formed by the interaction of morphine with methyl sulfate. It has no accepted medicinal value in the United States.

▶ **MORPHINE *N*-OXIDE**
Schedule I

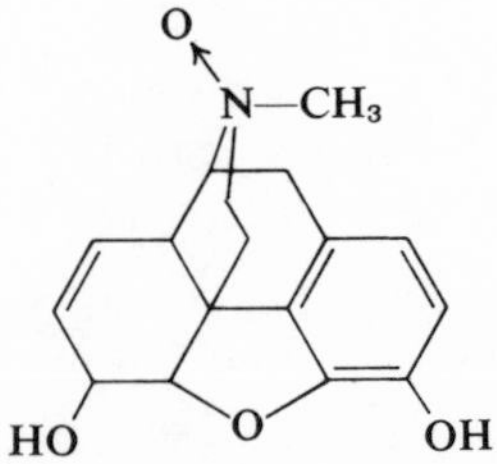

Synonyms: Genomorphine, morphine aminoxide, *N*-oxymorphine.

Pharmaceutical Preparations: Morphine *N*-oxide is not found in any pharmaceutical preparations sold in the United States.

General Comments: See **MORPHINE.**

Biochemistry: See **MORPHINE.**

Toxicology–Pharmacology: Morphine *N*-oxide is the product of peroxide oxidation of morphine. It has no accepted medicinal value in the United States. Morphine *N*-oxide is more active than morphine.

▶ **MYROPHINE**
Schedule I

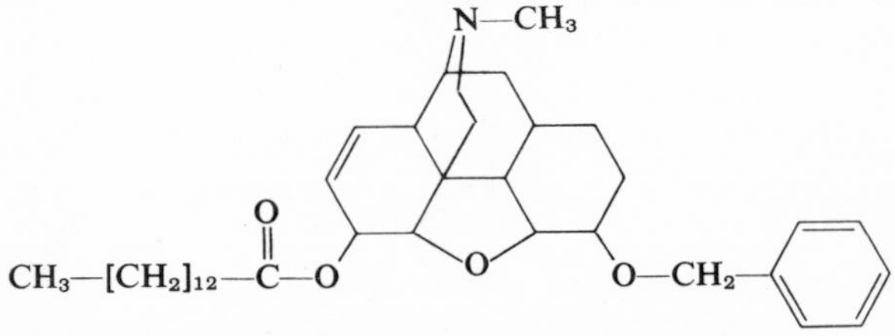

Synonyms: Mycicodine, myristylbenzylmorphine, 3-benzyloxy-7,8-dehydro-4,5-epoxy-*N*-methyl-6-myristoyloxymorphinan.

Pharmaceutical Preparations: Myrophine is not found in any pharmaceutical preparations sold in the United States.

General Comments: None.

Biochemistry: Unknown.

Toxicology–Pharmacology: Myrophine is a semisynthetic narcotic analgesic that has no medicinal usage in the United States.

▶ **NALORPHINE**
Schedule III

$$N{-}CH_2{-}CH{=}CH_2$$

HO   O   OH

Synonyms: N-allylnormorphine, N-allyl-7,8-dehydro-4,5-epoxy-3,6-dihydroxy-morphinan.
Pharmaceutical Preparations: Injections for hospital use.
General Comments: None.
Biochemistry: Nalorphine and morphine have the same absolute configuration (see **MORPHINE**). Thus, the stereochemical features of these two drugs are not related to their activity. Their activity is more related to a competitive action for the receptor site by agonists and antagonists.
Toxicology–Pharmacology: Nalorphine has many actions similar to those of the structurally related alkaloid, morphine. It also, however, has the ability to antagonize many of the actions of morphine and other narcotics. It is used principally to counteract the severe respiratory depression from overdosage with narcotics, and may be used to diagnose addiction to narcotics.

In the absence of a narcotic, nalorphine acts like a narcotic, reducing respiratory volume, lowering body temperature, constricting the pupils of the eyes, and acting as an antitussive. It has some analgesic effects, but also produces dysphoria, preventing its use for this purpose. When administered with or in the presence of a narcotic, nalorphine prevents or abolishes many of the narcotic actions. Intravenous injection of 5–10 mg nalorphine in a narcotic-depressed patient increases respiratory rate and volume within a minute or two. It tends to restore blood pressure, abolishes the pupillary constriction, and counteracts gastrointestinal spasm. It is therefore a specific antidote to overdosage with morphine and its derivatives, methadone, meperidine, and other synthetic narcotic derivatives.

When given to patients addicted to narcotics, nalorphine precipitates severe abstinence symptoms. Nalorphine is absorbed rapidly after subcutaneous administration, with maximal levels appearing in the brain within 15–20 minutes. After oral administration, it is poorly absorbed, requiring 120 mg to produce the same effect as 3–4 mg subcutaneously administered.

As nalorphine has low abuse potential since it does not have significant euphoric effects, and is used primarily in treatment of narcotic overdose, toxic reactions and death from overdose are rare.

▶ **NARCOBARBITAL**
Schedule III

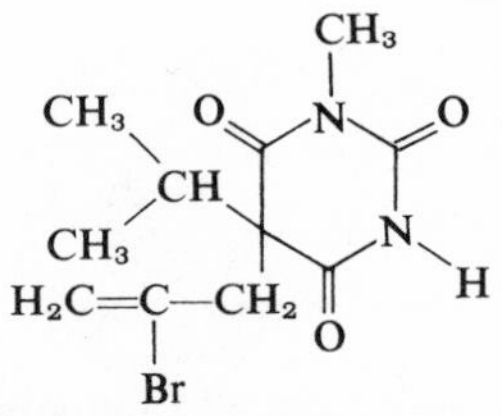

Synonyms: Enibomal, 5-(2-bromoallyl)-5-isopropyl-1-methyl-barbituric acid.
Pharmaceutical Preparations: Narcobarbital is not found in any pharmaceutical preparations sold in the United States.
General Comment: Narcobarbital is a Schedule III drug because it is a "derivative of barbituric acid."
Biochemistry: Similar to that of hexobarbital and butyallylonal.
Toxicology–Pharmacology: Narcobarbital is a very short-acting barbiturate, used to induce rapid anesthesia. Its actions are similar to those of hexobarbital and thiopental. It may be given in doses of up to 1000 mg intravenously (Clarke, 1969).

▶ **NEALBARBITAL**
Schedule III

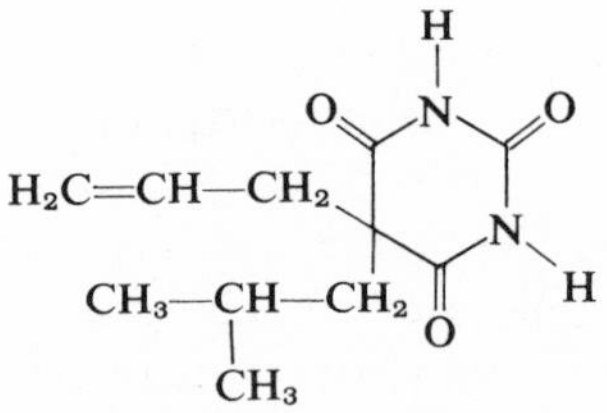

Synonyms: Alneobarbital, nealbarbitone, neallymalu, 5-allyl-5-neopentyl-barbituric acid.
Pharmaceutical Preparations: Nealbarbital is not found in any pharmaceutical preparations sold in the United States.
General Comment: Nealbarbital is a Schedule III drug because it is "a derivative of barbituric acid."
Biochemistry: Similar to that of amobarbital and secobarbital.

Toxicology–Pharmacology: Nealbarbital is an intermediate-acting barbiturate with actions similar to those of amobarbital. It may be used as a sedative–hypnotic medication.

▶ **NICOCODEINE**
Schedule I

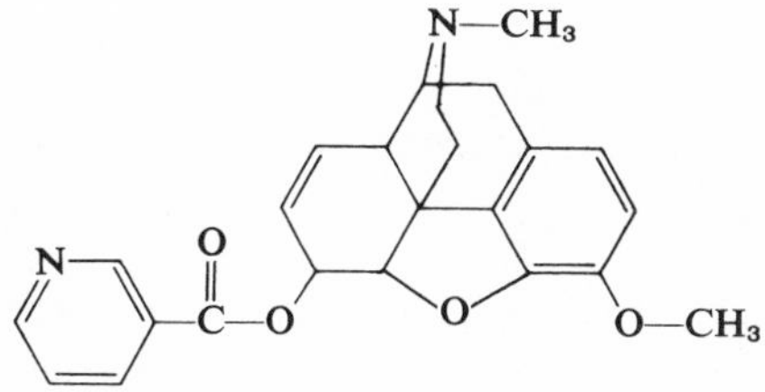

Synonyms: 6-Nicotinoylcodeine, 7,8-dehydro-4,5-epoxy-3-methoxy-*N*-methyl-6-nicotinoyl-oxymorphinan.
Pharmaceutical Preparations: Nicocodeine is not found in any pharmaceutical preparations sold in the United States.
General Comments: None.
Biochemistry: Unknown.
Toxicology–Pharmacology: Nicocodeine is a semisynthetic narcotic analgesic with antitussive properties. It has no accepted medicinal value in the United States.

▶ **NICOMORPHINE**
Schedule I

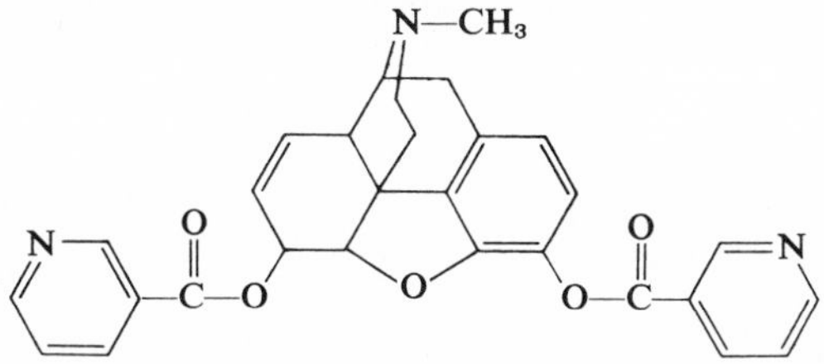

Synonyms: 3,6-Dinicotinylmorphine, nicophin, 7,8-dehydro-4,5-epoxy-*N*-methyl-3,6-di(nicotinoyl)morphinan.
Pharmaceutical Preparations: Nicomorphine is not found in any pharmaceutical preparations sold in the United States.
General Comments: Nicomorphine is a semisynthetic narcotic analgesic that has no accepted medicinal value in the United States.
Biochemistry: Unknown.
Toxicology–Pharmacology: Unknown.

▶ **NIKETHAMIDE**
Dangerous Drug

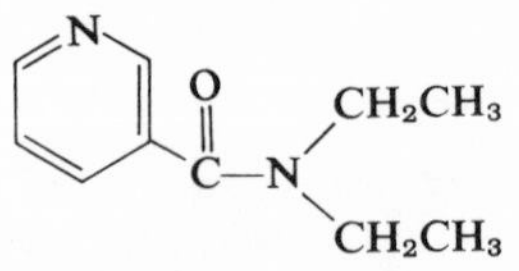

Synonyms: Aminocordine, cardinamide, diethylamide nicotinic acid, nicethamidum, nicorine, nikethylamide, pyridine-3-carboxydiethylamide.
Pharmaceutical Preparations: Coramine^R (Ciba)—Ampules. Oral solution: 25 percent by weight.
General Comments: Nikethamide is a central stimulant used medicinally to overcome central nervous system depression and circulatory failure. It is classified in this text as a Dangerous Drug because all pharmaceutical preparations require a prescription and bear the legend "Caution: Federal law prohibits dispensing without a prescription."
Biochemistry: Nikethamide is a *N*,*N*-diethylbenzamide with analeptic properties. Of all these compounds studied, those with 3-(lower alkoxyl)-4-hydroxy substitutions are most active (Cherniack and Young, 1964).
Toxicology–Pharmacology: Nikethamide is an analeptic drug, having primarily respiratory stimulant actions. It is used to counteract the respiratory depressant actions of narcotic drugs and the general depressants having respiratory depressant actions. Its efficacy in treatment of barbiturate poisoning is in doubt, however.

In higher doses, it stimulates higher motor centers, causing convulsions. Toxicity is first manifested by anxiety, nausea, and vomiting. No alarming or lasting side effects have been observed, however.

▶ **NITRAZEPAM**
Schedule IV

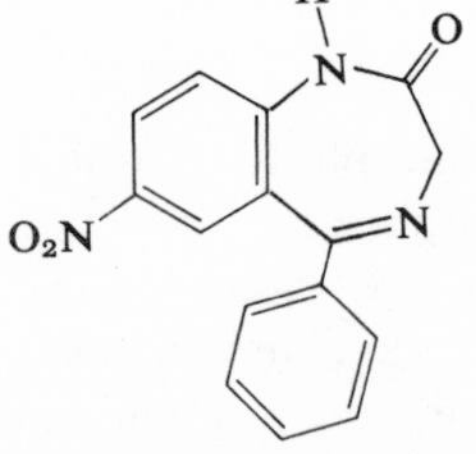

Synonym: 1,2-Dihydro-7-nitro-2-oxo-5-phenyl-3*H*-1,4-benzodiazepine.

Pharmaceutical Preparations: Nitrazepam is not found in any pharmaceutical preparations sold in the United States.

General Comment: Nitrazepam is a benzodiazepine tranquilizer.

Biochemistry: Similar to that of diazepam.

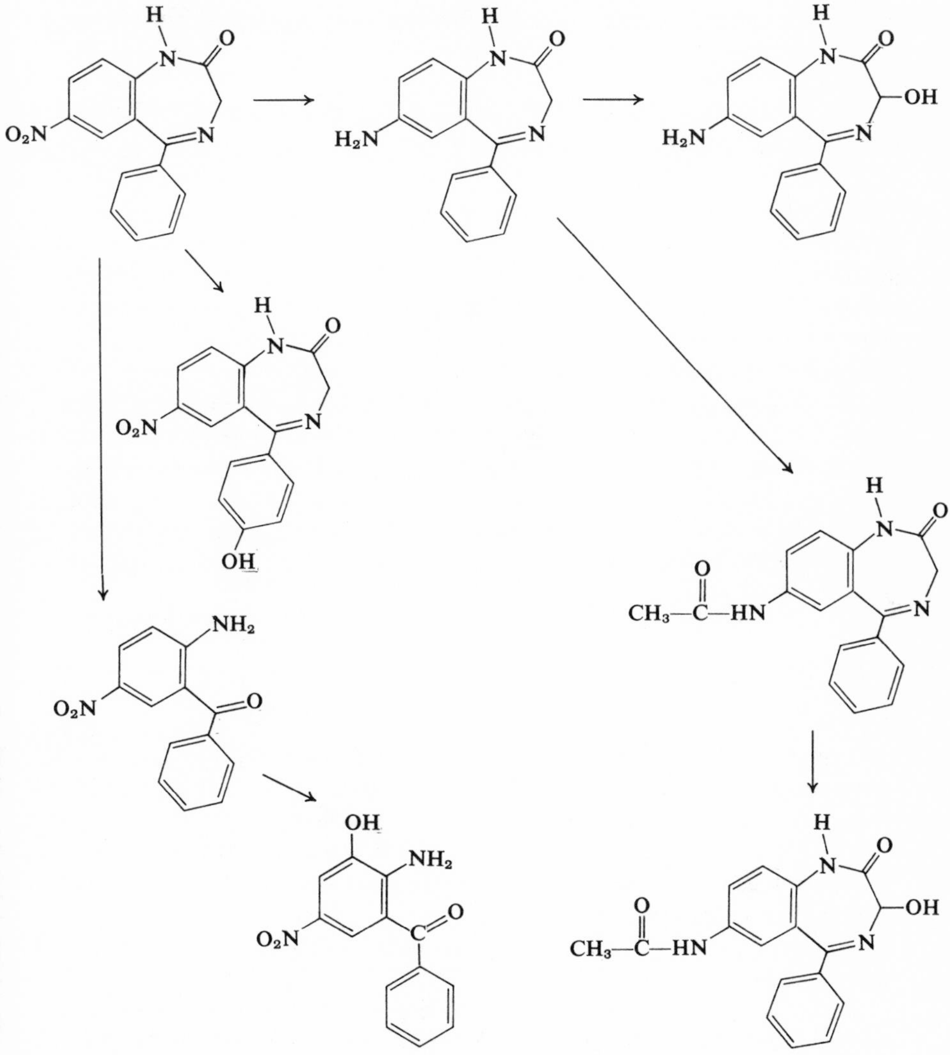

Toxicology–Pharmacology: Nitrazepam is a rapidly acting nonbarbiturate hypnotic, marketed in Europe under the trade name Mogadon^R. It has muscle-relaxant and anticonvulsant properties similar to the related compounds, chlordiazepoxide and diazepam. The principal use of nitrazepam is in the treatment of neuroses and anxiety. Nitrazepam usually induces sleep with a dosage of 10 mg.

Nitrazepam is metabolized to 7-amino nitrazepam, 7-acetamide nitrazepam, and 7-amino-3-hydroxy-2-amino-5-nitro benzophenone, which appear in the urine (Beyer and Sadie, 1969). About 23 percent of a dose is excreted in the urine within 48 hours of administration. Only 4.8 percent is excreted unchanged (Clarke, 1969).

At 6 hours after a 4-mg dose of nitrazepam, a plasma concentration of 0.004 mg/dl was observed (Reider, 1965). In a fatality from nitrazepam injection, a blood concentration of 0.90 mg/dl was reported (Baselt and Cravey, 1977).

▶ **NITROGLYCERIN**
Noncontrolled Substance
Encountered in Excepted Substances

$$CH_2—O—NO_2$$
$$CH—O—NO_2$$
$$CH_2—O—NO_2$$

General Comments: Nitroglycerin is a vasodilator drug that has direct action on arterioles and venules, resulting in a fall in blood pressure within 1–3 minutes following sublingual administration. It is encountered in excepted substances, and the following table shows the minimum drug/nitroglycerin ratios:

Drug	Drug/Nitroglycerin Ratio
Allobarbital	1/0.01
Butabarbital	1/0.02 with pentaerythritol tetranitrate, 0.67
Secobarbital	1/0.02 with pentaerythritol tetranitrate, 1.0

Toxicology–Pharmacology: Nitroglycerin has a direct vasodilating action on arterioles and venules, resulting in a fall in blood pressure within 1–3 minutes following sublingual administration. There is a flushing of the face, a throbbing headache, and an increase in cardiac rate induced by the fall in blood pressure. It is eliminated from the body very rapidly, and its effect is over within 30 minutes. It is used for patients with angina pectoris, in whom it is believed to improve myocardial oxygenation, marked increase in blood flow, and decrease in cardiac work.

Due to its relaxing effect on smooth muscle, it has been used for spasm of the biliary tract, gastrointestinal tract, and ureters, and for bronchospasm.

Toxic effects include throbbing headache, intense abdominal cramps with nausea and vomiting, and psychic disturbances. In severe cases, respiration may be slow and labored. The pulse slows and becomes dicrotic, and paralysis and clonic convulsions occur prior to death. Toxic effects may occur from inhalation of dust as well as by ingestion.

▶ **NORACYMETHADOL**
Schedule I

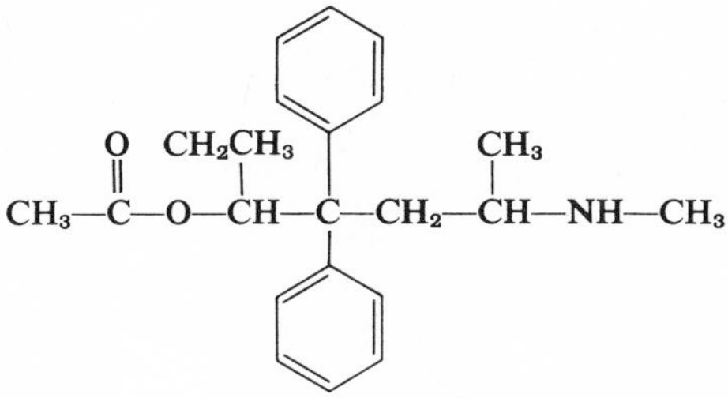

$$CH_3-\overset{\overset{\displaystyle O}{\|}}{C}-O-\overset{\overset{\displaystyle CH_2CH_3}{|}}{CH}-\overset{|}{C}-CH_2-\overset{\overset{\displaystyle CH_3}{|}}{CH}-NH-CH_3$$

Synonym: (±)-1-Ethyl-4-methylamino-2,2-diphenylpentylacetate.
Pharmaceutical Preparations: Noracymethadol is not found in any pharmaceutical preparations sold in the United States.
General Comment: Noracymethadol is a synthetic narcotic analgesic related to methadone that has no accepted medicinal value in the United States.
Biochemistry: Unknown.
Toxicology–Pharmacology: Unknown.

▶ **NORLEVORPHANOL**
Schedule I

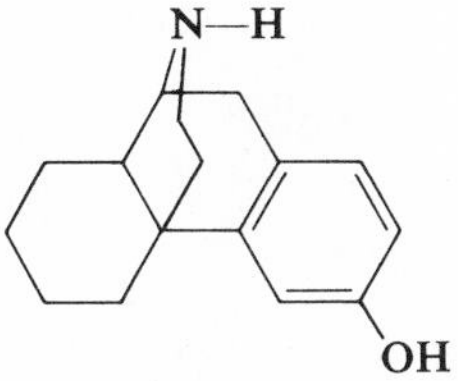

Synonym: (−)-3-Hydroxymorphinan.
Pharmaceutical Preparations: Norlevorphanol is not found in any pharmaceutical preparations sold in the United States.
General Comments: Norlevorphanol is a derivative (and also a metabolite) of

levorphanol, which is a Schedule II narcotic analgesic. Norlevorphanol has no accepted medicinal value in the United States.
Biochemistry: Unknown.
Toxicology–Pharmacology: Unknown.

▶ **NORMETHADONE**
Schedule I

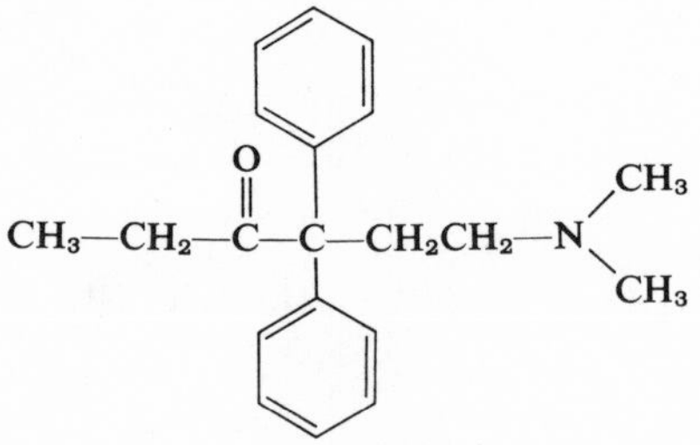

Synonyms: Phenyldimazone, 6-dimethylamino-4,4-diphenylhexan-3-one.
Pharmaceutical Preparations: Normethadone is not found in any pharmaceutical preparations sold in the United States.
General Comments: Normethadone is a derivative of methadone and is a synthetic narcotic analgesic and antitussive. It has no accepted medicinal value in the United States.
Biochemistry: Unknown.
Toxicology–Pharmacology: Unknown.

▶ **NORMORPHINE**
Schedule I

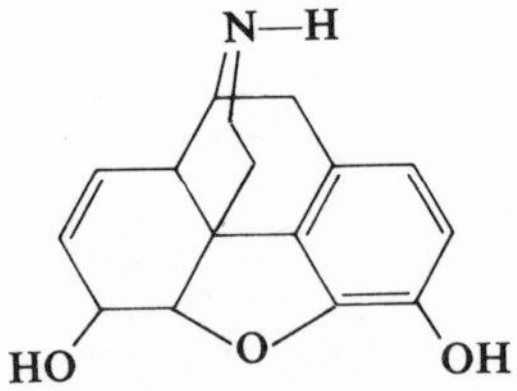

Synonyms: *N*-demethylmorphine, desmethylmorphine, 7,8-dehydro-4,5-epoxy-3,6-dihydroxy-morphinan.
Pharmaceutical Preparations: Normorphine is not found in any pharmaceutical preparations sold in the United States.

General Comments: Normorphine is a derivative (and a metabolite) of morphine. It has no accepted medicinal value in the United States.
Biochemistry: Unknown.
Toxicology–Pharmacology: Unknown.

▶ **NORPIPANONE**
Schedule I

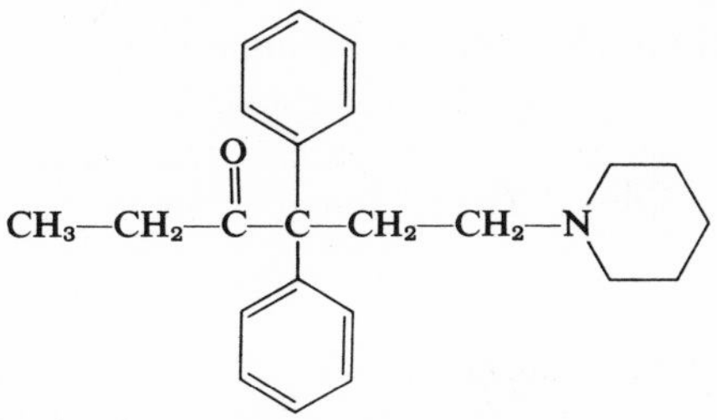

Synonym: 4,4-Diphenyl-6-(1-piperidyl)-3-hexanone.
Pharmaceutical Preparations: Norpipanone is not found in any pharmaceutical preparations sold in the United States.
General Comment: Norpipanone is a synthetic narcotic analgesic with no accepted medicinal value in the United States.
Biochemistry: Unknown.
Toxicology–Pharmacology: Unknown.

▶ **NORPSEUDOEPHEDRINE**
Noncontrolled Substance

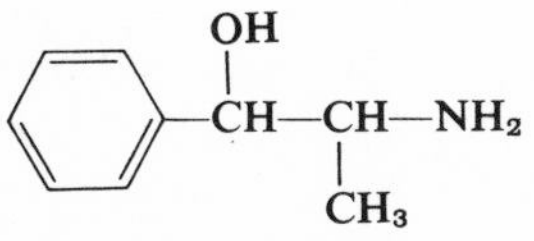

General Comments: Norpseudoephedrine is a sympathomimetic alkaloidal amine that has well-documented central stimulant properties. It is found naturally occurring in the leaves of a small tree (or shrub), *Catha edulis* Forsk. (Family *Celastraceae*), which is native to tropical East Africa.

The leaves are chewed habitually by many people in East Africa and the Arabian countries, or they make a tea from the leaves called khat or Abyssinian tea to alleviate the sensations of hunger and fatigue. Authorities disagree as to the safety of this practice. The Committee on Addiction-Producing

Drugs of the World Health Organization does not classify norpseudoephedrine as a drug producing habituation or addiction, but the French government considers it a narcotic.

▶ **OPIUM**

Schedule II—Opium is listed under Schedule II as opium and any salt, compound, derivative, or preparation of opium, including: (A) raw opium; (B) opium extracts; (C) opium fluid extracts; (D) powdered opium; (E) granulated opium; (F) tincture of opium; (G) opium poppy—defined as "the plant of the species *Papaver somniferum* L. except its seeds"; (H) opium straw—defined as "all parts, except the seeds, of the opium poppy, after mowing." The isoquinoline alkaloids of opium are exempt from control.

or

Schedule III for any material, compound, mixture, or preparation containing not more than 500 mg opium per 100 ml or per 100 g, or not more than 25 mg per dosage unit, with one or more active nonnarcotic ingredients in recognized therapeutic amounts

or

Schedule V for any compound, mixture, or preparation containing not more than 15 mg opium per 29.5729 ml, or per 28.35 g, that also contains one or more nonnarcotic active medicinal ingredients in sufficient proportion to confer on the compound, mixture, or preparation valuable medicinal qualities other than those possessed by the opium alone

Pharmaceutical Preparations

Schedule II

Pantopon^R (Roche)—Ampules: each 1 ml containing 20 mg opium alkaloids

B&O^R Supprettes (Webcon)—Suppositories: 15a, each suppository containing 30 mg powdered opium and 15 mg belladonna extract; 16a, each suppository containing 60 mg powdered opium and 15 mg belladonna extract

Schedule III

B.P.P.^{R}-Lemmon (Lemmon)—Tablets: yellow, containing 1.2 mg powdered opium

Diban^R (Robins)—Tablets: containing 12 mg powdered opium and 0.24 mg atropine

KBP/O^R Capsules (Cole)—Capsules: each containing 3.24 mg powdered opium

Schedule V

Donnagel^R-PG (Robins)—Each 30 cc (one fluid ounce) containing 24 mg powdered opium and 0.12 mg belladonna alkaloids

Parepectolin^R (Rorer)—Suspension: each fluid ounce containing 15 mg opium

The official pharmacopoeias standardize morphine content in opium at

9.5–12.0 percent (10 percent average). Commercial grades of opium contain morphine at 9–16 percent.

General Comments: None.

Biochemistry: There have been more than 25 different alkaloids isolated and identified from opium and its extracts. There are three major alkaloidal types: (1) the bridged phenanthrene type; (2) the isoquinoline alkaloids; (3) the berberine alkaloids.

1. The Bridged Phenanthrene Type

    a. Morphine

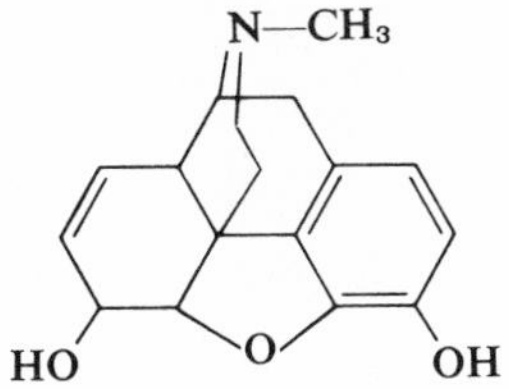

    Morphine is discussed under its own heading.

    b. Codeine

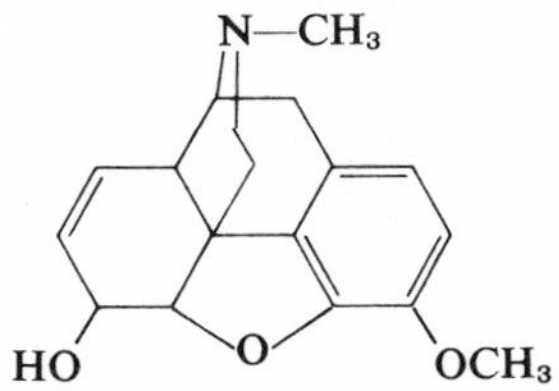

    Codeine is discussed under its own heading.

    c. Thebaine

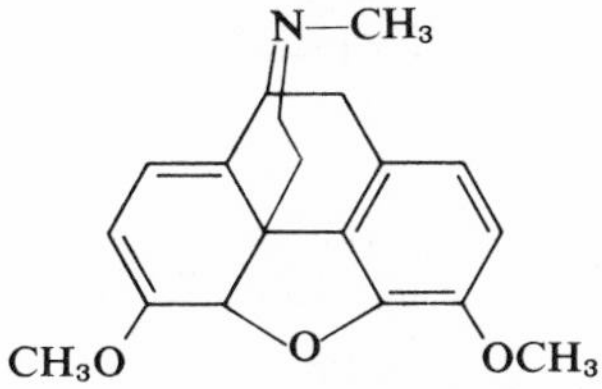

    Thebaine is discussed under its own heading.

    d. Sinomenine

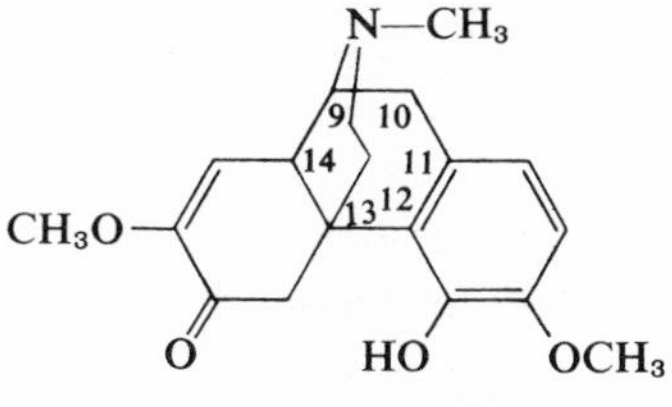

Sinomenine is structurally very similar to morphine, but stereochemically it is different. The configuration at the isometric centers, C-9, C-13, and C-14, is the mirror image of those in morphine. Sinomenine has very few systemic analgesic properties. Its toxicity, measured by the LD_{50} (oral administration), is 580 mg/kg.

e. Apomorphine

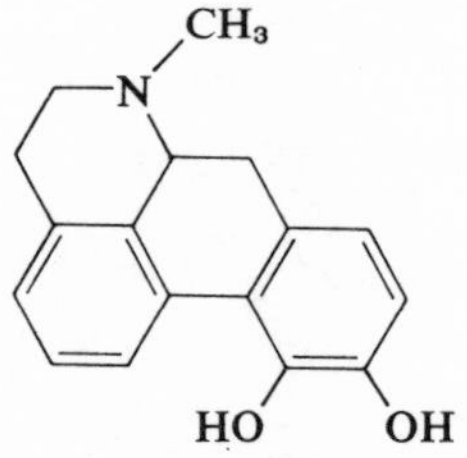

Apomorphine is discussed under its own heading.

2. *The Isoquinoline Alkaloids*
    a. Papaverine

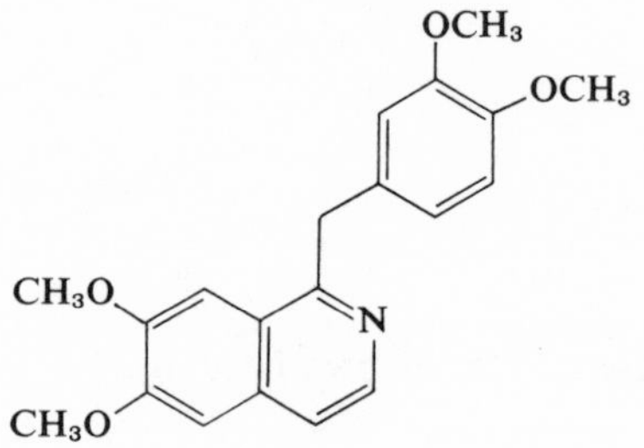

Papaverine is discussed under its own heading.

b. Laudanosine

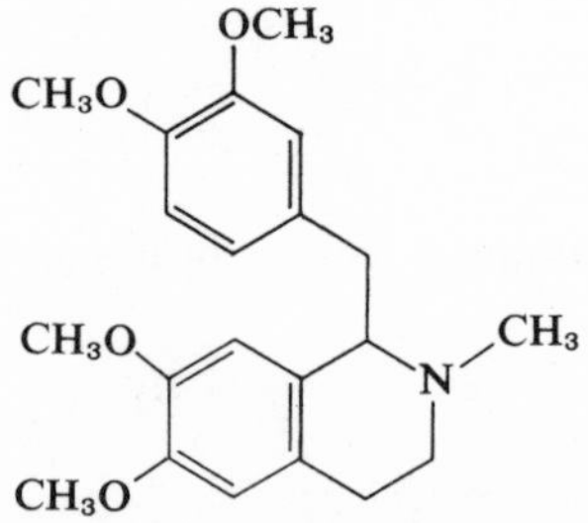

This alkaloid occurs to the extent of less than 0.1 percent in opium. It has also been synthetically produced by the reduction of papaverine.

c. Laudanine

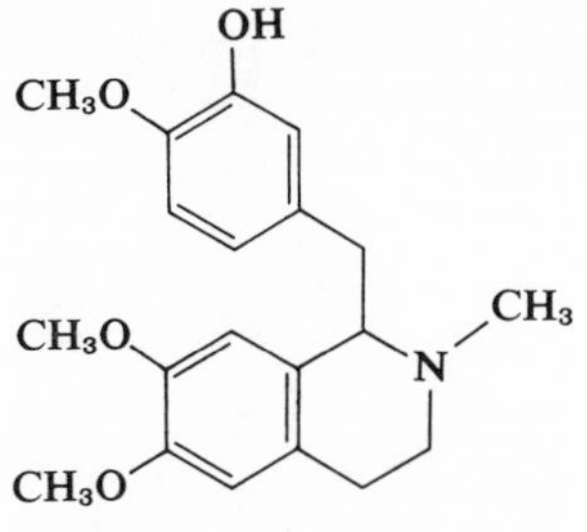

The structure of laudanine was determined by Spath. It was determined that laudanine, as the natural alkaloid in opium, is in the racemic form (Spath, 1920).

d. Noscapine (narcotine)

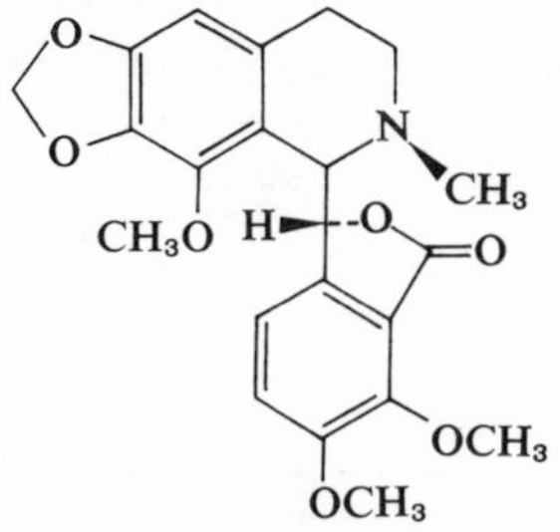

Noscapine is an alkaloid that was isolated from opium in 1804. It has been found present in opium up to the extent of 10 percent. Noscapine is a good cough suppressant. The naturally occurring isomer of noscapine is the α-isomer, positioned at C-1. Under the influence of the base, the α-noscapine is isomerized to β-noscapine.

3. *The Berberine Alkaloids*

The berberine alkaloids do not contain an isoquinoline nucleus, but are closely related to berberine.

a. Protopine

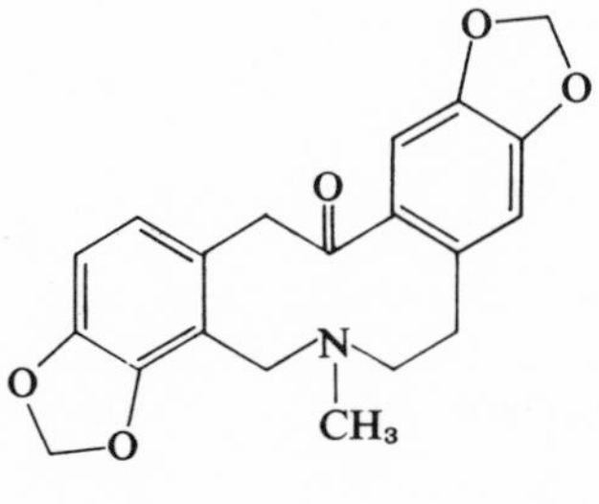

Protopine was first isolated from opium in 1871. Protopine is found in all genera of the family *Papaveraceae* that have been thoroughly examined. However, in opium it is present only in minute amounts.

b. Cryptopine

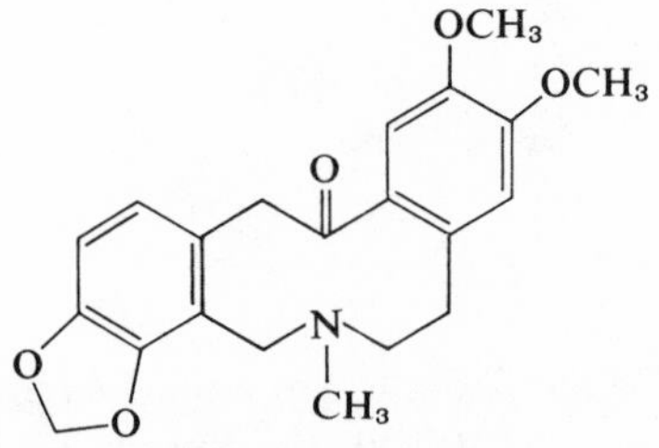

Cryptopine was first isolated from opium in 1867 and its structure elucidated in 1926. Like protopine, it has antifibrillatory properties.

Metabolism: The major metabolite of morphine is the phenolic glucuronide plus a diglucuronide of both OH groups. Codeine conjugates at the allylic OH as the major metabolite with equal amounts of *N*- and *O*-dealkylation.

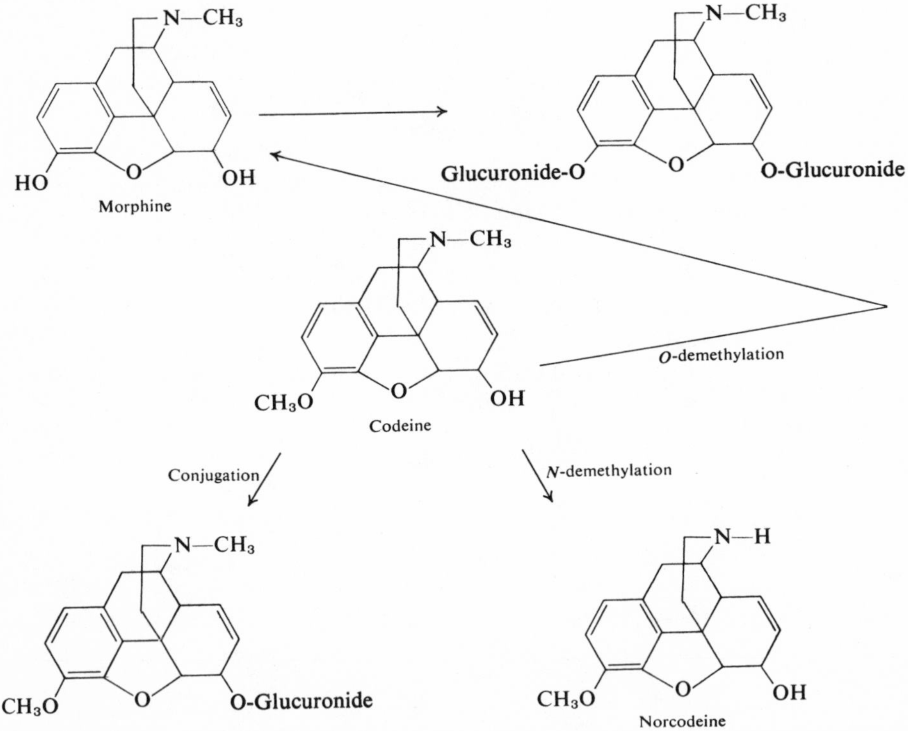

Biosynthesis: The basic biosynthetic reactions in opium are relatively simple. Papaverine is the result of the condensation of alanine or tyrosine. Norlaudanosoline is probably an intermediate in this reaction:

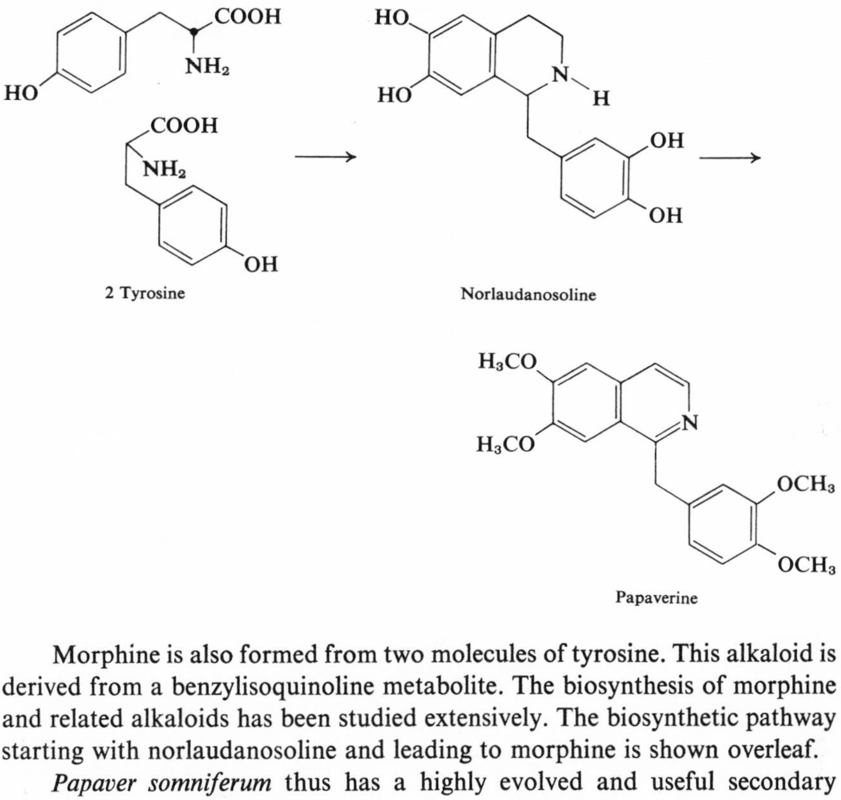

2 Tyrosine   Norlaudanosoline

Papaverine

Morphine is also formed from two molecules of tyrosine. This alkaloid is derived from a benzylisoquinoline metabolite. The biosynthesis of morphine and related alkaloids has been studied extensively. The biosynthetic pathway starting with norlaudanosoline and leading to morphine is shown overleaf.

Papaver somniferum thus has a highly evolved and useful secondary metabolism that culminates in morphine. *Papaver bracheatum*, a thebaine-producing poppy, appears to lack any significant demethylation capability. This feature may be useful in a medicinal source for codeine without relying on *P. somniferum*.

The opium alkaloids are formed in various cells of the poppy and excreted into the lactiferous ducts.

The isolated latex is capable of alkaloid biosynthesis in the presence of suitable precursors and cofactors, as well as metabolic destruction of morphine.

Toxicology–Pharmacology: Opium is the air-dried milky exudate obtained by incising the unripe capsules of *Papaver somniferum* Linne (Family Papaveraceae). Due to its long history as a cultivated species, several varieties of *P. somniferum* exist. Thus, the taxonomy of this plant is extremely complicated.

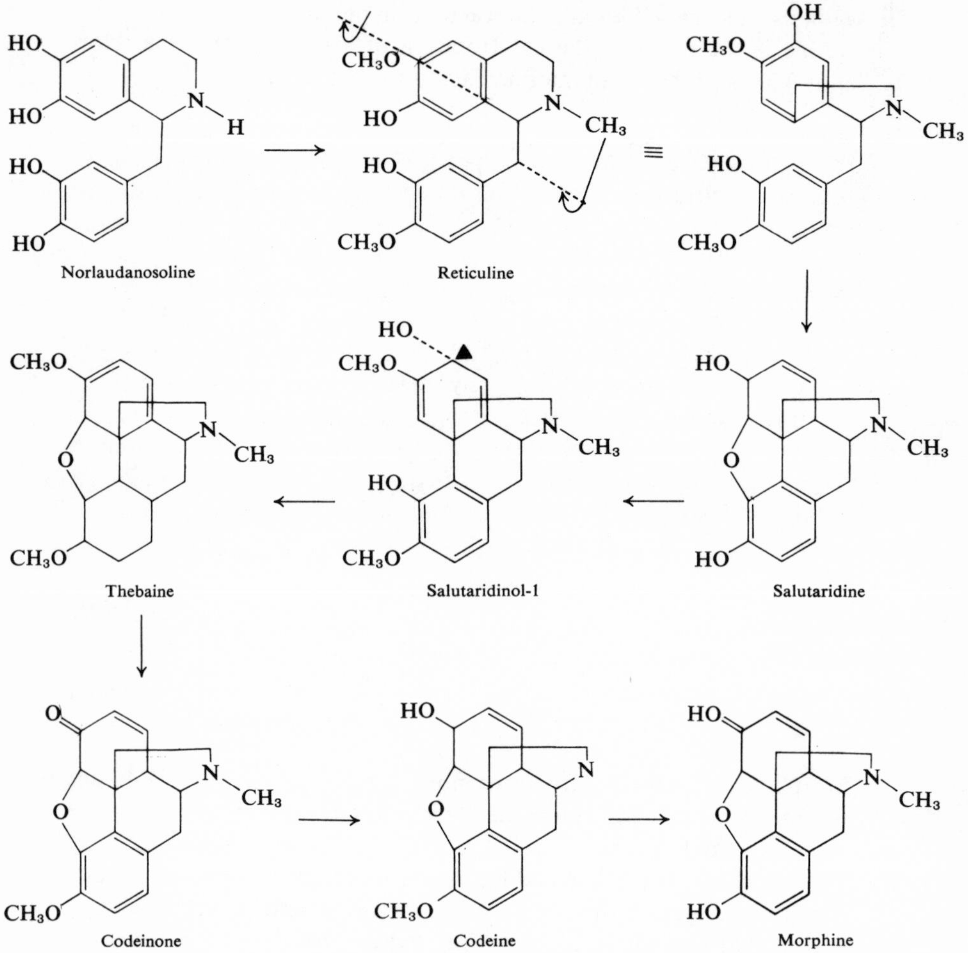

Norlaudanosoline → Reticuline ≡ (structure)

Thebaine ← Salutaridinol-1 ← Salutaridine

Codeinone → Codeine → Morphine

The term "opium" stems from the Greek word "opion," meaning poppy juice. *Papaver* is the Latin name for poppy, and *somniferum* is the Latin word meaning to produce sleep.

The opium poppy is an annual herb with large individual flowers varying in color from white to pink or purple. The color of its seed ranges from blue-black or gray to yellow-white or rose-brown.

Opium itself is rarely used today in therapeutics, its extracted and purified alkaloids being used instead. The most common application for opium is as a tincture (alcohol solution) given to control diarrhea. The benzylisoquinoline alkaloids, papaverine, narcotine, and narceine, have little effect, although narcotine may antagonize the respiratory depression induced by morphine. The predominant actions of opium are due to the phenanthrene alkaloids, morphine and codeine. Given as the mixture, in small doses, opium has little of the anesthetic and hypnotic properties of the pure alkaloids and synthetic narcotics.

In larger doses, opium produces euphoric sensations and drowsiness. In toxic doses, the most prominent symptom is sleep, accompanied by slowed respiration. As intoxication progresses, respiration becomes slower, more shallow, and irregular, and the skin becomes cyanotic. The pupils become smaller, as with other narcotic drug overdose, and coma followed by respiratory arrest may occur.

As little as 30 mg opium may be fatal, although tolerant individuals may ingest many times this dose without any effect. Opium poisoning may be treated by administration of narcotic antagonists, such as nalline and naloxone, to antagonize the respiratory depressant effect. Evacuation of the stomach must be accomplished by stomach tube, since opium inhibits vomiting, and emesis cannot be induced. Potassium permanganate solution can be used as a stomach lavage fluid, as it oxidizes morphine.

▶ **OXAZEPAM**
Schedule IV

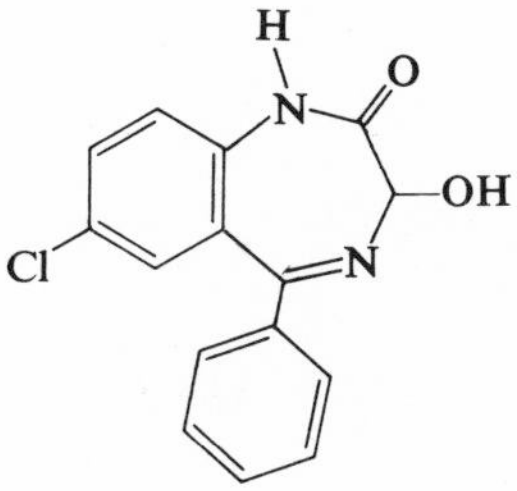

Synonym: 7-Chloro-1,3-dihydro-3-hydroxy-5-phenyl-2H-1,4-benzodiazepin-2-one.

Pharmaceutical Preparations

Serax^R (Wyeth)—Capsules, containing oxazepam: pink and white, 10 mg; red and white, 15 mg; maroon and white, 30 mg. Tablets: containing oxazepam, white, 15 mg.

General Comments: Oxazepam is a tranquilizer structurally and pharmacologically related to chlordiazepoxide and diazepam. It has sedative and anticonvulsant actions, but has little skeletal muscle relaxant activity.

Biochemistry: Similar to that of diazepam.

Toxicology–Pharmacology: Oxazepam is a tranquilizer with actions similar to those of diazepam and chlordiazepoxide. It has sedative and anticonvulsant actions, but little skeletal muscle relaxant actions as do the other benzodiazepines. It is used to treat patients with anxiety, tension, and irritability, but is not used in psychotic states.

It has a low incidence of side effects, although drowsiness is a common effect. Nausea, dizziness, hypotension, and slurred speech are among some of the less common side effects. It has synergetic effects that may cause a dangerous depression when it is combined with alcohol or other depressant or sedative medications.

Overdose is characterized by depression and drowsiness, but as the benzodiazepines do not seriously depress respiration, death from oral overdose is rare.

Oxazepam induces a dangerous potentiation of action when alcohol and/ or other psychotropic drugs are used concomitantly.

Therapeutic blood concentrations of oxazepam have been reported to be 0.09–0.14 mg/dl 2 hours after single oral dosages of 45 mg (Knowles and Ruelius, 1972). In one nonfatal case of overdose of oxazepam, a blood concentration of 0.05 mg/dl was found 18 hours after ingestion (Shimkin and Shaivitz, 1966).

▶ OXYCODONE
Schedule II

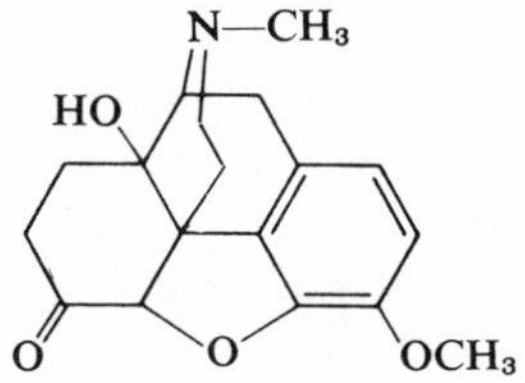

Synonyms: Dihydrohydroxycodeinon, 7,8-dihydro-14-hydroxycodeinon, dihydrone, oxycone, thecodin, 4,5-epoxy-14-hydroxy-3-methoxy-N-methyl-6-oxomorphinan.

Pharmaceutical Preparations

Percodan[R] (Endo)—Tablet: yellow, scored, containing 4.5 mg oxycodone hydrochloride, 0.38 mg oxycodone terephthalate, 224 mg aspirin, 160 mg phenacetin, and 32 mg caffeine

Percodan-Demi[R] (Endo)—Tablet: pink, scored, containing 2.5 mg oxycodone hydrochloride, 0.19 mg oxycodone terephthalate, 224 mg aspirin, 160 mg phenacetin, and 32 mg caffeine

General Comments: Oxycodone is a semisynthetic narcotic that is a derivative of morphine. It is pharmacologically related to hydrocodone in its sedative, analgesic, and antitussive properties.

Biochemistry: Similar to that of hydromorphone and oxymorphone. Also see **HYDROMORPHINOL.**

Toxicology–Pharmacology: Oxycodone is a synthetic narcotic derivative of morphine, having typical narcotic properties of sedation, analgesia, and antitussive actions. Its addiction potential is less than that of morphine. It is effective orally, and is used primarily as an analgesic.

Due to the euphoric properties characteristic of the narcotic drugs, oxycodone may be abused. Overdosage is characterized by respiratory depression and coma. It may be treated by use of narcotic antagonists such as nalline or naloxone.

▶ **OXYMORPHONE**
Schedule II

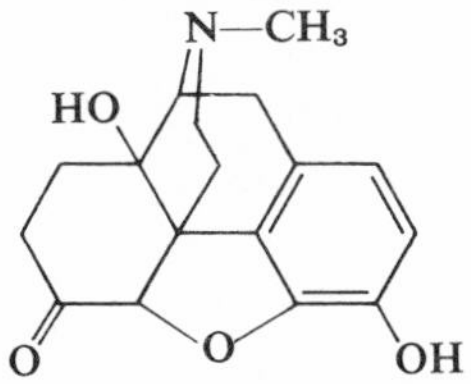

Synonyms: Dihydrohydroxymorphinone, 7,8-dihydro-14-hydroxymorphinone, dimorphone, oximorphone, oxydimorphone, 4,5-epoxy-3,14-dihydroxy-N-methyl-6-oxomorphinan.

Pharmaceutical Preparations: Oxymorphone is not frequently found in pharmaceutical preparations sold in the United States.

Biochemistry: Oxymorphone is produced by controlled demethylation of oxycodone. Both oxycodone and oxymorphone have a high physical-dependence potential. Also see **HYDROMORPHINOL.**

Toxicology–Pharmacology: Oxymorphone is a potent narcotic analgesic, being approximately ten times as potent as morphine. Since it also has an even higher euphoric action, it has a high addictive liability.

As little as 1 mg may be an effective analgesic dose, but with 1.5–2.0 mg, the outward effects are similar to those with 12 mg morphine sulfate.

The primary side effect with oxymorphone is respiratory depression, and caution must be used in debilitated or older patients when prescribing oxymorphone. Overdosage with oxymorphone is characterized by respiratory depression and coma, and can be treated with narcotic antagonists such as nalline or naloxone.

▶ **OXYPERTINE**
Dangerous Drug

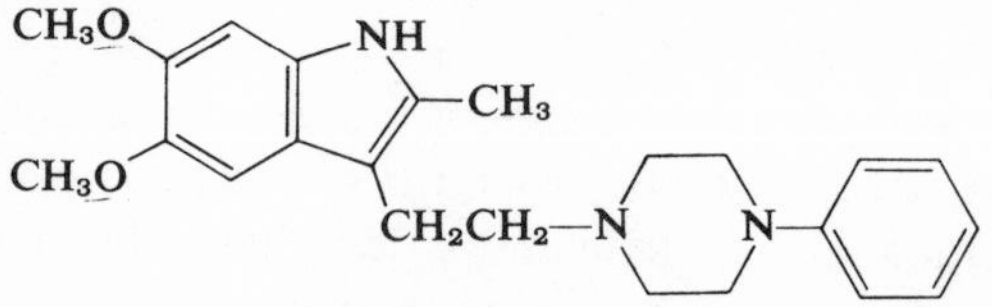

Synonym: 5,6-Dimethoxy-2-methyl-3-[2-(4-phenylpiperazin-1-yl)ethyl]indole.
Pharmaceutical Preparations: Oxypertine is not found in any pharmaceutical preparations sold in the United States.
General Comment: Oxypertine is a tranquilizer and is therefore classified in this text as a Dangerous Drug.
Biochemistry: Oxypertine is an antipsychotic agent with activity resembling that of the phenothiazines and butyrophenones. At low doses, it possesses many of the properties of the phenothiazines; however, it acts like reserpine by depleting monoamines. Oxypertine is the prototype of the indolylalkyl-phenylpiperazines.
Toxicology–Pharmacology: Oxypertine is a tranquilizer that has been used to treat schizophrenia and nervous disorders. The dose may be up to 300 mg per day.

▶ **OXYPHENCYCLIMINE**
Noncontrolled Substance
Encountered in Excepted Substances

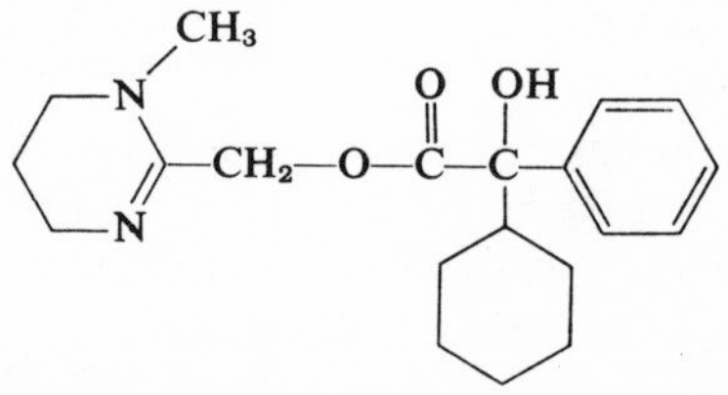

General Comments: Oxyphencyclimine is a parasympatholytic drug with atropine-like actions. It is encountered in phenobarbital preparations that are classified as excepted in a phenobarbital/oxyphencyclimine minimum ratio of 1/0.4.
Toxicology–Pharmacology: Oxyphencyclimine is an anticholinergic drug, with actions similar to those of atropine. Its actions on the gastrointestinal tract are to inhibit secretion of gastric juices and to inhibit the motility of the stomach and intestines. It is used in the treatment of peptic ulcer, spastic colon, gastritis, duodenitis, and hiatus hernia.

Untoward side effects include dryness of the mouth, blurred vision, constipation, and urinary retention. With high doses, central nervous system stimulation may occur.

▶ **PAPAVERINE**
Noncontrolled Substance

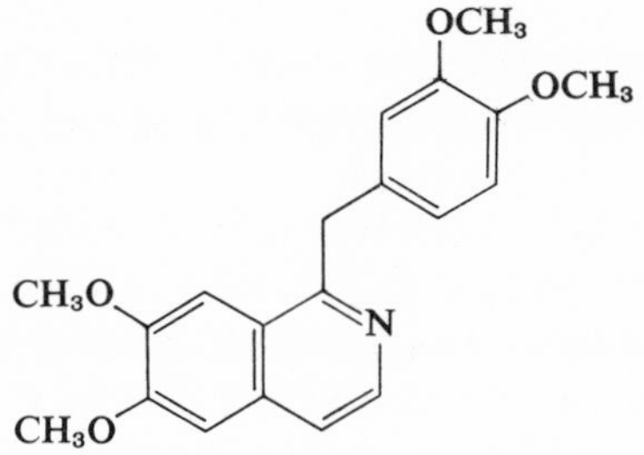

General Comments: Papaverine is an isoquinoline alkaloid of opium that was first discovered in 1848. It lacks the narcotic properties of morphine, but does have properties to relax smooth muscles.

Toxicology–Pharmacology: Papaverine is one of the alkaloids of opium, occurring in a concentration of about 1 percent. Papaverine lacks the narcotic properties of morphine, and has as its chief action the antagonism of smooth muscle spasm. It relaxes the smooth muscle of the intestinal and biliary tracts, bronchial tree, ureters, and blood vessels. It has been used to treat coronary artery disease and relieve pain from cardiac infarction when given intravenously. Some deaths have been reported, however.

It is given intramuscularly in a dose range of 30–60 mg, and orally in a dose of 60–200 mg.

It is short-acting, with a biological half-life of 100 minutes. It is metabolized to glucuronide conjugates, principally 4'-hydroxy-papaverine, which are excreted in the urine (Axelrod, 1958).

▶ **PARALDEHYDE**
Schedule IV

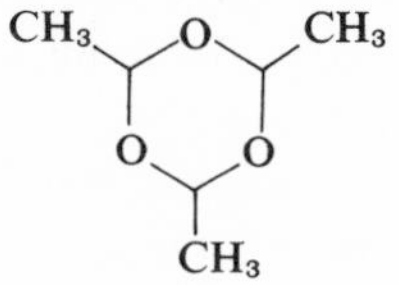

Synonym: Paracetaldehyde.

Pharmaceutical Preparations: Hospital preparations.
General Comments: Paraldehyde is a cyclic acetal of acetaldehyde. It was introduced as a medicinal agent in 1882.
Biochemistry: See Toxicology–Pharmacology below.
Toxicology–Pharmacology: Paraldehyde is a fast-acting hypnotic drug, inducing sleep within 10–30 minutes, and lasting 4–8 hours. It does not have analgesic effects, nor does it effect marked changes in the respiration, circulation, or sensibility. In large doses, it produces a deep coma. It is used to control insomnia, excitement, delirium, and convulsions. Its primary usefulness today is in treatment of delirium tremens, and to control excitement in psychiatric conditions. Continued use of paraldehyde can result in tolerance and addiction, similar to that experienced with alcohol.

Paraldehyde decomposes with time to yield toxic decomposition products. Fatalities have resulted from use of decomposed solutions. Paraldehyde is much more toxic in patients with lung and liver disease, and death from respiratory depression can occur after overdose.

After a 10-ml intramuscular injection of paraldehyde, maximum blood concentrations of 7.70 mg/dl were obtained in 70 minutes. The usual therapeutic blood concentration range is from 3.4 to 15.0 mg/dl (Maes *et al.*, 1969). The approximate lethal blood concentration is 50 mg/dl.

▶ **PECAZINE**
Dangerous Drug

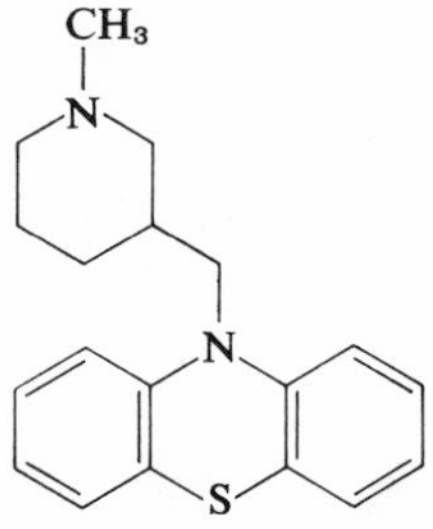

Synonyms: Mepazine, 10-(1-methylpiperid-3-ylmethyl)-phenothiazine.
Pharmaceutical Preparations: Pecazine is not found in any pharmaceutical preparations sold in the United States.
General Comment: Pecazine is a phenothiazine tranquilizer and is therefore classified in this text as a Dangerous Drug.
Biochemistry: Unknown.
Toxicology–Pharmacology: Unknown.

▶ **PEMOLINE**
Schedule IV

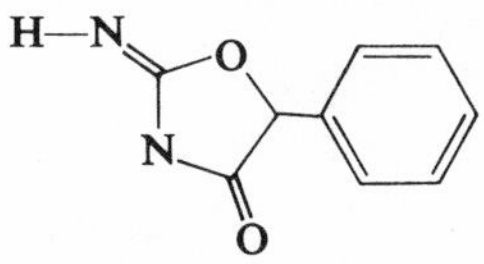

Synonyms: Phenilone, 5-phenylisohydantoin, 2-imino-4-oxo-5-phenyloxazo-lidine.

Pharmaceutical Preparations: Cylert^R (Abbott)—Tablets, scored, containing pemoline: yellow, 18.75 mg; orange, 37.5 mg; tan, 75 mg.

General Comments: None.

Biochemistry: See Toxicology–Pharmacology below.

Toxicology–Pharmacology: Pemoline is a central nervous system stimulant with pharmacological activity similar to that of other known stimulants but with minimal sympathomimetic effects. It is not structurally related to the amphetamines or methylphenidate.

Pemoline is used in treatment of children with psychological, educational, or social problems such as severe hyperactivity, short attention span, distractibility, emotional lability, and impulsiveness.

▶ **PENTAERYTHRITOL TETRANITRATE**
Noncontrolled Substance
Encountered in Excepted Substances

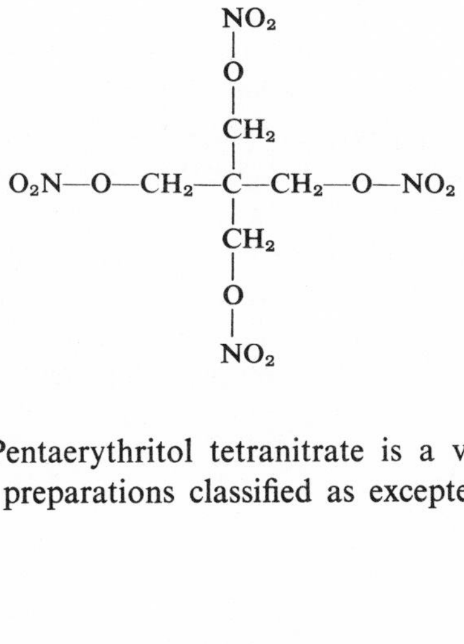

General Comments: Pentaerythritol tetranitrate is a vasodilator. It is encountered in various preparations classified as excepted preparations. The following table indicates the drug/pentaerythritol tetranitrate ratios encountered in these preparations:

Drug	Drug/Pentaerythritol Tetranitrate Ratio
Amobarbital	1/0.6
Butabarbital	1/0.75
Butabarbital	1/0.67 (with 0.02 nitroglycerine)
Secobarbital	1/1 (with 0.02 nitroglycerine)
Meprobamate	1/0.05
Mephobarbital	1/2 (with 3 ethaverine)
Phenobarbital	1/0.67

Toxicology–Pharmacology: Pentaerythritol tetranitrate is a vasodilator. It is used to reduce the frequency of attacks of angina pectoris, and to lessen the severity of anginal pain. Side effects may include headache, dizziness and weakness, and postural hypotension.

After oral administration, the drug acts within 30–60 minutes, and the effects persist 4–5 hours.

▶ **PENTAZOCINE**
Dangerous Drug

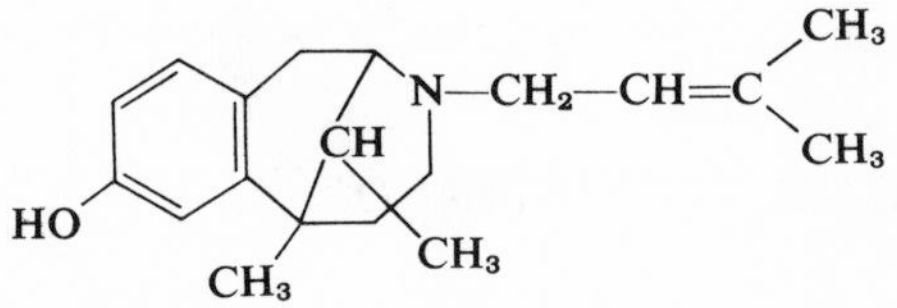

Synonym: 1,2,3,4,5,6-Hexahydro-8-hydroxy-6,11-dimethyl-3-(3-methylbut-2-enyl)-2,6-methano-3-benzazocine.
Pharmaceutical Preparations: Talwin^R (Winthrop)—Injection: each 1 ml containing 30 mg pentazocine lactate. Tablets: peach-colored, scored, containing 50 mg pentazocine (but as hydrochloride salt). Capsules: white, containing 12.5 mg pentazocine (but as hydrochloride salt) and 325 mg aspirin.
General Comments: Pentazocine is a synthetic analgesic. It is classified in this text as a Dangerous Drug, as all pharmaceutical preparations bear the legend "Caution: Federal law prohibits dispensing without a prescription."
Biochemistry: Pentazocine is a 6,7-benzomorphan derivative having the following molecular analgetic features (Schaumann, 1949): (1) benzene nucleus; (2) quaternary carbon atom attached to the nucleus; (3) tertiary nitrogen atom two methylene groups away from the quaternary carbon atom.

Synthetic procedures lead to either the α- or the β-(±)-(*cis*)-5-dialkyl compound. The β isomer has the greater analgetic potency, dependence liability, and toxicity.

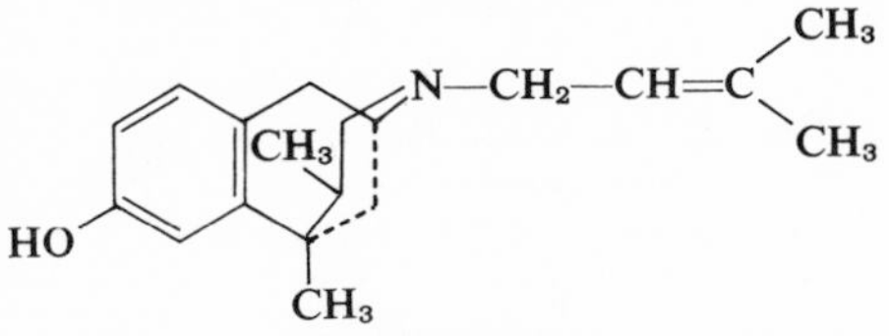

α-Pentazocine 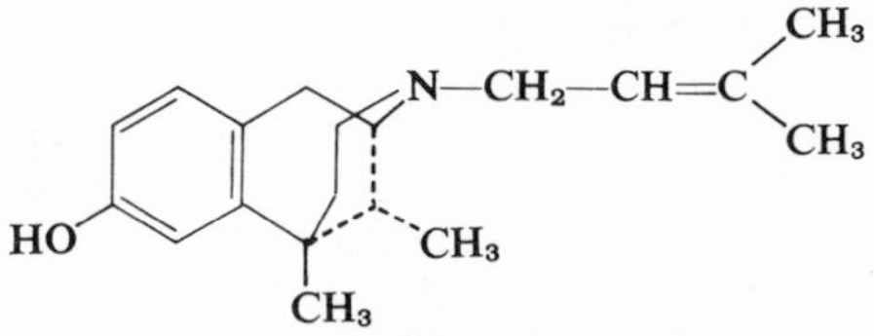   β-Pentazocine

Toxicology–Pharmacology: Pentazocine is a synthetic narcotic analgesic. It is about one third as effective as morphine on a weight basis in the relief of pain. Analgesia usually occurs within 15–20 minutes after an intramuscular injection, and lasts for about 3 hours. It is only about one fourth as effective if given orally, because of poor absorption from the gastrointestinal tract.

Tolerance and addiction may occur from the continued use of pentazocine, although its potential is not as great as with morphine. Pentazocine also is a mild narcotic antagonist, and withdrawal symptoms may be precipitated in narcotic addicts.

Overdose with pentazocine may occur, especially when it is used intravenously. Its respiratory depressant properties are not as great as those of other narcotics, and death by any means of administration is unusual. Overdose symptoms do not respond to treatment with the narcotic antagonist nalorphine, but naloxone may be used.

After administration of 45 mg intramuscularly, a plasma concentration of 0.012 mg/dl was observed (Berkowitz *et al.*, 1969). In four fatal overdoses by the oral route, blood concentrations ranged from 0.38 to 1.47 mg/dl (Garriott, 1977).

▶ **PENTHIENATE BROMIDE**
Noncontrolled Substance
Encountered in Excepted Substances

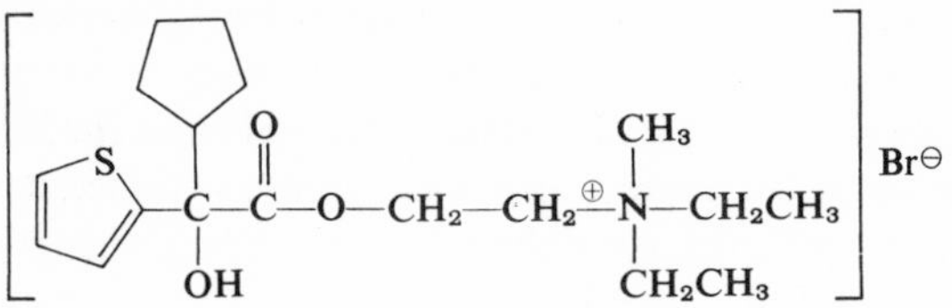

Penthienate bromide is an antimuscarinic drug that is a synthetic substitute for the belladonna alkaloids. It is encountered in various pharmaceutical preparations classified as excepted substances. The following table indicates the minimum drug/penthienate bromide ratio encountered in these excepted preparations:

Drug	Drug/Penthienate Bromide Ratio
Mephobarbital	1/0.15

Toxicology–Pharmacology: Penthienate bromide is a synthetic antimuscarinic drug, with properties similar to those of atropine. It is well absorbed after oral administration. It may be used to inhibit the effect of parasympathetic nervous system activity. General effects of penthienate are to inhibit salivation and sweating, diminish gastrointestinal motility and secretions, and produce mydriasis (dilation of the pupils of the eyes). Some conditions that may be treated by this agent are motion sickness, parkinsonism, and peptic ulcer.

Toxic doses produce dryness of the mouth, blurred vision, dizziness, tachycardia, tremor, and fatigue.

▶ **PENTOBARBITAL**
Schedule II

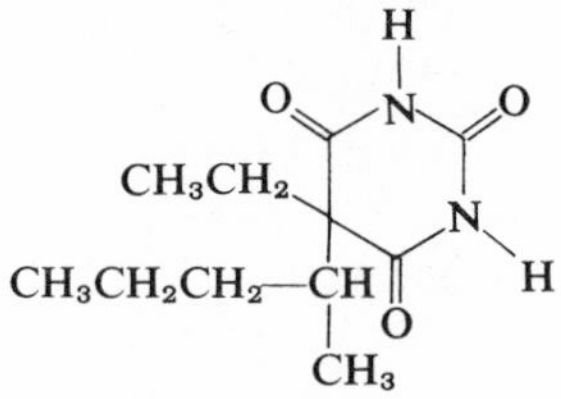

General Comments: The Controlled Substances Act states that Schedule III will apply to, unless listed in another schedule, any material, compound, mixture, or preparation that contains any quantity of pentobarbital having a potential for abuse associated with a depressant effect on the central nervous system, and that contains, in addition to pentobarbital, one or more active medicinal ingredients that are not scheduled substances. Also, any suppository dosage approved by the Food and Drug Administration that contains pentobarbital falls into Schedule III. In addition, any of the Schedule III preparations are subject to the excepted substances clause in Schedule III.

Synonyms: Pentobarbitone, ethaminal, 5-ethyl-5-(1 +methylbutyl)barbituric acid.

Pharmaceutical Preparations

Schedule II

Nebralin[R] (Dorsey)—Tablet: timed-release, containing 90 mg pentobarbital

Nembutal[R] Elixir (Abbott)—Elixir: each 5 ml containing 20 mg sodium pentobarbital

Nembutal[R] Gradumet (Abbott)—Tablets: blue, containing 100 mg sodium pentobarbital

Nembutal[R] Sodium (Abbott)—Capsules, containing sodium pentobarbital: yellow, 30 mg; clear and yellow, 50 mg; yellow, 100 mg. Injection: Each 1 ml containing 50 mg.

Schedule III

Emerset[R] (Arnar-Stone)—Suppositories: pink, containing 30 mg pentobarbital and 25 mg pyrilamine; green, containing 45 mg pentobarbital and 50 mg pyrilamine; blue, containing 100 mg pentobarbital and 50 mg pyrilamine

Nembutal[R] (Abbott)—Suppositories: containing 20, 30, 60, or 120 mg sodium pentobarbital

Also see Chapter 6.

General Comments: None.

Biochemistry: The two major metabolites of pentobarbital are the two optical isomers of hydroxypentobarbital. These metabolites account for a major portion of a dose of pentobarbital excreted in the urine. Minor metabolites are pentobarbital carboxylic acid and ketopentobarbital. A very small percentage is excreted as the unchanged drug (Kuntzman *et al.*, 1967).

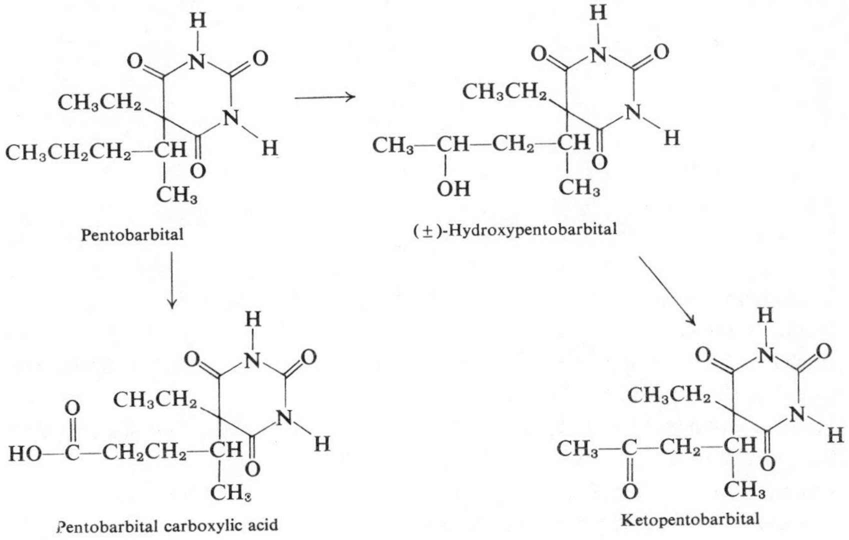

Pentobarbital

(±)-Hydroxypentobarbital

Pentobarbital carboxylic acid

Ketopentobarbital

Toxicology–Pharmacology: Pentobarbital is a widely used short- to inter-mediate-acting barbiturate. It is a sedative–hypnotic drug, and is employed primarily as a hypnotic in the treatment of insomnia. Its general effect, as with other derivatives of barbituric acid, is as a general depressant primarily on the central nervous system, but also to some extent on smooth muscles, skeletal muscles, and cardiac muscle. Ordinary doses have no effect on muscles of the cardiovascular system, but effect a sedation or general anes-thesia.

With overdose, all systems are depressed, and depression of the respirat-ory system may lead to death, if not treated. A usual hypnotic dose of pento-barbital is 100–200 mg. Lethal doses of pentobarbital ranged from 1.5 to 9.1 g, with the majority from 1.5 to 4.4 g (Cimbura et al., 1972).

After administration of 600 mg over a 3-hour period, maximum blood concentrations of 0.18–0.47 mg/dl were observed at 30 minutes after the last administration. After 18 hours, blood concentrations were 0.12–0.17 mg/dl (Parker et al., 1970).

In a study of 55 deaths from oral overdose of barbiturates, blood con-centrations of from 0.5 to 16.9 mg/dl were found, the average being 3.0 mg/dl (Baselt et al., 1975b).

▶ **PERICYAZINE**
Dangerous Drug

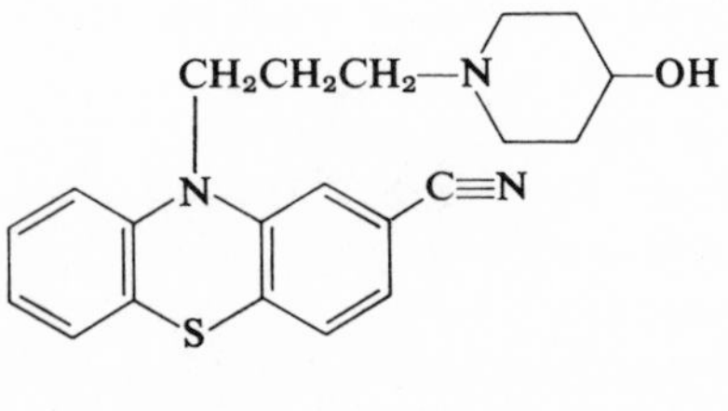

Synonyms: Propericeazine, 2-cyano-10-[3-(4-hydroxypiperidino)propyl]-phenothiazine.
Pharmaceutical Preparations: Pericyazine is not found in any pharmaceutical preparations sold in the United States.
General Comment: Pericyazine is a phenothiazine tranquilizer and is there-fore classified in this text as a Dangerous Drug.
Biochemistry: Unknown.
Toxicology–Pharmacology: Unknown.

▶ **PERPHENAZINE**
Dangerous Drug

$$CH_2CH_2CH_2-N \bigcirc N-CH_2CH_2-OH$$

Synonyms: Chlorpiprazine, 2-chloro-10-(3-[4-(2-hydroxyethyl)piperazin-1-yl]propyl)phenothiazine.

Pharmaceutical Preparations

Etrafon^R (Schering)—Tablets, sugar-coated: yellow, containing 20 mg perphenazine and 10 mg amitriptyline; orange, containing 4 mg perphenazine and 10 mg amitriptyline; pink, containing 2 mg perphenazine and 25 mg amitriptyline; red, containing 4 mg perphenazine and 25 mg amitriptyline

Triavil^R (Merck Sharp & Dohme)—Tablets, triangular, coated: orange, containing 2 mg perphenazine and 25 mg amitriptyline; yellow, containing 4 mg perphenazine and 25 mg amitriptyline; blue, containing 2 mg perphenazine and 10 mg amitriptyline; salmon, containing 4 mg perphenazine and 10 mg amitriptyline

Trilafon^R (Schering)—Tablets, sugar-coated, containing perphenazine: gray, 2, 4, 8, or 16 mg; white, 8 mg. Syrup: each 5 ml containing 2 mg perphenazine. Concentrate: each 5 ml containing 16 mg perphenazine. Injection: each 1 ml containing 5 mg perphenazine.

General Comment: Perphenazine is a phenothiazine tranquilizer and is therefore classified in this text as a Dangerous Drug.

Biochemistry: Similar to that of acetophenazine.

Toxicology–Pharmacology: Perphenazine is a substituted phenothiazine tranquilizer. Its tranquilizing actions are more potent than those of prochlorperazine or chlorpromazine. It is used as a tranquilizer for the treatment of psychomotor agitation associated with acute and chronic psychoses, such as schizophrenia, manic–depressive psychosis, and toxic psychosis. It is useful in the treatment of psychoneuroses in which anxiety, tension, and agitation predominate.

It is also very effective as an antiemetic in the control of nausea and vomiting. It does not have as much sedative or hypotensive actions as some of the other phenothiazines. Perphenazine, as a tranquilizer, has central depressant properties, and may have additive effects if taken with other depressant drugs or alcohol. It has a high therapeutic ratio, and lethal reactions are rare, even after large overdose.

After intramuscular administration of 100 mg, blood concentration averaged 0.005 mg/dl in 1 hour (Hansen, C. E., and Larsen, 1974).

▶ **PETHIDINE**
Schedule II

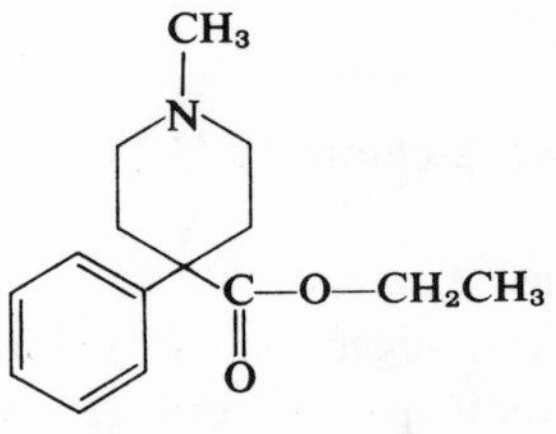

Synonyms: Meperidine, isonipecaine, ethyl-1-methyl-4-phenylpiperidine-4-carboxylate.

Pharmaceutical Preparations

Demerol^R (Winthrop)—Injection, containing pethidine hydrochloride: each 1 ml containing 25, 50, 75, or 100 mg. Tablets: containing pethidine hydrochloride, 50 or 100 mg. Elixir: each 5 ml containing 50 mg pethidine hydrochloride.

General Comments: None.

Biochemistry: Pethidine is a potent synthetic narcotic analgesic. Hydrolysis is the major metabolic reaction, with N-demethylation occurring to a lesser extent.

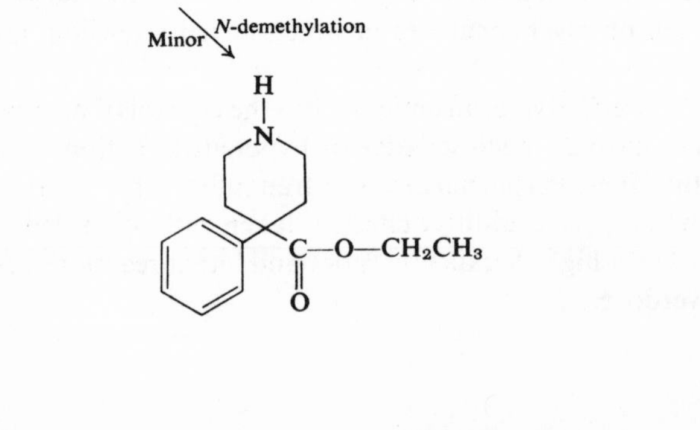

This drug was first prepared in 1939 by Eisleb and Schaumann among numerous piperidine derivatives (Eisleb and Schaumann, 1939).

Evidence for pethidine acting at the morphine receptor is given by the fact that it is antagonized by nalorphine and naloxone.

There are only small structural differences among prodine, desmethylprodine, and pethidine.

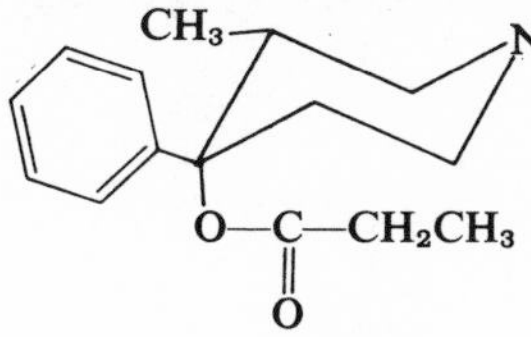

Prodine

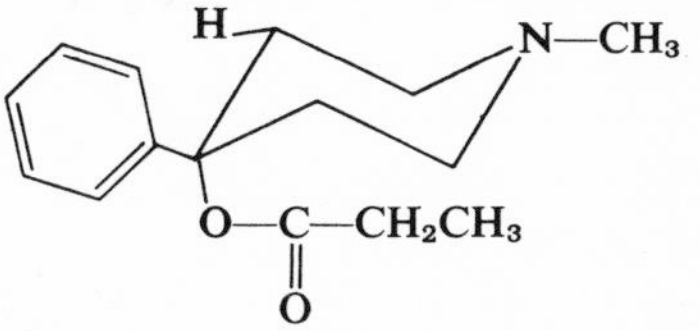

Desmethylprodine

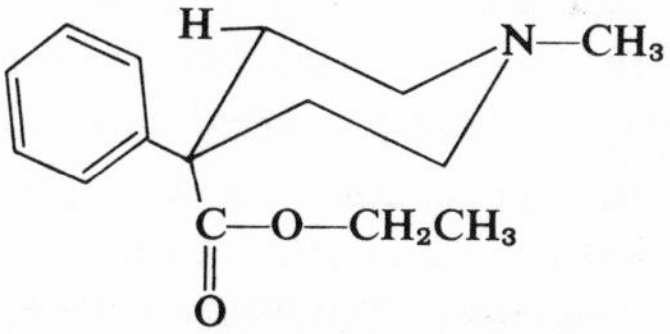

Pethidine

The reversal of the ester chain from desmethylprodine to pethidine gives a tenfold potency difference.

Quantum chemical calculations have been made of the electronic distribution and conformational behavior of pethidine using the PCILO method (Loew and Jester, 1975). A phenyl equatorial conformation was preferred over a phenyl axial one. (Also see **ALPHAPRODINE** and **BETAPRODINE**.)

Toxicology–Pharmacology: Pethidine (meperidine) is a frequently used synthetic narcotic analgesic with actions qualitatively the same as morphine. It is about one eighth to one tenth as potent as morphine in its analgetic actions, and has a shorter duration of action. It is rapidly absorbed from the gastrointestinal tract, so is effective when given orally or parentally. It usually reaches its peak analgetic effectiveness in about an hour, subsiding in 2–4 hours. Other narcotic actions, such as sedation, euphoria, and respiratory depression, are similar to those of morphine. It does not have any therapeutically useful antitussive, antidiarrhea, or local anesthetic actions.

Pethidine is used for its analgetic action when a short duration of analgesia is required. It is used in diagnostic procedures, and as preanesthetic medication in surgery. It has a sedative effect and relieves apprehension. It is also used postoperatively to relieve pain and restlessness.

As with other narcotic drugs, pethidine can cause habituation and addiction when used repeatedly. After overdose, respiratory depression is a major toxic effect, and coma and death may ensue.

The respiratory depression may be antagonized with nalorphine or levallorphan. At 1 hour after intravenous injection of 50 mg pethidine, serum levels of 0.018 mg/dl were obtained. After oral administration of 50 mg, maximum serum concentrations of 0.014 mg/dl were achieved in 2 hours (Stambough *et al.*, 1976). After a 100-mg intramuscular dose, maximum serum levels of 0.038 mg/dl were observed (Shih *et al.*, 1976).

In fatal overdose cases, blood concentrations of 0.30–1.00 mg/dl may be found.

▶ **PEYOTE**
Schedule I
General Comments: The provisions of the Controlled Substances Act relating to the possession and distribution of peyote do not apply to the use of peyote by members of the Native American Church in bona fide religious ceremonies of the church. However, persons who supply the church with the substance are required to register and maintain appropriate records of receipts and disbursements in accordance with rules promulgated by the director. The exemption granted to members of the Native American Church does not apply to a member with less than 25 percent Indian blood.

The Native American Church, having approximately 250,000 members throughout the United States and Canada, was legally organized in 1918 by several Indian religious groups. It originated in about 1880 when the use of peyote began to spread among certain tribes of plains Indians. The American Indians, having encountered peyote in northern Mexico, adopted this plant to use for a sacrament. They built a ceremony around its use by incorporating pagan and Christian ideas.

Biochemistry: The peyote cactus is one of the two species from the genus *Lophophora, Lophophora williamsii*. It grows in the deserts of central to northern Mexico and southern United States. Peyote is usually ingested by eating the dried brown tops of the cactus, called "buttons." After drying, the mescal buttons are very stable.

The most active hallucinogenic substance in peyote is mescaline, an alkaloidal derivative of phenylethylamine. Other phenylethylamine derivatives have been identified from peyote, such as *N*-acetylmescaline, tyramine, *N*-methyltyramine, hordenine (anhalin), candicine, and 3,4-dimethoxyphenyl-ethylamine (Lundstrom and Agurell, 1968; McLaughlin and Paul, 1966).

In addition, several tetrahydroisoquinoline alkaloids have been identified. These include alkaloids such as anhalamine, anhalanine, anhalonidine, *O*-methyl-anhalonidine, anhalidine, pellotine, and lophophorine (Kapadia and Fales, 1968).

Peyote intoxication may, and should, differ from mescaline intoxication, as the effects of the numerous other alkaloids found in the cactus will enter into the physiological action.

Toxicology–Pharmacology: The effects in man of the peyote cactus arise from ingestion of several "buttons," or tops of the peyote cactus (*Lophophora williamsii*). The most active component of the cactus is mescaline, but at least thirteen minor alkaloids have been identified, and no doubt contribute to the characteristic intoxication. Mescaline itself is a sympathomimetic amine related to amphetamine, and with similar actions.

Peyote induces a state of mental stimulation and visual hallucinations. The intoxication consists, first, of a period of contentment and hypersensitivity, followed by one of nervous calm and muscular sluggishness, during which typical colored visions occur. Flashes of color across the field of vision may occur, followed by visions consisting of geometric figures, scenes, and objects. The Indian user believes that the visions put him in contact with the spirit world. The visual hallucinations are often accompanied by auditory, taste, olfactory, and tactile hallucinations. Sensations of weightlessness, depersonalization, and alteration or loss of time perception are experienced. Users may ingest from 4 to more than 30 of the buttons. Although relatively large doses of mescaline given to rats cause death (LD_{50} 370 mg/kg) (Speck, 1957), no reports of death in humans from overdose have been made.

▶ **PHENACETIN**
Noncontrolled Substance

Toxicology–Pharmacology: Phenacetin is an antipyretic and analgesic drug. It does not reduce body temperature when it is normal, but does significantly lower it when it is abnormally elevated. It is effective in relieving mild to moderately severe pain due to headache, migraine, myalgias and neuralgias, and arthritis and rheumatism.

Phenacetin is deethylated in the body to acetaminophen, and this latter agent may contribute to the effect. It has been demonstrated, however, that phenacetin itself is effective, even when the metabolism has been inhibited. Phenacetin attains its maximal effects in 30 to 60 minutes, and is effective up to 3 hours after a single dose. With long-term use, nephropathies may occur.

Sideroblastic anemia was demonstrated in 7 of a series of 100 patients who misused phenacetin. The phenacetin was shown to be the sole cause of this condition (Popović *et al.*, 1973).

After a single 900-mg dose of phenacetin, a plasma concentration of 0.026 mg/dl was found in 1 hour. Concomitantly, the acetaminophen concentration was 0.77 mg/dl. After 4 hours, the phenacetin concentration was 0.007 mg/dl, with the acetaminophen value being 1.51 mg/dl (Garland *et al.*, 1977).

▶ **PHENADOXONE**
Schedule I

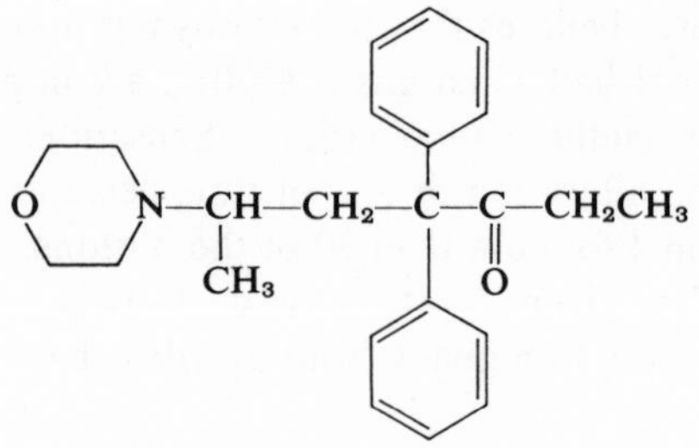

Synonyms: Heptazone, morphodone, 6-morpholine-4,4-diphenylheptan-3-one.
Pharmaceutical Preparations: Phenadoxone is not found in any pharmaceutical preparations sold in the United States.
General Comments: Phenadoxone is a synthetic narcotic analgesic structurally similar to methadone. It has no accepted medicinal value in the United States.
Biochemistry: Unknown.
Toxicology–Pharmacology: Unknown.

▶ **PHENAMPROMIDE**
Schedule I

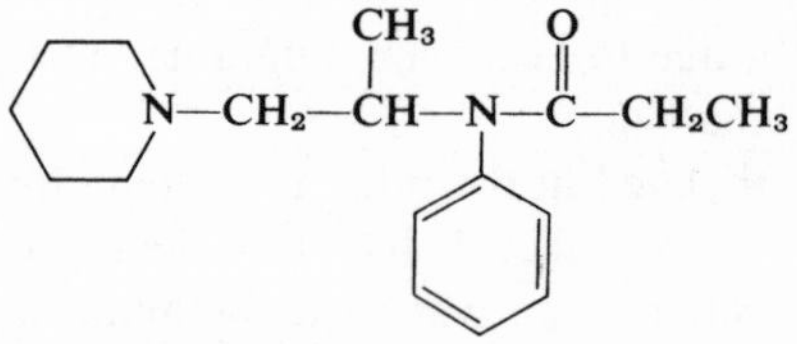

Synonym: *N*-(1-methyl-2-piperidinoethyl)propionanilide.

Pharmaceutical Preparations: Phenampromide is not found in any pharmaceutical preparations sold in the United States.

General Comments: Phenampromide is a synthetic narcotic analgesic that was prepared by structurally modifying methadone. It has no accepted medicinal value in the United States.

Biochemistry: Phenampromide was synthesized in 1959 as a nitrogen analogue of methadone in which the quaternary carbon atom with one attached phenyl group is replaced by nitrogen. The result was a drug with a potency comparable to that of pethidine and having dependence liability (Wright *et al.*, 1959).

Toxicology–Pharmacology: Similar to that of pethidine.

▶ **PHENAZOCINE**
Schedule II

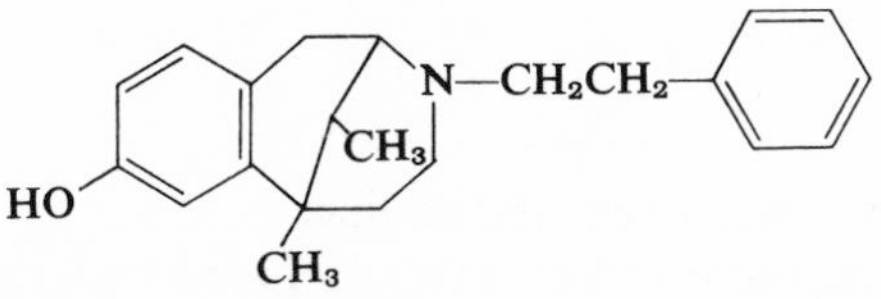

Synonyms: 1,2,3,4,5,6-Hexahydro-8-hydroxy-2,6-methano-6,11-dimethyl-3-phenethyl-3-benzazocine.

Pharmaceutical Preparations: Phenazocine is not frequently found in pharmaceutical preparations sold in the United States.

General Comments: None.

Toxicology–Pharmacology: Phenazocine is a synthetic narcotic analgesic with actions and uses similar to those of morphine. In humans, it has an analgesic potency of three to four times that of morphine. However, the degree of sedation produced by phenazocine is less than that produced by morphine or pethidine. Administered intravenously, its action is immediate. The duration of action ranges from 1 to 6 hours.

It is used to control severe pain, as an adjunct to anesthesia to reduce the amount of anesthetic required, for relief of postoperative emergence excitement and pain, and for relief of pain during labor and delivery. It produces the same amount of respiratory repression as does meperidine and morphine. Physical dependence appears to be milder and develop more slowly than with morphine and meperidine, but nevertheless it has a high addiction liability.

Overdose is characterized by respiratory depression. The effects may be counteracted by administering levallorphan or nalorphine.

▶ **PHENAZOPYRIDINE**
Noncontrolled Substance

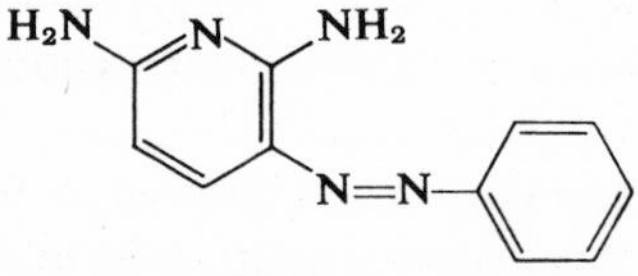

General Comments: Phenazopyridine is a urogenital analgesic that has been encountered in cases of drug abuse due to a "mistaken identity," as its name sounds similar to the names of some narcotics. It has no known actions on the central nervous system.

▶ **PHENCYCLIDINE**
Schedule II

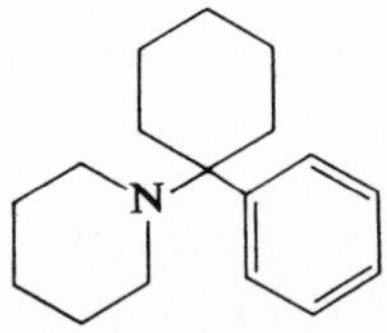

Synonym: 1-(1-Phenylcyclohexyl)piperidine.
Pharmaceutical Preparations: Veterinary preparations Sernyl[R] and Sernylan[R].
General Comments: Phencyclidine, a hallucinogen in humans, is legitimately manufactured as a veterinary anesthetic. It is also produced in clandestine laboratories and sold as PCP, Peace Pill, Hog, DOA, Dead on Arrival, Dust of Angels, and Angel Dust. The trip that it produces often includes feelings of weightlessness, diminishing body size, loss of comprehension of the immediate environment, and feelings of dying or being dead. It also intensifies overt or latent psychotic tendencies. A PCP trip can be very alarming, especially if it is unexpected. This can happen easily, since PCP is frequently sold as mescaline, LSD, or THC, or mixed with any of these or other drugs.

A physician at Detroit's Lafayette Clinic noted that the drug was so powerful his hospital was forced to discontinue tests of it when it could not find enough subjects who were willing to try it twice.

Phencyclidine was first observed as a drug of abuse in 1967. At this time, this drug was marketed as Sernylan[R] by Parke-Davis & Co. as a veterinary prescription drug for use in anesthesia of animals.
Biochemistry: See Toxicology–Pharmacology below.
Toxicology–Pharmacology: The use of phencyclidine in humans is known only in the sense of drug abuse, as there are no legitimate preparations approved for human use. Its continued popularity as a street drug, however, results in frequent encounters of this drug by the toxicologist, both in submitted street samples and in blood or urine of drug abusers.

After oral administration of phencyclidine, effects begin within 15 minutes, and may last from several hours to as long as several days. The duration of the action is prolonged with increasing dosage. It is rapidly metabolized to inactive products, and is excreted in the urine primarily as the mono-4-hydroxy piperidine conjugate (Domino, 1964). Phencyclidine is an analgesic with sympathomimetic and central nervous system stimulant and depressant properties. With low doses, such effects as nystagmus, miosis, blurred vision, ataxia, tremors, muscle weakness, slurred speech, and drowsiness may occur. Psychological effects include amnesia, anxiety, body-image distortion, euphoria, depersonalization, and disordered thought processes. Increased pulse rate and blood pressure are also common. Hallucinations are rare (Liden *et al.*, 1975).

After overdose of phencyclidine, drowsiness, nystagmus, miotic pupils, elevated blood pressure, increased deep tendon reflexes, ataxia, anxiety, and agitation are observed. In more severe cases, seizures, spasticity, and opisthotonos may occur, in addition to deep coma and respiratory depression. Treatment is symptomatic, although the spasmicity and agitation respond well to diazepam (Liden *et al.*, 1975).

In four fatalities involving deaths from overdose of phencyclidine, blood concentrations of 0.23, 0.05, 0.50, and 0.40 mg/dl were found, while in seven cases of death from other causes, but in which phencyclidine was detected, concentrations of 0.029–0.106 mg/dl were found (Reynolds, 1976).

▶ **PHENDIMETRAZINE**
Schedule III

Synonym: (+)-3,4-Dimethyl-2-phenylmorpholine.
Pharmaceutical Preparations
Bacarate[R] (Tutag)—Tablet: containing 35 mg phendimetrazine tartrate
Bontril[R] PDM (Carnick)—Tablet: containing 35 mg phendimetrazine tartrate
Melfiat[R] (Reid-Provident)—Tablet: containing 35 mg phendimetrazine tartrate
Melfiat[R] Unicelles (Reid-Provident)—Capsule: timed-release, containing 105 mg phendimetrazine tartrate
Obe-Nil[R] TR (Thera-Medic)—Capsules: timed-release, containing 105 mg phendimetrazine tartrate

Plegine^R (Ayerst)—Tablet: containing 35 mg phendimetrazine tartrate
Statobex^R (Lemmon)—Tablet: green, oblong, containing 35 mg phendimetrazine tartrate
Statobex-D^R (Lemmon)—Tablet, white with green specks, oblong. Capsules: green and white. Both contain 70 mg phendimetrazine tartrate.
Trimstat^R (Laser)—Tablet: tan, containing 35 mg phendimetrazine tartrate
Trimtabs^R (Mayrand)—Tablet: containing 35 mg phendimetrazine tartrate
General Comments: None.
Biochemistry: The tartrate salt of phendimetrazine is a white, odorless, crystalline powder, having a bitter taste. It is contraindicated when monoamine oxidase inhibitors are being used.
Toxicology–Pharmacology: Phendimetrazine is a sympathomimetic amine, having qualitatively the same general effects as amphetamine. It is marketed for use as an anorexiant, to be used in the management of simple obesity resulting from overeating. Usual dosage for this effect is 17–70 mg, two or three times daily.

In addition to its appetite suppressant actions, it acts as a general central nervous system stimulant. These actions result in nervousness, dizziness, and insomnia, and may cause tachycardia, elevation of blood pressure, and palpitation infrequently. Phendimetrazine is commonly encountered in drug confiscations, and is often taken by injecting a solution of the drug intravenously. Abuse patterns of this drug may be similar to those described for amphetamine.

After oral administration of a 35-mg single dose to five adults, serum concentrations were 0.009 mg/dl in 1 hour. After 2 hours, the concentrations were 0.0045 mg/dl, indicating a very short half-life of 1 hour (Hundt *et al.*, 1975).

▶ **PHENELZINE**
Dangerous Drug

$$\langle\!\!\!\!\!\bigcirc\!\!\!-CH_2CH_2-NH-NH_2$$

Synonym: 2-Phenethylhydrazine.
Pharmaceutical Preparations: Nardil^R (Warner-Chilcott)—Tablets: orange-coated, containing 15 mg phenelzine (prepared as phenelzine sulfate).
General Comment: Phenelzine is an antidepressant and monoamine oxidase inhibitor that is classified in this text as a Dangerous Drug under the "legend drug" provision because all pharmaceutical preparations containing phenelzine require a prescription and bear the label "Caution: Federal law prohibits dispensing without a prescription."

Biochemistry: Many types of compounds, such as hydrazines, are inhibitors of monoamine oxidase (MAO), the enzyme responsible for deamination of a variety of amines, including catecholamines and serotonin. These agents produce many effects other than MAO inhibition, but inhibition of this enzyme itself results in a number of pharmacological responses.

Several mechanisms have been considered responsible for the anti-hypertensive effect of MAO inhibitors. These include ganglionic blockade, decreased responsiveness of the peripheral vascular system to norepinephrine, and blockade of norepinephrine transport at sympathetic nerve endings. The lack of significant adrenergic and ganglionic blockade in the hypotensive action of most MAO inhibitors is generally accepted.

Toxicology–Pharmacology: Phenelzine is a MAO inhibitor, having anti-depressant actions. It is used primarily in patients with endogenous depression and depressed effective psychosis. It is not effective in depressions that are reactive in origin, in schizophrenic pseudodepressions, or in organic syndromes of the brain. Remissions in patients responding to the drug usually occur within a week or two. Improved mood, better appetite, and improved sleep are observed in many patients.

Effects of overdose with phenelzine may include agitation, hallucinations, hyperreflexia, hyperpyrexia, and convulsions. Chronic toxicity with MAO inhibitors is a more serious problem. A variety of toxic effects have been reported, including hepatotoxicity, excessive central nervous system stimulation, convulsions, and orthostatic hypotension. The interactions of MAO inhibitors with other drugs and chemicals are well recognized. A severe toxic episode may be precipitated if such agents as amphetamine or other stimulants, certain cheeses, beer, wine, chicken liver, yeast, or pickled herring are ingested during the course of therapy. These reactions are due to decreased metabolism of tyramine or other sympathomimetic amines, resulting in enhanced effects in the body. Other drugs having adverse reactions with MAO inhibitors include antidepressants such as imipramine, adrenaline, ephedrine, phenylpropanolamine, narcotics, antihistamines, cocaine, procaine, atropine, and chloroquine.

▶ **PHENIRAMINE**
Noncontrolled Substance

General Comment: Pheniramine is an antihistaminic drug that is encountered in cases of drug abuse.

Toxicology–Pharmacology: Pheniramine is an antihistaminic drug. Its therapeutic usefulness results from its ability to antagonize the actions of histamine. The primary uses are to reduce the intensity of allergic and anaphylactic reactions. The most useful effect is to antagonize the constrictive effect of histamine on the respiratory smooth muscle. It also antagonizes the vasoconstrictor and vasodilator effects of histamine. Thus, the edema resulting from increased capillary permeability in skin reactions to histamine release as well as the bronchoconstriction resulting from a variety of conditions may be effectively treated by pheniramine. Certain conditions resulting in itching of the skin may be treated by antihistamines. Common side effects of pheniramine and other antihistamines are drowsiness and dryness of the mouth.

▶ **PHENMETRAZINE**
Schedule II

Synonym: 3-Methyl-2-phenylmorpholine.

Pharmaceutical Preparations: Preludin^R (Boehringer Ingelhein)—Tablets: pink, square, scored "BI-42," containing 25 mg phenmetrazine hydrochloride; white, round, "BI-79," containing 50 mg phenmetrazine hydrochloride; pink, round, "BI-62," containing 75 mg phenmetrazine hydrochloride.

General Comments: None.

Biochemistry: Phenmetrazine, an off-white, crystalline powder, was first prepared by cyclizing α-[1-[(2-hydroxyethyl)amino]ethyl]benzyl alcohol with the aid of strong sulfuric acid. The drug is contraindicated in coronary artery disease, hyperthyroidism, hypertension, agitation, emotional instability, and when there is a record of drug abuse. It should not be given at the same time as monoamine oxidase inhibitors.

Toxicology–Pharmacology: Phenmetrazine is a sympathomimetic amine with actions qualitatively similar to those of amphetamine. Its appetite suppressant actions are more pronounced in relationship to its central stimulant actions, when compared to amphetamine. It is therefore the drug of choice for management of simple obesity resulting from overeating.

Phenmetrazine also stimulates the central nervous system, producing hyperexcitability, euphoria, and insomnia. Although this effect is mild when compared with those of amphetamine, it accounts for the popularity of this drug on the black market. It is frequently taken by injection, by which route the central stimulation and euphoria are more pronounced.

After a single oral dose of 75 mg phenmetrazine, plasma levels of 0.007 mg/dl were found at 1 hour. The maximum occurred at 2 hours with 0.013 mg/dl. The concentrations declined thereafter with a half-life of about 10 hours (Quinn *et al.*, 1967). In one death from intravenous injection, a blood level of 0.40 mg/dl was found (Norheim, 1973).

▶ **PHENOBARBITAL**
Schedule IV

Synonyms: Phenobarbitone, fenobarbital, phenemalum, phenylethylmalonyl-urea, 5-ethyl-5-phenylbarbituric acid.

Pharmaceutical Preparations

Belap^R (Lemmon)—Tablets: No. 2, green, scored, "HB," containing 30 mg phenobarbital and 8 mg belladonna extract

Chardonna^R (Rorer)—Tablet: containing 20 mg phenobarbital and 5 mg belladonna alkaloids

Eskabarb^R Spansule (Smith Kline & French)—Capsules: containing 65 or 97 mg phenobarbital

Luminal^R (Winthrop)—Powder for injection; or Ampules, each 1 ml containing 130 mg phenobarbital

Phazyme-PB^R (Reed & Carnrick)—Tablet: yellow, containing 16.25 mg phenobarbital

Sedadrops^R (Merrell-National)—Drops, each 1 ml containing 24 mg phenobarbital and 0.27 mg homatropine methylbromide

Solfoton^R (Poythress)—Tablets, Capsules, or Sugar-Coated Tablets; each containing 16 mg phenobarbital

Also see Chapter 6.

General Comments: None.

Biochemistry: The major pathway for the metabolism and deactivation of phenobarbital is the oxidation of the aromatic ring to give p-hydroxypheno-barbital and o-hydroxyphenobarbital. These primary metabolites have been found with the unchanged drug in the urine of humans poisoned with pheno-barbital (Curry, 1955; Algeri and McBay, 1956). It is only partly conjugated as the sulfate, not the glucuronide (Butler, 1956).

Phenobarbital   p-Hydroxyphenobarbital   o-Hydroxyphenobarbital

Toxicology–Pharmacology: Phenobarbital is one of the oldest and most use-ful barbiturates. It is a long-acting barbiturate, but has actions stronger than those of barbital. It has been used since the early 1900s for treating grand mal epilepsy, and is probably the safest drug for this purpose. It is also used to produce mild and relatively prolonged sedation.

Phenobarbital is primarily a central nervous system (CNS) depressant, as are the other barbiturate derivatives. Due to its long-acting property, having a half-life of up to 72 hours, it is ideal for use as a sedative when mild, prolonged sedation is required, as in some anxiety and tension states, hyper-tension, functional gastrointestinal disorders, and preoperative apprehension. It is used most extensively in treatment of seizure disorders, such as grand mal epilepsy, and is effective in preventing seizures if the proper blood concentra-tion is maintained.

Overdose from phenobarbital results in CNS and respiratory depression. Due to the long-acting nature and depressant properties milder than those of other barbiturate derivatives, larger doses can be tolerated. The estimated LD_{50} for phenobarbital is 6.0 g vs. 1.6 g for pentobarbital.

The therapeutic range of blood concentrations for control of seizures may be from 1.0 to 4.5 mg/dl. Each patient must be titrated to determine the optimal effective dosage. In most cases, blood concentrations in excess of 4.5 mg/dl will be associated with signs of overdose, depending on individual tolerance.

In ten patients given repeated daily 200-mg oral doses for seizure control, blood concentrations of 1.6–4.8 mg/dl were achieved (Plaa and Hine, 1960). In a series of five deaths from phenobarbital intoxication, the blood concen-tration ranged from 7.8 to 11.6 mg/dl (Baselt and Cravey, 1977).

▶ **PHENOMORPHAN**
Schedule I

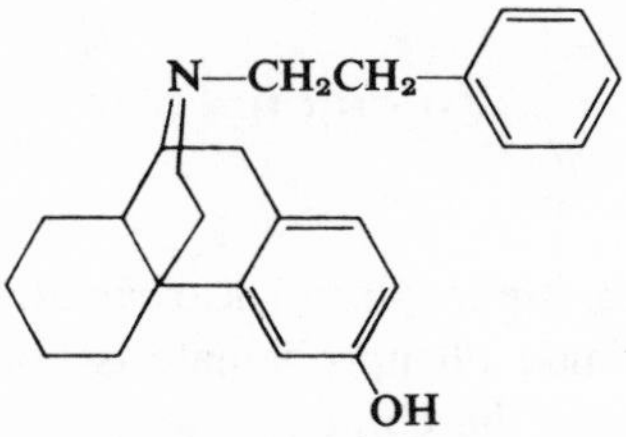

Synonym: 3-Hydroxy-*N*-phenethylmorphinan.
Pharmaceutical Preparations: Phenomorphan is not found in any pharmaceutical preparations sold in the United States.
General Comments: Phenomorphan is a synthetic narcotic analgesic structurally related to racemorphan and racemethorphan. It has no accepted medicinal value in the United States.
Biochemistry: Unknown.
Toxicology–Pharmacology: Unknown.

▶ **PHENOPERIDINE**
Schedule I

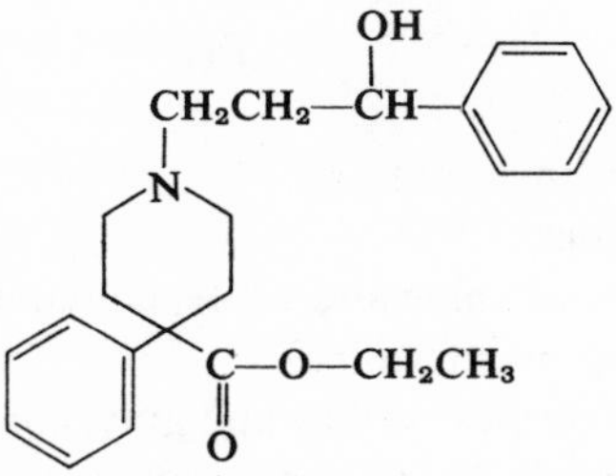

Synonyms: Phenopridine, ethyl-1-(3-hydroxy-3-phenylpropyl)-4-phenylpiperidine-4-carboxylate.
Pharmaceutical Preparations: Phenoperidine is not found in any pharmaceutical preparations sold in the United States.
General Comments: Phenoperidine is a synthetic narcotic analgesic in the piperidine series and is structurally related to pethidine. It has no accepted medicinal value in the United States.
Biochemistry: Unknown.
Toxicology–Pharmacology: Unknown.

▶ **PHENPROBAMATE**
Dangerous Drug

$$\text{C}_6\text{H}_5-\text{CH}_2\text{CH}_2\text{CH}_2-\text{O}-\overset{\displaystyle \text{O}}{\overset{\displaystyle \|}{\text{C}}}-\text{NH}_2$$

Synonyms: Proformiphen, 3-phenylpropylcarbamate.
Pharmaceutical Preparations: Phenprobamate is not found in any pharmaceutical preparations sold in the United States.
General Comment: Phenprobamate is a muscle relaxant and tranquilizer. Being a tranquilizer, it is classified in this text as a Dangerous Drug.
Biochemistry: Phenprobamate is in the same chemical group as meprobamate. The metabolism of phenprobamate is a deactivating mechanism, as 67 percent of an oral dose is converted into hippuric acid (Schatz and John, 1966). Some hydroxylation of the phenyl group also occurs.
Toxicology–Pharmacology: Similar to that of meprobamate.

▶ **PHENTERMINE**
Schedule IV

$$\text{C}_6\text{H}_5-\text{CH}_2-\overset{\displaystyle \text{CH}_3}{\underset{\displaystyle \text{CH}_3}{\overset{\displaystyle |}{\underset{\displaystyle |}{\text{C}}}}}-\text{NH}_2$$

Synonym: Dimethylphenethylamine.
Pharmaceutical Preparations
Fastin[R] (Beecham)—Capsule: blue and white, containing 30 mg phentermine hydrochloride (24 mg phentermine)
Ionamin[R] (Pennwalt)—Capsules: yellow and gray, containing 15 mg phentermine; yellow, containing 30 mg phentermine
General Comments: Phentermine has been encountered in illicit preparations mixed with methamphetamine. Since phentermine is structurally similar to methamphetamine, detection of methamphetamine may be difficult without employing special laboratory procedures.
Biochemistry: Similar to that of methamphetamine.
Toxicology–Pharmacology: Phentermine is isomeric with methamphetamine. Like other amphetamine drugs, phentermine is used as an anorexian in the management of simple obesity resulting from excessive caloric intake. It is a sympathomimetic amine, having actions similar to those of amphetamine, although with less central nervous system stimulant actions. The usual dose

regimen is 8 mg three times daily. Untoward effects with phentermine may include dryness of the mouth, insomnia, nervousness, and headache.

In one case of a woman having died from other causes, who was taking 40 mg of slow-release phentermine daily, a blood concentration of 0.09 mg/dl was detected (Price, 1974). In another case, probably involving abuse, a truck driver killed in an accident was found to have a blood concentration of 0.46 mg/dl phentermine. In six medical examiner cases believed to have been taking therapeutic doses of phentermine, blood concentrations were 0.02 mg/dl in two cases, less than 0.01 mg/dl in two, and 0.07 and 0.08 mg/dl in the other two (Garriott, 1977).

▶ **1-PHENYLCYCLOHEXYLAMINE**
Schedule II

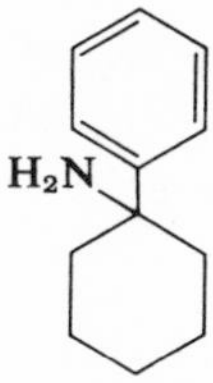

Synonyms: None found.
Pharmaceutical Preparations: 1-Phenylcyclohexylamine is not found in pharmaceutical preparations sold in the United States.
General Comments: 1-Phenylcyclohexylamine was added to Schedule II of the Controlled Substances Act on June 16, 1978. The premise for control of 1-phenylcyclohexylamine is under the precursor clause as it is a precursor of phencyclidine.
Biochemistry: Unknown.
Toxicology–Pharmacology: Unknown.

▶ **PHENYLEPHRINE**
Noncontrolled Substance

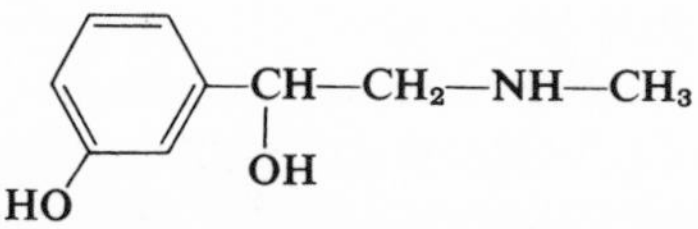

General Comment: Phenylephrine is a sympathomimetic amine structurally resembling epinephrine with pharmacological properties that resemble those of norepinephrine.

▶ **PHENYLPROPANOLAMINE**
Noncontrolled Substance

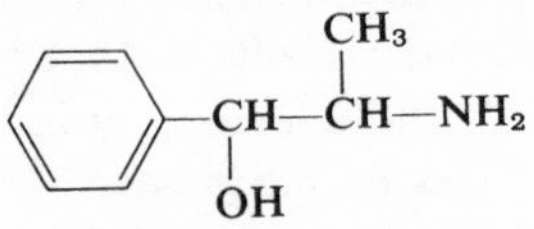

$$\text{C}_6\text{H}_5-\underset{\underset{\text{OH}}{|}}{\text{CH}}-\underset{\underset{\text{CH}_3}{}}{\text{CH}}-\text{NH}_2$$

Toxicology–Pharmacology: Phenylpropanolamine is a sympathomimetic amine related structurally and pharmacologically to both ephedrine and amphetamine.

When applied locally, phenylpropanolamine constricts capillaries and shrinks swollen mucous membranes. Thus, it is an ingredient of many formulations used for treatment of nasal allergies.

Phenylpropanolamine has little central stimulant actions compared with amphetamine. Its primary actions are vasoconstriction in nasal mucous membranes, and thereby effective decongestion of nasal passages. It is also used extensively in over-the-counter anorexiant preparations. Untoward effects include insomnia, nervousness, restlessness, tachycardia, headache, and nausea.

▶ **PHENYLPROPYLMETHYLAMINE**
Noncontrolled Substance

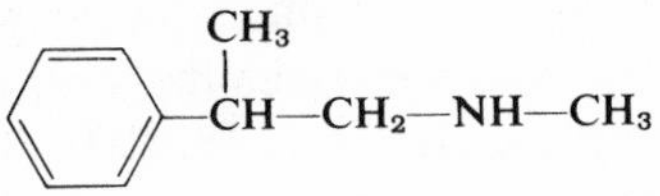

$$\text{C}_6\text{H}_5-\underset{\underset{\text{CH}_3}{}}{\text{CH}}-\text{CH}_2-\text{NH}-\text{CH}_3$$

Toxicology–Pharmacology: Phenylpropylmethylamine is a sympathomimetic amine with actions similar to those of phenylpropanolamine. It is primarily used as a nasal decongestant.

▶ **PHENYTOIN**
Dangerous Drug

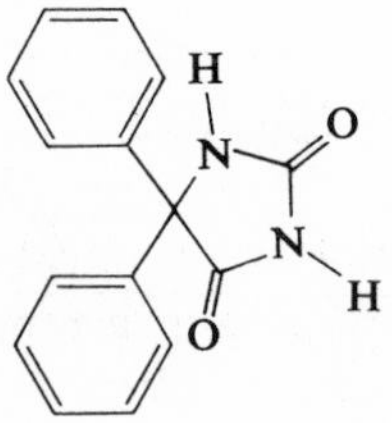

Synonyms: Diphenylhydantoin, phenantonium, 5,5-diphenylhydantoin.

Pharmaceutical Preparations

Dilantin[R]—Capsules: white with red band, imprinted "PD 362," containing 100 mg phenytoin sodium; white with red band, imprinted "PD 365," containing 30 mg phenytoin sodium; white with red band, imprinted "PD 375," containing 100 mg phenytoin sodium and 16 mg phenobarbital; white with blue band imprinted "PD 531," containing 100 mg phenytoin sodium and 32 mg phenobarbital. Tablet: yellow, triangular, imprinted "PD 007" (Infatabs[R]), containing 50 mg phenytoin sodium. Suspension: containing 125 mg or 30 mg phenytoin sodium.

Diphenyl[R] 250 (TM) (Drug Industries)—Capsule: Blue and white, containing 250 mg diphenylhydantoin

Ekko[R] (Fleming)—Capsules, containing diphenylhydantoin: Sr., 250 mg; Jr., 100 mg; III, 50 mg

General Comment: Phenytoin is an anticonvulsant that is classified in this text as a Dangerous Drug under the "legend drug" provision since all pharmaceutical preparations containing phenytoin require a prescription and bear the label "Caution: Federal law prohibits dispensing without a prescription."

Biochemistry: Diphenylhydantoin (phenytoin) is well absorbed when administered orally. The biological half-life in human plasma is about 24 hours. Like phenobarbital, the principal pathway of metabolism is by oxidative hydroxylation. Not more than 5 percent of the administered dose is excreted in the intact form. About 50 percent is excreted as the conjugated p-hydroxyphenytoin glucuronide:

Phenytoin   Aromatic oxygenation →   p-Hydroxyphenytoin

Phenytoin was first prepared in 1908 (Biltz, 1908). It was evaluated in 1938 with respect to anticonvulsant activity (Merritt and Putnam, 1938).

Toxicology–Pharmacology: Phenytoin, which is more commonly referred to as Dilantin[R], or diphenylhydantoin, is an anticonvulsant drug. It was introduced into medicine for the symptomatic treatment of epilepsy in 1938. It has specific antiseizure activity, and does not act as a sedative as do phenobarbital and other anticonvulsant medications. It apparently inhibits the spread of the epileptic discharge through the brain, possibly by promoting the release of sodium from neurons. It is often administered in combination with phenobarbital to effect complete control of seizures in some forms of epilepsy. It has also been found to be sometimes effective for relief of vascular headache, as migraine, and of trigeminal neuralgia.

The usual adult dose is 100 mg, orally three times daily. In some patients, up to 600 mg per day may be required. Blood concentrations in patients with good seizure control, but with no signs of toxicity, varied from 0.23 to 2.90 mg/dl, with a mean of 0.98 mg/dl. In 12 patients showing signs of diphenyl-hydantoin toxicity, concentrations ranged from 2.40 to 4.30 mg/dl, with 11 of these being in excess of 3.00 mg/dl. Serious toxicity is therefore seldom seen with concentrations lower than 3.00 mg/dl (Bock and Sherwin, 1971). As phenytoin does not exert a significant degree of central nervous system depression, death from overdose of this drug is rarely seen. In one case report of a child comatose after phenytoin overdose, a blood concentration of 11.20 mg/dl was found (Tenckhoff *et al.*, 1968).

▶ **PHOLCODINE**
Schedule I

Synonyms: Morpholinylethylmorphine, 7,8-dehydro-4,5-epoxy-6-hydroxy-*N*-methyl-3-(2-morpholinoethoxy)morphinan.
Pharmaceutical Preparations: Pholcodine is not found in any pharmaceutical preparations sold in the United States.
General Comment: Pholcodine is a semisynthetic narcotic that has no accepted medicinal value in the United States.
Biochemistry: Unknown.
Toxicology–Pharmacology: Pholcodine is a semisynthetic narcotic and anti-tussive structurally related to codeine. It is a drug well known in England and France, but not in the United States. It is more potent but less toxic than codeine.

Pholcodine is claimed to have a high degree of therapeutic effectiveness in both acute and chronic cough. Respiratory depression is less with pholcodine than with codeine, and pholcodine is not constipating. It is considered a relatively nonaddicting drug.

▶ **PIMINODINE**
Schedule II

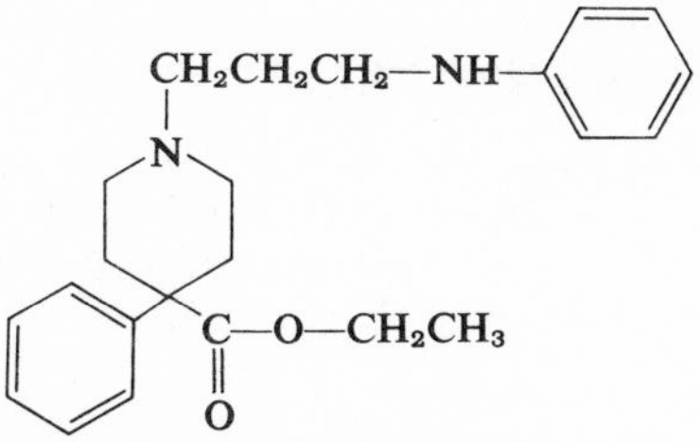

Synonyms: Anopridine, ethyl-1-(3-anilinopropyl)-4-phenylpiperidine-4-car-boxylate.
Pharmaceutical Preparations: Piminodine is not frequently found in pharmaceutical preparations sold in the United States.
General Comments: None.
Biochemistry: Unknown.
Toxicology–Pharmacology: Piminodine is a synthetic narcotic analgesic, related structurally to meperidine. It has an analgesic potency approximately equivalent to that of morphine, and about five times more potent than meperidine. Its hypnotic and sedative effects are less than with morphine, and consequently it does not produce marked drowsiness when analgesic doses are given.

Its addiction potential is similar to that of morphine. Untoward effects include nausea and vomiting, respiratory depression, and lightheadedness. Its actions may be counteracted by use of the narcotic antagonists nalorphine or levallorphan.

Usual dose, if given orally, is 25–50 mg every 4–6 hours. If given parentally, 10–20 mg is given every 4 hours.

▶ **PIPAMPERONE**
Dangerous Drug

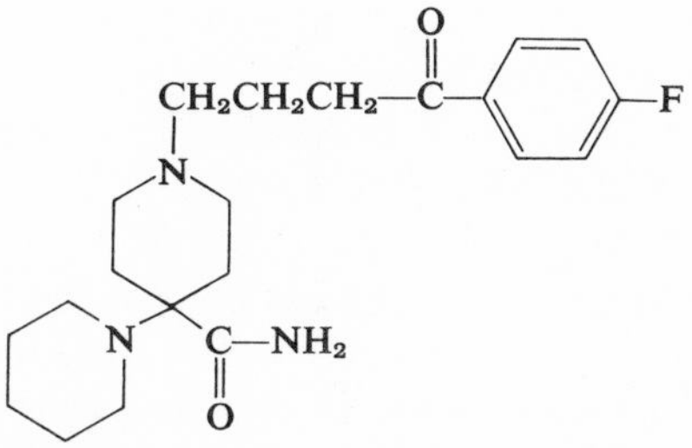

Synonyms: Floropipamide, 1-[3-(4-fluorobenzoyl)propyl]-4-piperidino-piper-dine-4-carboxamide.
Pharmaceutical Preparations: Pipamperone is not found in any pharmaceutical preparations sold in the United States.

General Comment: Pipamperone is a tranquilizer and is therefore classified in this text as a Dangerous Drug.
Biochemistry: Unknown.
Toxicology–Pharmacology: Unknown.

▶ **PIPENZOLATE BROMIDE**
Noncontrolled Substance
Encountered in Excepted Substances

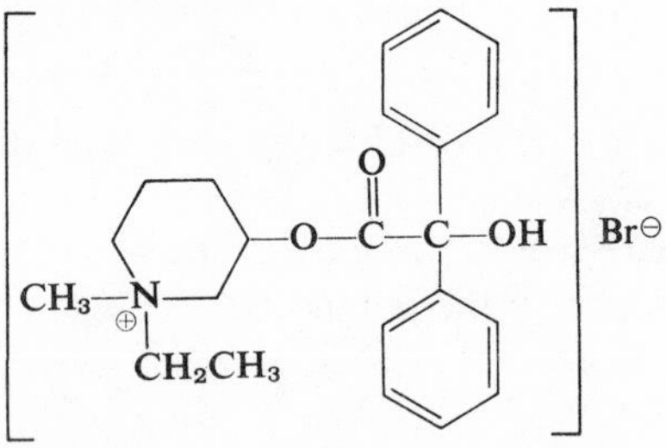

General Comments: Pipenzolate bromide is a parasympatholytic drug. It is an ingredient in several formulations containing phenobarbital that are classified as excepted preparations. The minimum phenobarbital/pipenzolate bromide ratio found in such preparations is 1/3.12.
Toxicology–Pharmacology: Pipenzolate bromide is a synthetic quaternary nitrogen compound having anticholinergic properties similar to those of atropine. Its primary actions are to decrease gastrointestinal motility and inhibit gastric secretions. It is employed mainly for adjunctive treatment of peptic ulcer.

Side effects include dryness of the mouth and blurring of vision, urinary retention, constipation, tachycardia, and dizziness. The usual adult dose is 20–25 mg per day.

▶ **1-PIPERIDINOCYCLOHEXANECARBONITRILE**
Schedule II

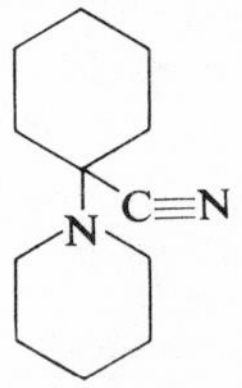

Synonym: 1-PCC.
Pharmaceutical Preparations: 1-Piperidinocyclohexanecarbonitrile is not found in pharmaceutical preparations sold in the United States.
General Comments: 1-Piperidinocyclohexanecarbonitrile was added to Schedule II of the Controlled Substances Act on June 16, 1978. The premise

for control of 1-piperidinocyclohexanecarbonitrile is under the precursor clause as it is a precursor of phencyclidine.
Biochemistry: Unknown.
Toxicology–Pharmacology: Unknown.

▶ **PIPERIDOLATE BROMIDE**
Noncontrolled Substance
Encountered in Excepted Substances

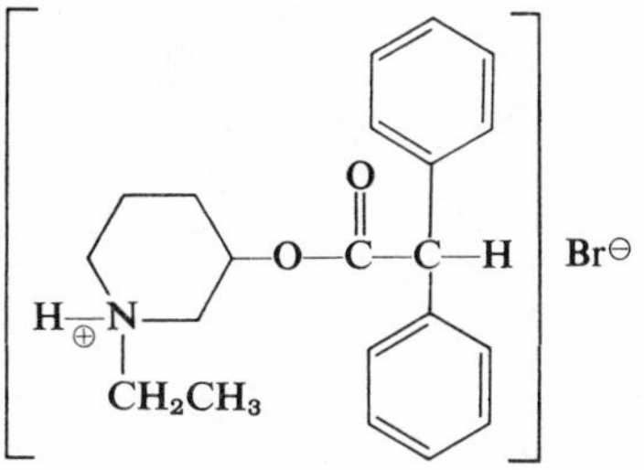

General Comments: Piperidolate bromide is a parasympatholytic drug. It is an ingredient in several formulations containing phenobarbital that are classified as excepted preparations. The minimum phenobarbital/piperidolate bromide ratio found in such preparations is 1/3.12.

Toxicology–Pharmacology: Piperidolate is a synthetic tertiary amine, related structurally and pharmacologically to pipenzolate bromide. It is an anticholinergic agent, and antagonizes acetylcholine chiefly at the cholinergic nerve endings. It does not have ganglionic blocking action or inhibit transmission to skeletal muscle.

Its chief therapeutic action is to inhibit motility of the gastrointestinal tract. It is therefore useful in functional management of gastrointestinal disorders in which there is pain, spasm, and hypermotility.

The usual adult dose is 50 mg, given orally four times a day.

▶ **PIPETHANATE**
Dangerous Drug

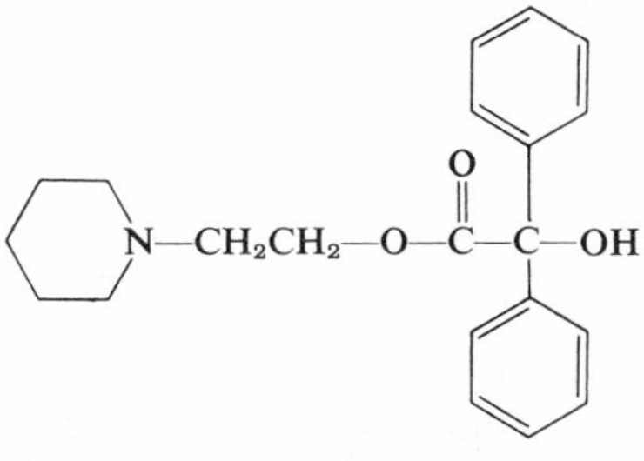

Synonyms: Pentamethate, piperilate, 2-piperidinoethylbenzilate.
Pharmaceutical Preparations: Pipethanate is not found in any pharmaceutical

preparations sold in the United States. Outside the United States, it is marketed as Sycotrol^R.

General Comment: Pipethanate is a tranquilizer and is therefore classified in this text as a Dangerous Drug.

Biochemistry: Similar to that of dicyclomine.

Toxicology–Pharmacology: Similar to that of dicyclomine.

▶ **PIPRADROL**
Noncontrolled Substance

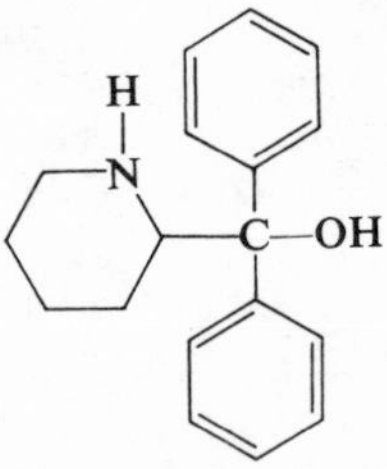

General Comments: Pipradrol is a central nervous system stimulant. Its action appears to be mostly in the upper brainstem and the septal area. It has been used as a stimulant in treating reactive depressions that are not attended by pronounced anxiety or compulsive behavior.

Pipradrol is not controlled unless it is contained in a pharmaceutical preparation that requires a prescription; then it is classified as a Dangerous Drug.

Toxicology–Pharmacology: Pipradrol is reported to be of therapeutic efficacy in cases of depression that are not attended by pronounced anxiety or compulsive behavior. It should not be used in endogenous depression, since anxiety may be aggravated. Untoward effects include hyperexcitability, nausea, insomnia, and mild anorexia.

▶ **PIRITRAMIDE**
Schedule I

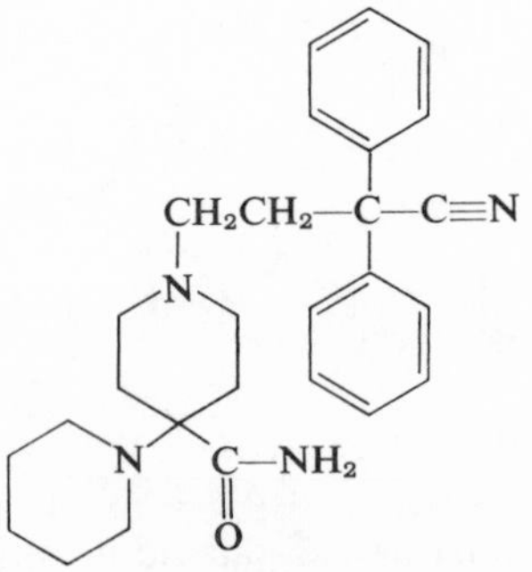

Synonyms: Pirinitramide, 1-(3-cyano-3,3-diphenylpropyl)-4-piperidinopiperidine-4-carboxyamide.

Pharmaceutical Preparations: Piritramide is not found in any pharmaceutical preparations sold in the United States.

General Comment: Piritramide is a synthetic narcotic analgesic that has no accepted medicinal value in the United States.

Biochemistry: Unknown.

Toxicology–Pharmacology: Unknown.

▶ **POLDINE METHYLSULFATE**
Noncontrolled Substance
Encountered in Excepted Substances

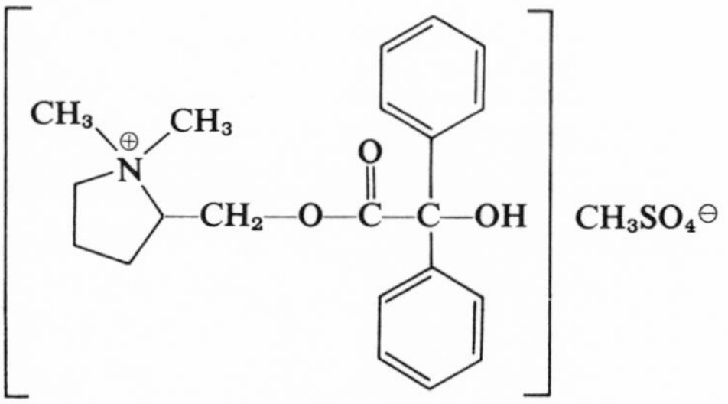

General Comments: Poldine methylsulfate is a parasympatholytic drug. It is an ingredient in several formulations containing butabarbital that are classified as excepted preparations. The minimum butabarbital/poldine methylsulfate ratio found in such preparations is 1/0.26.

Toxicology–Pharmacology: Poldine methylsulfate is a synthetic quaternary nitrogen anticholinergic agent. Its actions are qualitatively similar to those of atropine. Its primary effects are to inhibit motility of the gastrointestinal and urinary tracts. It also diminishes secretions of the salivary glands, gastrointestinal tract, and pancreas.

It is employed primarily as an adjunct in the management of peptic ulcer and gastrointestinal disorders associated with hyperacidity, hypermotility, and spasm. Side effects include dryness of the mouth, blurred vision, dizziness, tachycardia, and urinary hesitancy or retention. The dose range is 12–16 mg, given orally before meals and at bedtime.

▶ **PRAZEPAM**
Schedule IV

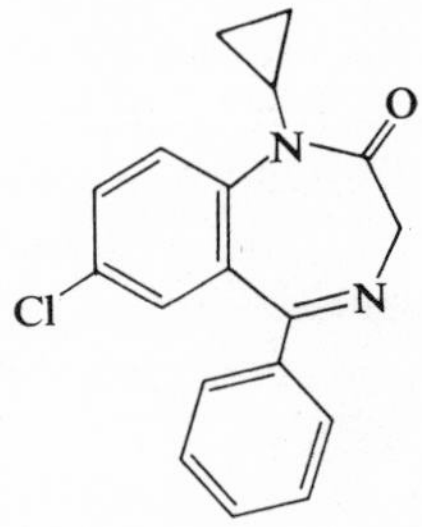

Synonym: 7-Chloro-1-(cyclopropylmethyl)-1,3-dihydro-5-phenyl-2H-1,4-ben-zodiazepin-2-one.
Pharmaceutical Preparations: Verstran[R] (Warner/Chilcott).
General Comment: Prazepam is a benzodiazepine tranquilizer that was added to Schedule IV of the Controlled Substances Act in December 1976.
Biochemistry: Prazepam is metabolized by N-dealkylation (Di Carlo *et al.*, 1970).

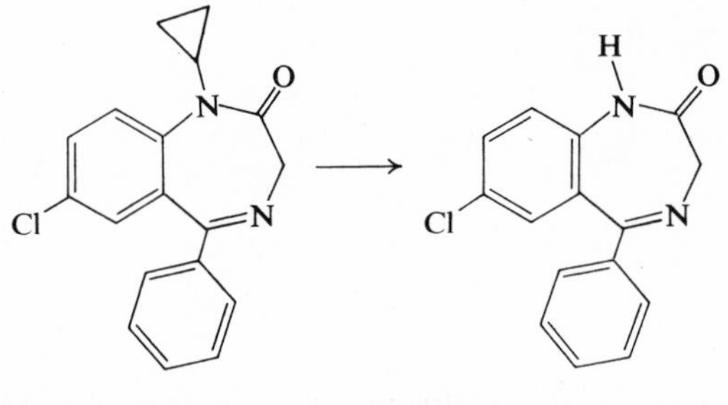

Toxicology–Pharmacology: Somewhat similar to that of diazepam.

▶ **PROBANTHINE**
Noncontrolled Substance
Encountered in Excepted Substances

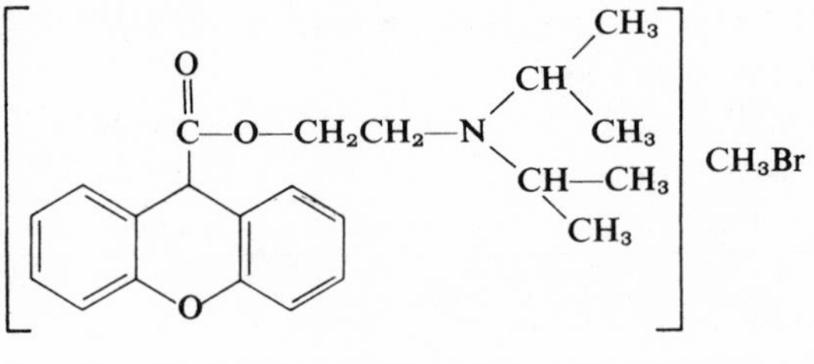

General Comments: Probanthine is a synonym coined from the pharmaceutical preparation Probanthine[R] (Searle) containing propantheline bromide. It is a parasympatholytic drug that is an ingredient in several formulations containing phenobarbital that are classified as excepted preparations. The minimum phenobarbital/probanthine ratio found in such preparations is 1/0.5.

Toxicology–Pharmacology: Probanthine (propantheline bromide) is an anticholinergic drug, having the antisecretary and antispasmodic actions characteristic of the other anticholinergic drugs. Its principal action is to inhibit the cholinergic mediation of impulses at the neuromuscular junction, particularly at the meuromuscular junction.

By inhibiting the motility of the gastrointestinal and genitourinary tracts, and diminishing secretion, it is useful in the treatment of peptic ulcer, chronic hypertrophic gastritis, and other disorders involving hypermotility of the gastrointestinal tract.

Untoward effects include dryness of the mouth, blurring of vision, urinary retention, and dryness of the skin.

It may be given orally or parenterally. The average oral dose is 15 mg, taken three times daily with meals, and 30 mg at bedtime.

▶ **PROBARBITAL**
Schedule III

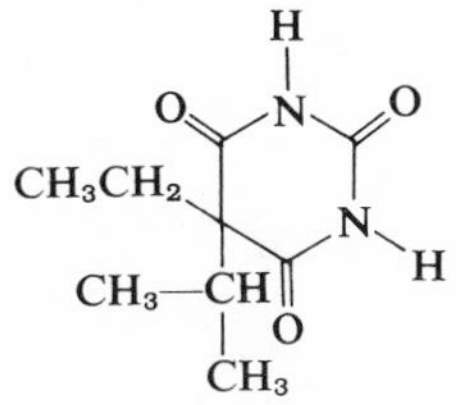

Synonym: 5-Ethyl-5-isopropylbarbituric acid.

Pharmaceutical Preparations: Probarbital is not found in any pharmaceutical preparations sold in the United States.

General Comment: Probarbital is an intermediate-acting barbiturate with actions similar to those of amobarbital.

Biochemistry: Similar to that of amobarbital.

Toxicology–Pharmacology: Similar to that of amobarbital.

▶ **PROCAINE**
Dangerous Drug

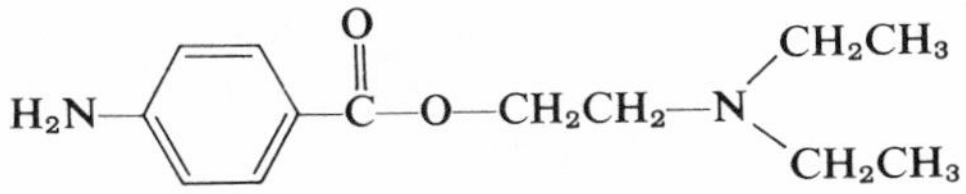

Synonyms: Allocaine, ethocaine, syncaine, 2-diethylaminoethyl-*p*-amino-benzoate

Pharmaceutical Preparations

Novocain^R (Winthrop)—Injection: 2 percent or 1 percent

Novocain^R (Winthrop)—Injection for spinal anesthesia; 10 percent

General Comments: Procaine is a local anesthetic that is classified as a Dangerous Drug in this text except ointments and creams for topical application containing not more than two and one half percent ($2\frac{1}{2}\%$) strength. All other pharmaceutical preparations containing procaine require a prescription and bear the legend "Caution: Federal law prohibits dispensing without a prescription."

Procaine is encountered in cases of drug abuse in many areas of the country as a common adulterant in illicit heroin samples.

Biochemistry: Procaine has a very short biological half-life, being hydrolyzed rapidly by an esterase, forming *p*-aminobenzoic acid and diethylaminoethanol:

Procaine

p-Aminobenzoic acid

Diethylaminoethanol

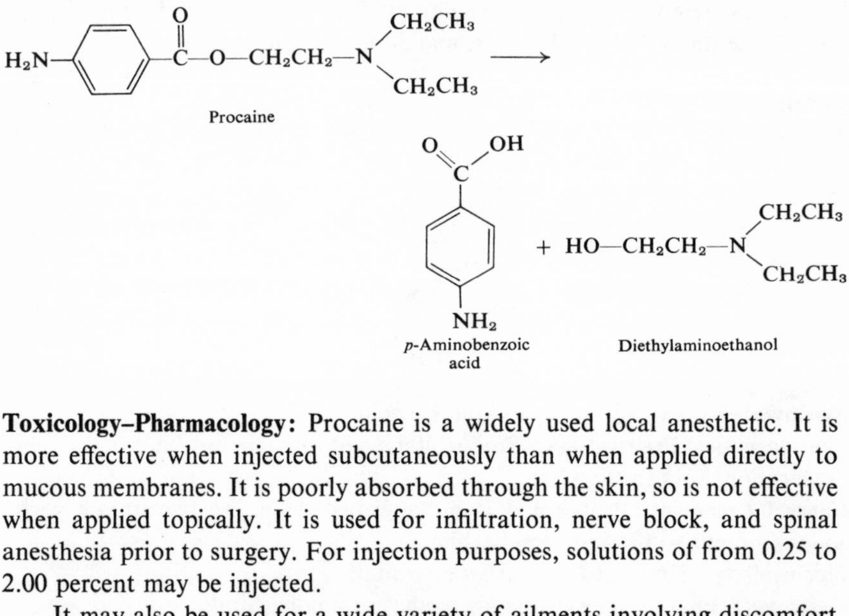

Toxicology–Pharmacology: Procaine is a widely used local anesthetic. It is more effective when injected subcutaneously than when applied directly to mucous membranes. It is poorly absorbed through the skin, so is not effective when applied topically. It is used for infiltration, nerve block, and spinal anesthesia prior to surgery. For injection purposes, solutions of from 0.25 to 2.00 percent may be injected.

It may also be used for a wide variety of ailments involving discomfort and pain. It is also used as an antiarrhythmic agent, being injected intravenously for this purpose. Procainamide is more commonly used for this purpose, however. Rapid intravenous injection of high doses can, however, result in stimulation of the central nervous system, followed by depression and death.

Procaine is commonly encountered in illicit drug preparations, and is frequently used as a diluent for heroin.

In an adult given 2000 mg procaine intravenously over a period of 2 hours, a plasma concentration of 0.02 mg/dl was found 15 minutes following the injection. Concomitantly, 0.27 mg of the major metabolite, diethylaminoethanol, was found. After 1 hour, no procaine was found, but 0.17 mg/dl of the metabolite was found (Brodie *et al.*, 1948).

▶ **PROCHLORPERAZINE**
Dangerous Drug

Synonyms: Prochlorpemazine, 2-chloro-10-[3-(4-methylpiperazin-1-yl)-propyl]phenothiazine.

Pharmaceutical Preparations

Combid^R (Smith Kline & French)—Capsule: Containing 10 mg prochlorperazine maleate and 5 mg isopropamide

Compazine^R (Smith Kline & French)—Containing prochlorperazine maleate: Tablets: 5, 10, or 25 mg. Capsules: 10, 15, 30, or 75 mg. Ampules: each 1 ml containing 5 mg. Vials: each 1 ml containing 5 mg. Suppositories: $2\frac{1}{2}$, 5, or 25 mg. Syrup: each 5 ml containing 5 mg. Concentrate: each 1 ml containing 10 mg.

Eskatrol^R Spansule (Smith Kline & French)—See **AMPHETAMINE**

General Comment: Prochlorperazine is a phenothiazine tranquilizer, and is thus classified in this text as a Dangerous Drug.

Biochemistry: Approximately 35 percent of unchanged prochlorperazine is excreted in the feces in 24 hours after oral dose. After repeated dosage, tissue peak levels are reached in about 2 hours after administration.

The 4-methyl-1-piperazine group contributes significantly to the drug's potency.

Toxicology–Pharmacology: Prochlorperazine, like its prototype, chlorpromazine, is a psychotherapeutic agent believed to act at the subcortical level of the brain. It principally depresses the central nervous system. It is about five times more potent than chlorpromazine.

Prochlorperazine is used under the same circumstances as is chlorpromazine. It is useful in controlling emotional stress associated with serious somatic disorders, such as peptic ulcer, cardiac ailments, premenstrual tension, asthma, arthritis, and epilepsy. Anxious and agitated geriatric patients are improved, and it may be given to hospital patients to relieve anxiety and tension. It is especially effective in controlling the anxiety, agitation, tension, and confusion observed in schizophrenia, manic–depression, and various psychoses. It may also be used for treating acute intoxication and anxiety in chronic alcoholics.

Dosage is usually begun in adults at 5–10 mg, three or four times per day. The dosage may be increased as needed. In psychotic patients, this may reach 50–150 mg daily.

In four nonfatal overdoses, serum concentrations of 0.12–0.16 mg/dl were found (Tompsett, 1968).

▶ **PROHEPTAZINE**
Schedule I

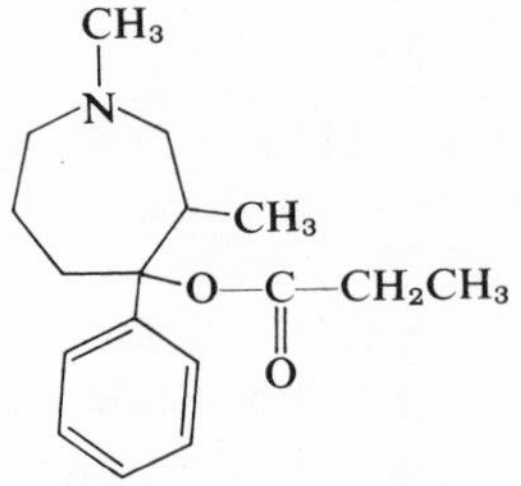

Synonyms: Dimepheprimine, propyl-1,3-dimethyl-4-phenyl-1-azacyclohep-tane-4-carboxylate.
Pharmaceutical Preparations: Proheptazine is not found in any pharmaceutical preparations sold in the United States.
General Comment: Proheptazine is a synthetic narcotic analgesic that has no accepted medicinal value in the United States.
Biochemistry: Unknown.
Toxicology–Pharmacology: Unknown.

▶ **PROLINTANE**
Noncontrolled Substance

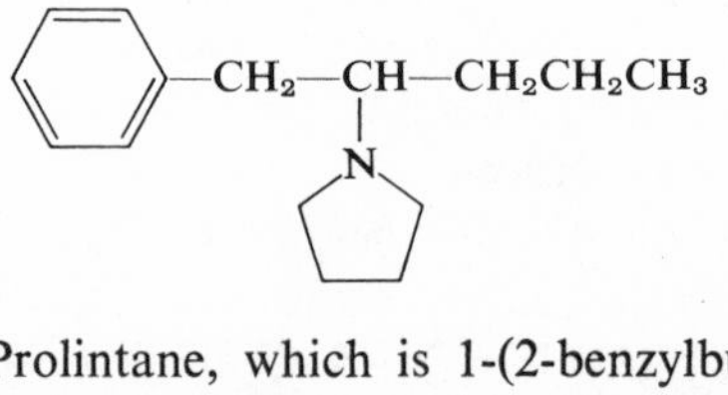

General Comments: Prolintane, which is 1-(2-benzylbutyl)pyrrolidine, is a central stimulant drug that is not accepted for medicinal use in the United States. It has been used in England.

▶ **PROMAZINE**
Dangerous Drug

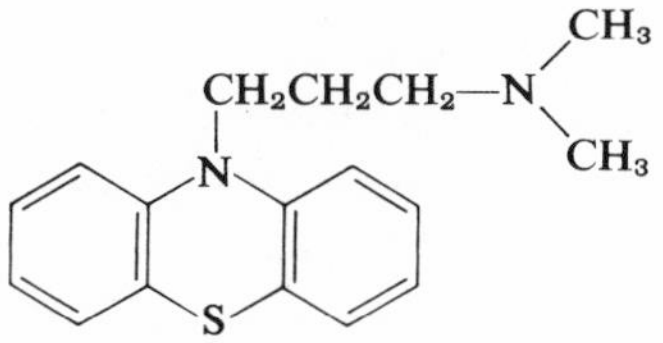

$$CH_2CH_2CH_2-N\begin{smallmatrix}CH_3\\CH_3\end{smallmatrix}$$

Synonym: 10-(3-Dimethylaminopropyl)phenothiazine.

Pharmaceutical Preparations: Sparine[R] (Wyeth)—Not available.

General Comment: Promazine is a phenothiazine tranquilizer, and as such is classified in this text as a Dangerous Drug.

Biochemistry: Promazine was first synthesized in the early 1940's in a search for antimalarial drugs.

The primary metabolic pathway is sulfoxide formation. Secondary metabolism is *N*-dealkylation.

Toxicology–Pharmacology: The action of promazine is very similar to that of chlorpromazine. In addition to its tranquilizing action, promazine has antiemetic, analgesic-potentiating, and anesthetic-potentiating actions.

Promazine is used primarily in treating acute and chronic abnormalities of the central nervous system characterized by emotional disturbances and hyperactivity.

It is used in agitated psychoses, neurotic anxiety, psychological stress, and alcoholism. It may also be used in senile psychoses and in behavior disorders of disturbed or mentally retarded children.

Doses of up to 50 or 150 mg may be given initially, and this may be increased up to a daily dose of 1 g, in severe cases.

▶ **PROMETHAZINE**
Noncontrolled Substance

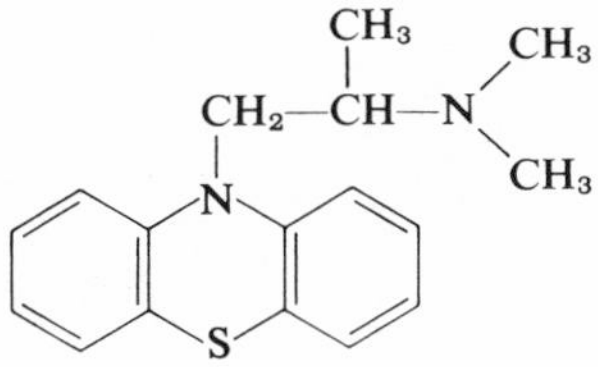

$$CH_2-CH-N\begin{smallmatrix}CH_3\\CH_3\end{smallmatrix}$$
$$\quad\ \ |CH_3$$

General Comments: Promethazine is an antihistaminic drug that is encountered in cases of drug abuse probably because of the similarity of its name to the names of certain tranquilizers. It is not controlled unless it is contained in a pharmaceutical preparation requiring a prescription. In such a case, it would be considered a Dangerous Drug under the legend drug provision.

Toxicology–Pharmacology: Promethazine is an antihistaminic drug. It has, in addition, sedative and antiemetic effects. It may be used in the treatment of allergic conditions, as a sedative to effect sleep, or to provide surgical or obstetric sedation. It is also effective in prevention and treatment of motion sickness, and in management of the nausea and vomiting associated with surgical operations and pregnancy. It is also a potent local anesthetic agent.

Adult dosage for sedation is 25–50 mg orally. For motion sickness, 25 mg orally may be given.

▶ **PROMETHESTROL DIPROPIONATE**
Noncontrolled Substance
Encountered in Excepted Substances

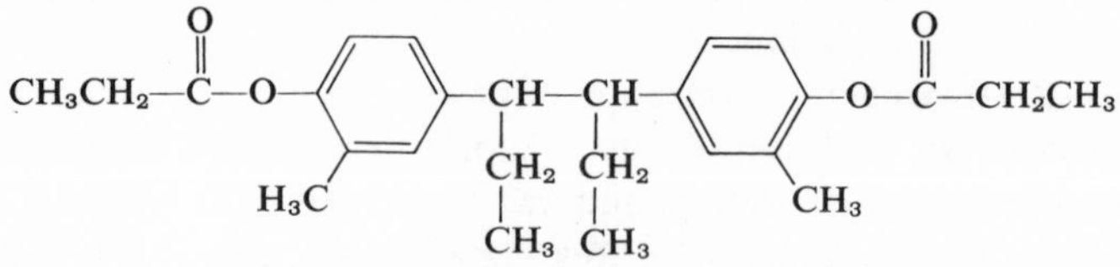

General Comments: Promethestrol dipropionate is an estrogen with actions and uses similar to those of diethylstilbestrol and other synthetic estrogens. It is encountered in formulation containing phenobarbital that are classified as excepted preparations. The minimum phenobarbital/promethestrol dipropionate ratio found in such preparations is 1/0.06.

▶ **PROPERIDINE**
Schedule I

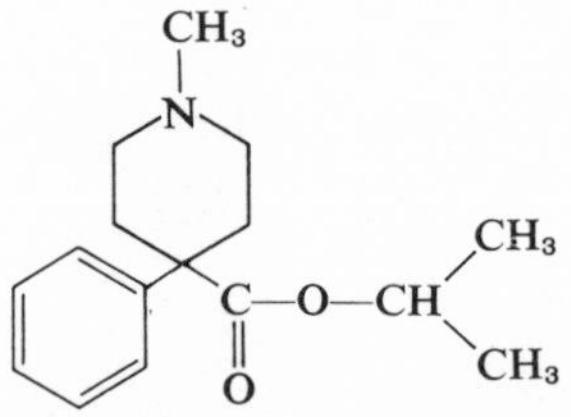

Synonyms: Gevelina, ipropethidine, isopedine, isopropyl-1-methyl-4-phenyl-piperidine-4-carboxylate.

Pharmaceutical Preparations: Properidine is not found in any pharmaceutical preparations sold in the United States.

General Comments: Properidine is a synthetic narcotic analgesic of the piperidine type. It is similar to ketobemidone and anileridine, among others. Properidine has no accepted medicinal value in the United States.
Biochemistry: Unknown.
Toxicology–Pharmacology: Unknown.

▶ **PROPIOMAZINE**
Dangerous Drug

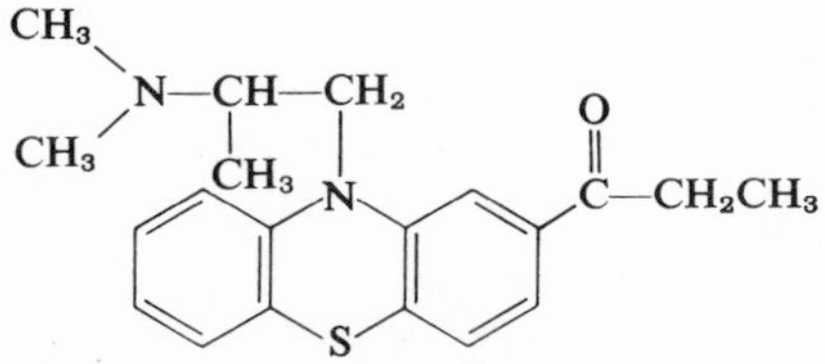

Synonym: 10-(2-Dimethylaminopropyl)-1-propionylphenothiazine.
Pharmaceutical Preparations: Propiomazine is not found in pharmaceutical preparations sold in the United States.
General Comment: Propiomazine is a phenothiazine tranquilizer, and as such is classified in this text as a Dangerous Drug.
Biochemistry: Similar to that of promethazine.
Toxicology–Pharmacology: Propiomazine is structurally similar to promethazine, and like promethazine, it has antihistaminic, sedative, and antiemetic actions. Its central nervous system depressant action is, however, more potent than that of promethazine.

It is used mainly for its sedative effect, which is more rapidly attained and of shorter duration than that of promethazine. It is used to provide nighttime, surgical, or obstetrical sedation.

Untoward effects include dryness of the mouth, moderate elevation of blood pressure, and rarely, hypotension or tachycardia. The drug should be given with caution to ambulatory patients, and patients should be cautioned against driving motor vehicles, due to the drowsiness and dizziness that occur.

The usual adult dose is 20 mg, administered intramuscularly.

▶ **PROPIRAM**
Schedule I

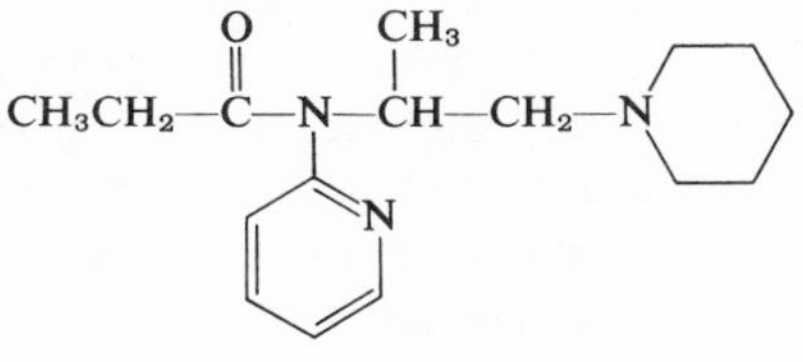

Synonym: N-(1-methyl-2-piperidinoethyl)-N-2-pyridyl-propionamide.

Pharmaceutical Preparations: Propiram is not found in any pharmaceutical preparations sold in the United States.

General Comment: Propiram is a synthetic narcotic analgesic that has no accepted medicinal value in the United States.

Biochemistry: Unknown.

Toxicology–Pharmacology: Unknown.

▶ **PROPOXYPHENE**
Schedule IV

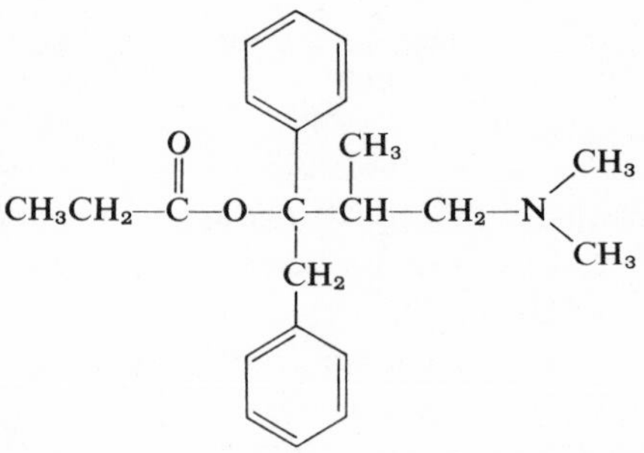

$$CH_3CH_2-\overset{\overset{\displaystyle O}{\|}}{C}-O-\overset{\overset{\displaystyle C_6H_5}{|}}{\underset{\underset{\displaystyle CH_2}{|}}{C}}-\overset{\overset{\displaystyle CH_3}{|}}{CH}-CH_2-N\overset{\diagup CH_3}{\diagdown CH_3}$$

Synonym: α-4-Dimethylamino-3-methyl-1,2-diphenylbut-2-yl-propionate.

Pharmaceutical Preparations

Darvocet-N[R] (Lilly)—Tablets: containing 50 or 100 mg propoxyphene napsylate and 325 mg acetaminophen

Darvon[R] (Lilly)—Capsules, containing propoxyphene hydrochloride: "HO2," light-pink, 32 mg; "HO3," light-pink, 65 mg

Darvon[R] Compound (Lilly)—Capsules, containing propoxyphene hydrochloride, aspirin, phenacetin, and caffeine: light pink and light gray, 32, 227, 162, and 32.4 mg, respectively, of above substances. Compound 65; red and light gray, containing 65 mg propoxyphene, plus same as above.

Darvon[R] with A.S.A. (Lilly)—Capsules: red and light pink, containing 65 mg propoxyphene hydrochloride and 325 mg aspirin

Darvon-N[R] (Lilly)—Suspension: each 5 ml containing 50 mg propoxyphene napsylate. Tablet: containing 100 mg propoxyphene napsylate.

Darvon-N[R] with A.S.A. (Lilly)—Tablets: orange, containing 100 mg propoxyphene napsylate and 325 mg aspirin

Dolene[R] (Lederle)—Capsule: containing 65 mg propoxyphene hydrochloride

Dolene[R] Compound-65 (Lederle)—Capsule: containing 65 mg propoxyphene hydrochloride, 227 mg aspirin, 162 mg phenacetin, and 32.4 mg caffeine

Dolene[R] AP-65 (Lederle)—Tablet: containing 65 mg propoxyphene hydrochloride and 650 mg acetaminophen

Repro[R] Compound-65 (Reid-Provident)—Capsule: pink and black, containing 65 mg propoxyphene hydrochloride with aspirin, phenacetin, and caffeine

SK-65[R] (Smith Kline & French)—Capsule: "SKF-463," gray and white, containing 65 mg propoxyphene hydrochloride

SK-65[R] Compound (Smith Kline & French)—Capsule: "SKF-467," gray and orange, containing 65 mg propoxyphene hydrochloride, 227 mg aspirin, 162 mg phenacetin, and 32.4 mg caffeine

Stereo-Darvon[R] with A.S.A. (Lilly)—Tablet: turquoise, coated, "C37," containing 32 mg propoxyphene hydrochloride, 0.25 mg paramethasome, and 500 mg aspirin

Unigesic-A[R] (Upjohn)—Tablet: white, "UPJOHN-771," containing 65 mg propoxyphene hydrochloride and 325 mg aspirin

Wygesic[R] (Wyeth)—Tablet: green, oblong, "WYETH-85," containing 65 mg propoxyphene hydrochloride and 650 mg acetaminophen

General Comment: Propoxyphene is an analgesic that was added to Schedule IV in February 1977.

Biochemistry: Propoxyphene is widely used as a "nonnarcotic" analgesic—but this is questionable as to addictive potential. It is very closely related to methadone in structure. About 10 percent is excreted unchanged with N-demethylation as the major metabolic route. Chronic use of propoxyphene leads to appearance of the cyclic metabolite:

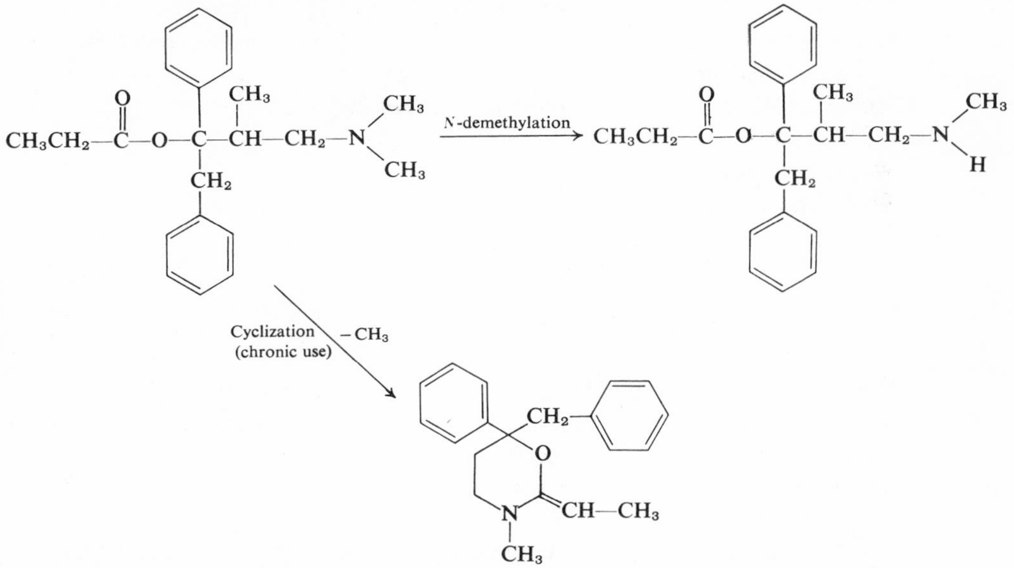

Toxicology–Pharmacology: Propoxyphene is structurally related to methadone. Propoxyphene is used therapeutically as an analgesic, often in

combination with aspirin. It is one of the most commonly prescribed drugs in the United States. It is used to provide relief in mild to moderate pain, whether acute, chronic, or recurrent.

Propoxyphene is effective when administered orally. Although closely related to methadone structurally, it has little addictive liability and only mild narcotic actions. It has been used in very high doses to suppress the heroin abstinence syndrome, however (Nash *et al.*, 1975). Overdose with propoxyphene has been successfully treated by administration of the narcotic antagonists naloxone, levallorphan, and nalorphine (Kersh, 1973).

Propoxyphene is generally supplied as either the hydrochloride salt or, more recently as the napsylate. The napsylate preparation is less soluble in water, and is probably absorbed somewhat more slowly.

Toxic effects of propoxyphene, usually after overdose, include mental confusion, muscle fasciculations, respiratory depression, coma, or convulsions. The respiratory depression can be counteracted with narcotic antagonists.

Propoxyphene is now one of the most frequent causes of death from drug overdose, being exceeded only by alcohol or barbiturates. In some localities, it is even the primary cause of drug-induced deaths.

Therapeutic concentrations of propoxyphene in plasma may range from 0.024 to 0.075 mg/dl after chronic daily administration of 195 mg. The corresponding norpropoxyphene (main metabolite) concentrations were 0.59–3.01 mg/dl (Verebely and Inturresi, 1973).

In fatal intoxications, blood concentrations of propoxyphene of greater than 0.10 mg/dl are usually found. In suicide cases involving ingestion of large doses of propoxyphene, concentrations of 0.20–1.00 mg/dl are usually found (Baselt *et al.*, 1975a; Sturner and Garriott, 1973).

▶ **PROPYLHEXEDRINE**
Noncontrolled Substance

$$\text{CH}_2-\overset{\overset{\displaystyle CH_3}{|}}{\text{CH}}-\text{NH}-\text{CH}_3$$

General Comments: Propylhexedrine, closely related to amphetamine, produces the same vasoconstrictive and decongestant effects on the mucous membranes as amphetamine does. It has, however, less intense vasoconstrictor action, and its central stimulating effect is considerably less than that of amphetamine.

Propylhexedrine replaced amphetamine as a volatile nasal decongestant when amphetamine was misused for its central stimulant effects. At present, propylhexedrine is being similarly abused. These nasal decongestants are being taken apart, the propylhexedrine removed from the cotton by syringe, and the solution injected. Unfortunately, several deaths have occurred due to this practice.

Toxicology–Pharmacology: Propylhexedrine is a sympathomimetic amine, related structurally to amphetamine. Its primary actions are to exert vasoconstrictive and decongestant effects on the mucous membranes. Although effective as a vasoconstrictor, its central nervous stimulant actions is only one twelfth that of amphetamine (Anlage, 1973).

When inhaled, as directed, very low quantities of propylhexedrine (approximately 0.5 mg) are absorbed, and less than 0.001 mg/dl may be detected in the blood. However, abusers who inject the solution eluted from the cotton of the inhaler may inject 250 mg or more of this substance. In five cases of death occurring as a result of this practice, blood concentrations of from 0.03 to 0.25 mg/dl were found (Di Maio and Garriott, 1977b).

Oral ingestion of 250 mg of the drug in a nonfatal intoxication caused palpitation, headache, chest pain, shock, and myocardial infarction in a 22-year-old man (Marsden and Sheldon, 1972).

▶ **PROTHIPENDYL**
Dangerous Drug

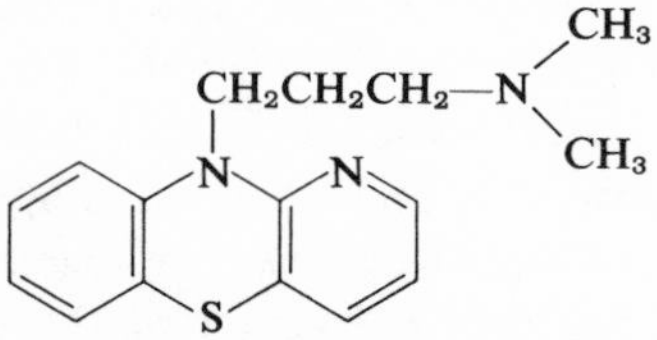

Synonyms: Phrenotropin, 9-(3-dimethylaminopropyl)-10-thia-1,9-diazaanthracene.

Pharmaceutical Preparations: Prothipendyl is not found in any pharmaceutical preparations sold in the United States.

General Comment: Prothipendyl is a tranquilizer and is therefore classified in this text as a Dangerous Drug.

Biochemistry: Unknown.

Toxicology–Pharmacology: Unknown.

▶ **PROTOKYLOL**
Noncontrolled Substance

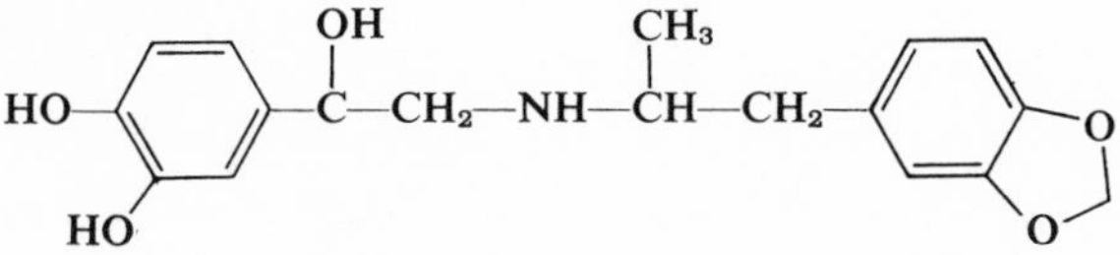

General Comments: Protokylol is not controlled unless it is contained in a pharmaceutical preparation that requires a prescription, such as Ventaire[R] (Marion). Such a preparation would be classified as a Dangerous Drug by the legend drug provision.

Toxicology–Pharmacology: Protokylol is a long-acting sympathomimetic amine, similar in structure and actions to those of isoproterenol. It selectively effects bronchodilation, and is effective when given orally. It reduces the frequency and severity of asthmatic attacks, and is used primarily in treatment of asthma. When inhaled, its effects are immediate, and may last for 3–6 hours.

▶ **PSEUDOEPHEDRINE**
Noncontrolled Substance

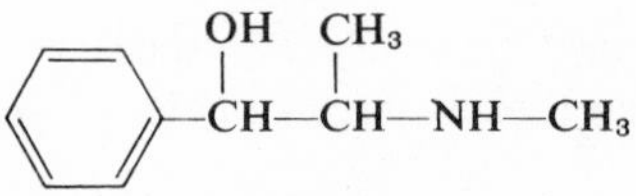

General Comments: Ephedrine contains two asymmetric carbon atoms, so that four optically active isomers and two racemic mixtures may exist. The most active, pharmacologically, is the *l*-isomer, *l-ephedrine*. A mixture of *l*-ephedrine with *d-ephedrine* is known as *racephedrine*, which is used in medicine and known as *ephedrine*. The other pair of optical isomers are known as *l-pseudoephedrine* and *d-pseudoephedrine*, or together as (±) *pseudoephedrine*. Pseudoephedrine has only a fraction of the pressor activity of the ephedrine counterpart.

Toxicology–Pharmacology: Pseudoephedrine has qualitatively the same actions as does ephedrine. It has only a fraction of the pressor effect that ephedrine has, but does have significant bronchodilator and decongestant actions. It is effective when taken orally, and may exert this effect for 4 hours or more.

▶ **PSILOCIN**
Schedule I

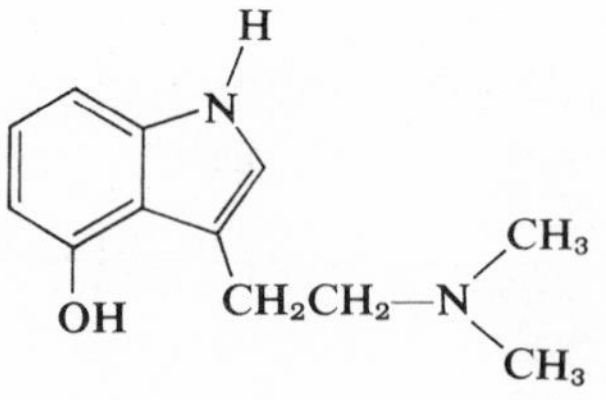

Synonyms: 4-Hydroxydimethyltryptamine,   3-(2-dimethylaminoethyl)-4-hydroxyindole.

Pharmaceutical Preparations: Psilocin is not found in any pharmaceutical preparations sold in the United States.

General Comment: Psilocin is an indole alkaloid that has no accepted medicinal value in the United States.

Biochemistry: See Toxicology–Pharmacology under **PSILOCYBIN.**

▶ **PSILOCYBIN**
Schedule I

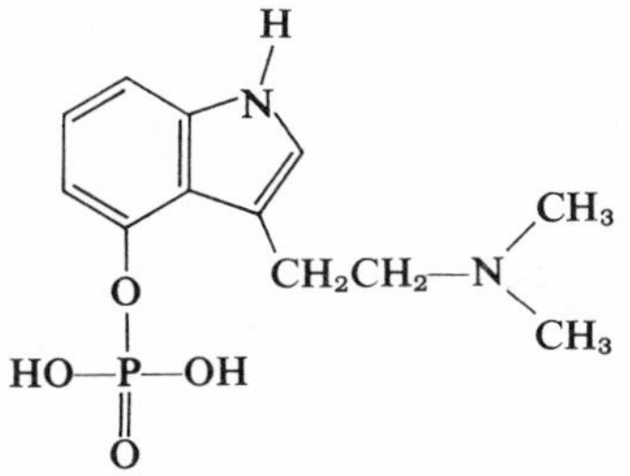

Synonyms: 4-Phosphoryloxy-*N*,*N*-dimethyltriptamine,   3-(2-dimethylamino-ethyl)indol-4-yl dihydrogen phosphate.

Pharmaceutical Preparations: Psilocybin is not found in any pharmaceutical preparations sold in the United States.

General Comment: Psilocybin is an indole alkaloid that has no accepted medicinal value in the United States.

Biochemistry: See Toxicology–Pharmacology below.

Toxicology–Pharmacology: Psilocybin is psilocin that is phosphorylated on the 4-hydroxy group. It is the primary hallucinogenic substance from the *Psilocybe* mushrooms, and is found in certain other genera such as *Panaeolus* and *Stropharia*.

The oral dose required in man to produce hallucinations similar to those produced by LSD is 4–8 mg. It elicits the same symptoms as the consumption of about 2 g of dried mushroom. The time course of psilocybin and psilocin reactions is shorter than that of LSD or mescaline reactions. Psilocin is approximately 1.4 times as potent as psilocybin. Psilocybin is 2.5 times less toxic than mescaline, but has a psychotomimetic effect 50 times higher.

Also see **PSILOCIN, 6-HYDROXYDIMETHYLTRYPTAMINE,** and **7-HYDROXYDIMETHYLTRYPTAMINE.**

Symptoms of the psilocybin mushroom intoxication include muscular relaxation, flaccidity, and mydriasis in the early stages, followed by a period of emotional disturbance such as hilarity and difficulty in concentration. At this point, visual and auditory hallucinations usually appear. Following this is a period of lassitude and mental and physical depression, with alteration of time and space perception (Schultes and Hofmann, 1973). The effects may peak in about 1–1$\frac{1}{2}$ hours, and may subside in about 6 hours. The effects of psilocybin are identical to those of the mushrooms.

Psilocybin has a low toxicity, with an LD_{50} in mice of 280 mg/kg. It is therefore 2.5 times less toxic than mescaline, but 50 times more powerful as a psychotomimetic in human beings (Hofmann, 1961). Its effects on the autonomic nervous system include pupillary dilatation. In animals, reduced motor activity is observed (Cerletti, 1959).

▶ **QUINIDINE**
Noncontrolled Substance

General Comments: Quinidine is an alkaloid found in various species and hybrids of *Cinchona* and in *Remejia pedunculata* Fluckiger (Family *Rubiaceae*).

It is an optical isomer of quinine and was first described in 1848 by Van Heyningen. The use of *Cinchona* alkaloids for artial fibrillation dates back to 1749 (Goodman and Gilman, 1970).

Toxicology–Pharmacology: The pharmacological actions of quinidine are similar to those of quinine. In high concentration, it has general protoplasmic poison properties as does quinine, and is as potent as quinine as an antimalarial.

The main use for quinidine, however, is as an antiarrhythmic agent. It was found to be about twice as effective as quinine or cinchonine in suppressing cardiac arrhythmias. It is of primary usefulness in fresh atrial fibrillation, ventricular tachycardia, and postthyroidectomy atrial flutter or fibrillation. It is also commonly used in relatively old atrial flutter and fibrillation, premature ventricular beats, and atrial fibrillation occurring during myocardial infarction.

The adverse effects of quinidine are similar to those of quinine. Cinchonism, manifested by ringing in the ears, obtunding of the hearing, and blurring of vision, may occur. Hypotension may also occur. Quinidine poisoning may result in diastolic arrest of the heart. Manifestations of hypersensitivity include fever, urticaria, and purpura.

After oral administration of 400-mg doses to adults, plasma concentrations of 0.34 mg/dl were observed at 1 hour, and the maximum of 0.40 mg/dl occurred at 2 hours. After 6 hours, the plasma value was 0.24 mg/dl, and 24 hours later was 0.04 mg/dl (Goldberg, W. M., and Chakrabarti, 1964).

In a fatal overdose of quinidine, a blood concentration of 4.5 mg/dl was found at death, 28 hours after the ingestion (Baselt and Cravey, 1977).

▶ **QUININE**
Noncontrolled Substance

General Comments: Until World War II, quinine was the most important drug available for the control of malaria, but it was largely replaced by more effective and less toxic synthetic antimalarial agents.

Quinine has been encountered as an adulterant in illicit heroin samples. This is more common on the east coast of the United States than in the southwest section.

Quinine is a levorotatory stereoisomer of quinidine.

Toxicology–Pharmacology: Quinine is one of the alkaloids obtained from the bark of the cinchona species. It was extensively used for the control of malaria prior to World War II, but has largely been replaced by more effective and less toxic synthetic antimalarials. As some of the strains of the malaria organism have become resistant to the newer drugs, quinine is still used for the purpose, however. Quinine has also had considerable use as an analgesic for headache, myalgia, neuralgia, and other conditions but salicylates have been found to be far more effective. It has also antipyretic actions by virtue of the peripheral vasodilatation, mediated via the central nervous system. Quinine also has some antiarrhythmic actions on the heart, but is less effective than its isomer, quinidine.

Untoward effects of quinine are referred to as "cinchonism." Up to 300 mg per day can be taken without any adverse effects, but 600 mg per day causes mild symptoms in many people. The most common of these is ringing in the ears, often accompanied with a sensation of fullness in the head, dulling of the sense of hearing, and blurred vision. Giddiness and staggering may occur. In overdose, severe headache, delirium, stupor, deafness and blindness, dilated pupils, convulsions, paralysis, and finally collapse and coma may occur.

After ingestion of 540 mg quinine in 11 adults, average plasma concentrations of 0.182 mg/dl were found at 2 hours, and 0.171 mg/dl was found at 8 hours (Hall *et al.*, 1973).

In a case of death from overdose of an unknown quantity of quinine, a blood concentration of 2.20 mg/dl was found. In another case, 1.20 mg/dl was found after ingestion of 61 capsules containing 5 g quinine each (Winek *et al.*, 1974).

▶ **RACEPHEDRINE**
Noncontrolled Substance
General Comment: Racephedrine is a mixture of the *d-* and *l-*isomers of ephedrine. See **EPHEDRINE** for discussion.

▶ **RACEMETHORPHAN**
Schedule II

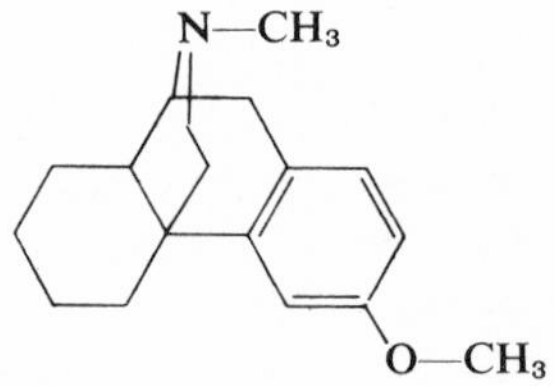

Synonyms: (±)-3-Methoxy-*N*-methylmorphinan, methorphan.
Pharmaceutical Preparations: Racemethorphan is not found in any pharmaceutical preparations sold in the United States.
General Comments: None.
Biochemistry: See Toxicology–Pharmacology below.
Toxicology–Pharmacology: Racemethorphan (methorphan) is the methyl analogue of racemorphan. It is a mixture of the *dextro* and *levo* isomers of methorphan. Dextromethorphan has no narcotic and analgesic properties, but it is frequently found in pharmaceutical preparations for its antitussive (cough-suppressant) actions [e.g., Robitussin[R] (Robins)]. It is not subject to control. Levomethorphan, on the other hand, is a narcotic analgesic and is subject to control. (See **DEXTROMETHORPHAN** and **LEVOMETHORPHAN** for additional discussion.)

▶ **RACEMORAMIDE**
Schedule I

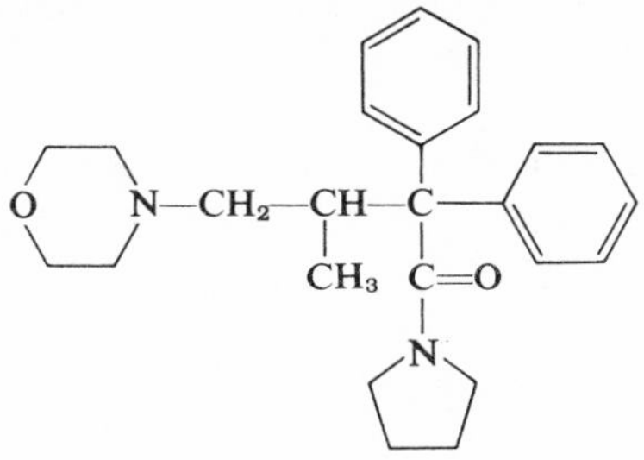

Synonyms: ($\pm$)-1-(3-Methyl-4-morpholino-2,2-diphenylbutyryl)pyrrolidine, moramide.
Pharmaceutical Preparations: Racemoramide is not found in any pharmaceutical preparations sold in the United States.
General Comments: None.
Biochemistry: See Toxicology–Pharmacology below.
Toxicology–Pharmacology: Racemoramide (moramide) is a synthetic narcotic analgesic that is a mixture of the *dextro* and *levo* isomers, dextromoramide and levomoramide. Moramide, which includes all isomers, has no accepted medicinal value in the United States. (See **DEXTROMORAMIDE** and **LEVOMORAMIDE** for additional discussion.)

▶ **RACEMORPHAN**
Schedule II

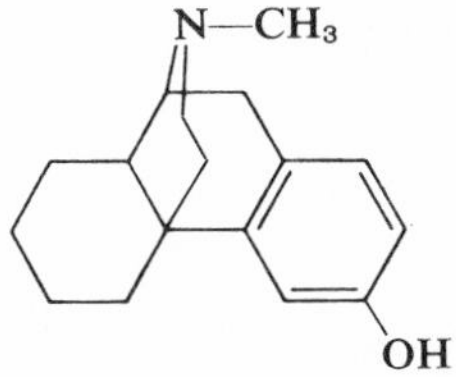

Synonyms: ($\pm$)-3-Hydroxy-*N*-methylmorphinan, morphan.
Pharmaceutical Preparations: See **LEVORPHANOL.**
General Comments: None.
Biochemistry: See Toxicology–Pharmacology below.
Toxicology–Pharmacology: Racemorphan is a mixture of *dextro* and *levo* isomers (dextrorphan and levorphanol, respectively). Dextrorphan, a nonnarcotic antitussive agent, is not subject to control. Levorphanol is five times

as potent an analgesic, on a weight basis, as morphine, and probably has more
sedative effect. It is subject to control under Schedule II, as is the mixture of
isomers, racemorphan. (See **DEXTRORPHAN** and **LEVORPHANOL** for
further discussion.)

▶ **RESCINNAMINE**
Dangerous Drug

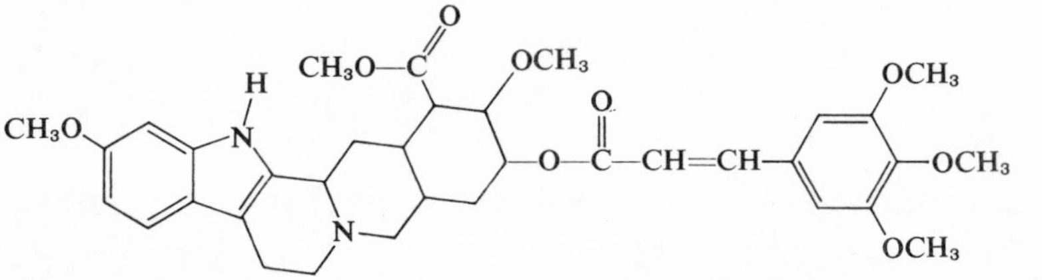

Synonym: Methyl-18-(3,4,5-trimethoxycinnamoyl)reserpate.
Pharmaceutical Preparations: Moderil^R (Pfizer)—Tablets, oval, scored:
yellow, "441," containing 0.25 mg rescinnamine; salmon, "442," containing
0.5 mg rescinnamine
General Comment: Rescinnamine is a tranquilizer, and as such is classified in
this text as a Dangerous Drug.
Biochemistry: See **RESERPINE.**
Toxicology–Pharmacology: Rescinnamine is an alkaloid occurring in
Rauwolfia serpentina and other *Rauwolfia* species. It is used as an antihyper-
tensive drug and tranquilizer.

The actions and uses of rescinnamine are essentially the same as those of
reserpine. It is used primarily for treatment of hypertension, having both
tranquilizing and antihypertensive effects. It may also be used for its tranquilizing action to treat anxiety, tension, nervousness, and irritability. See
also **RESERPINE.**

▶ **RESERPINE**
Dangerous Drug

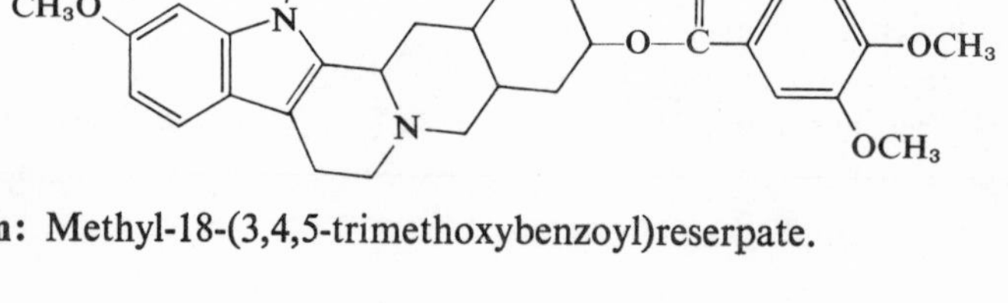

Synonym: Methyl-18-(3,4,5-trimethoxybenzoyl)reserpate.

Pharmaceutical Preparations

Butiserpazide[R] (McNeil)—Schedule III, Penalty Group 3, preparation: Tablets: green, containing 30 mg butabarbital, 25 mg hydrochlorothiazide, and 0.1 mg reserpine; orange, containing 30 mg butabarbital, 50 mg hydrochlorothiazide, and 0.1 mg reserpine

Diupres[R] (Merck Sharp & Dohme)—Tablets, pink, scored: "MSD-230," containing 250 mg chlorothiazide and 0.125 mg reserpine; "MSD-405," containing 500 mg chlorothiazide and 0.125 mg reserpine

Diutensen-R[R] (Mallinckrodt)—Tablet: containing 2.5 mg methychlothiazide and 0.1 mg reserpine

Dralserp[R] (Lemmon)—Tablet: orange, oblong, containing 25 mg hydralazine and 0.1 mg reserpine

Exna-R[R] (Robins)—Tablet: white, scored, containing 50 mg benzthiazide and 0.125 mg reserpine

Hydrochlorothiazide[R] with Reserpine (Philips & Roxane)—Tablets: containing 25 or 50 mg hydrochlorothiazide and 0.125 mg reserpine

Hydromox[R] (Lederle)—Tablet: yellow, scored, containing 50 mg quinethazone and 0.125 mg reserpine

Hydropres[R] (Merck Sharp & Dohme)—Tablets, green, scored: "MSD-53," containing 25 mg hydrochlorothiazide and 0.125 mg reserpine; "MSD-127," containing 50 mg hydrochlorothiazide and 0.125 mg reserpine

Hydrotensin-50[R] (Mayrand)—Tablet: containing 50 mg hydrochlorothiazide and 0.125 mg reserpine

Hydrotensin-Plus[R] (Mayrand)—Tablet: containing 15 mg hydrochlorothiazide, 25 mg hydralazine, and 0.1 mg reserpine

Metatensin[R] (Merrell-National)—Tablets: yellow, containing 2 mg trichloromethiazide and 0.1 mg reserpine; lavender, containing 4 mg trichloromethiazide and 0.1 mg reserpine

Naquival[R] (Schering)—Tablet: peach, scored, containing 4 mg trichloromethiazide and 0.1 mg reserpine

Rau-Sed[R] (Squibb)—Tablet: containing 0.25 mg reserpine

Regroton[R] (USV)—Tablet: pink, single-scored, containing 50 mg chlorthalidone and 0.25 mg reserpine

Renese-R[R] (Pfizer)—Tablet: blue, scored, containing 20 mg polythiazide and 0.25 mg reserpine

Salutensin[R] (Bristol)—Tablet: containing 50 mg hydroflumethiazide and 0.125 mg reserpine

Sandril[R] (Lilly)—Ampules: each ml containing 2.5 mg reserpine. Tablets: orange, "J99," containing 0.1 mg reserpine; green, "U29," containing 0.25 mg reserpine.

Ser-Ap-Es[R] (Ciba)—Tablet: dark salmon pink, containing 0.1 mg reserpine, 25 mg hydralazine, and 15 mg hydrochlorothiazide

Serpasil[R] (Ciba)—Tablets: white, scored, containing 1 mg reserpine; white, scored, containing 0.25 mg reserpine; white, containing 0.1 mg reserpine. Elixir: green, each 4 ml containing 0.2 mg reserpine. Vial: each 1 ml containing 2.5 mg reserpine.

Serpasil-Apresoline[R] (Ciba)—Tablets: yellow, containing 0.2 mg reserpine and 50 mg hydralazine; yellow, containing 0.1 mg reserpine and 25 mg hydralazine

Serpasil-Esidrix[R] (Ciba)—Tablets: light orange, containing 0.1 mg reserpine and 25 mg hydrochlorothiazide; light orange, containing 0.1 mg reserpine and 50 mg hydrochlorothiazide

General Comment: Reserpine is a tranquilizer, and as such is classified in this text as a Dangerous Drug.

Biochemistry: Naturally occurring reserpine is levorotatory, being one of 64 possible stereoisomers. Several other stereoisomers have been prepared by chemical isomerizations, but all have the *cis*-C-15, C-20 ring juncture (Schlittler and Bein, 1967).

Deserpidine is an alkaloid similar to reserpine only lacking the $11\text{-}OCH_3$ group. It has the same degree of hypotensive activity, central depression, and depletion of peripheral norepinephrine as reserpine. Thus, the $11\text{-}OCH_3$ has no value for pharmacological activity. However, other naturally occurring alkaloids differing from reserpine in the C-17 or C-18 stereoisomer have reduced antihypertensive activity or are completely inactive.

The specific stereochemistry at C-17 is not essential. However, a methoxyl group rather than a hydroxyl group is necessary. This is shown by the fact that raunescine, pseudoreserpine, and rescidine are much less active than deserpidine, reserpine, and rescinnamine. Rescinnamine exhibits less antihypertensive properties than reserpine. The ester group at C-18 is essential. By varying the C-18 ester group, the sedative and hypotensive activities vary. However, none of the derivatives increased activity over reserpine (Plummer *et al.*, 1954).

Modifications of the indole moiety of reserpine have produced substances with antihypertensive activity and minimal sedative properties. However, in each case, the C-, D-, and E-rings must not differ from those of reserpine (Lucas, 1963).

It may be noted here that yohimbine differs from reserpine in its stereochemistry at positions 3, 16, and 20, and lacks the 18-ester group.

Toxicology–Pharmacology: Reserpine is an alkaloid from the root of *Rauwolfia serpentina* Linne (Family Apocynaceae) and certain other species of *Rauwolfia*. It was first isolated in 1952 and is one of 20 alkaloids identified from *Rauwolfia*. The plant itself has been used for many centuries for treatment of hypertension, insomnia, and various mental disorders.

It is now used medicinally for its antihypertensive and tranquilizing actions. The tranquilizing and antipsychotic actions of reserpine were elicited around the same time as those of the phenothiazines. It was found that the latter group of drugs could be used with more effectiveness and easier control, and consequently, reserpine has not been as frequently used.

The mechanism of action of reserpine and related alkaloids was found to be depletion of serotonin and norepinephrine.

Presumably, these effects account for the effects of the drug. Reserpine toxicity is manifested by drowsiness and parasympathetic predominance, including bradycardia, excessive salivation, cutaneous vasodilatation, nausea, and diarrhea. Mental depression is often a serious adverse effect. Parkinsonism may also occur following large doses of reserpine.

Usual dosage for adults is 0.5–1.0 mg daily for 1 week, followed by maintenance dosage of 0.25–0.50 mg per day.

▶ **SALICYLATE**
Noncontrolled Substance

General Comment: Aspirin, acetylsalicylic acid, is commonly found in drug preparations that are subject to abuse.

Toxicology–Pharmacology: The group of salicylates includes derivatives of salicylic acid, including acetylsalicylic acid, salicylamide, sodium salicylate, and methyl salicylate. The antipyretic properties of willow bark were known to the ancients. This was found to contain salicin. Salicylic acid was prepared from salicin in 1838, and later, sodium salicylate.

The salicylates lower body temperature in febrile patients, and exert analgesic properties, by actions on the central nervous system. They are encountered in many over-the-counter preparations for use as antipyretics and analgesia for a wide variety of mild pain-producing disorders.

Due to their ready availability to the public, their use is extensive, and intoxications are not uncommon. After overdose, symptoms such as headache, dizziness, tinnitus (ringing in the ears), difficulty in hearing, mental confusion, and gastrointestinal irritation occur. Metabolic acidosis is the most serious complication of toxicity with salicylates.

After therapeutic administration of 1000-mg doses, maximum serum concentrations of 3.1–1.4 mg/dl were found in 20 adults, at the 2-hour interval

(Hollister and Kanter, 1965). Death from overdose may occur with blood concentrations in excess of 50 mg/dl. Intoxications commonly occur in children, although suicidal overdose in adults is also relatively common.

▶ **SCOPOLAMINE**
Noncontrolled Substance
Encountered in Excepted Substances

General Comments: Scopolamine belongs to the class of cholinergic blocking drugs, also known as parasympathetic blocking drugs. In general, it resembles atropine in its action on the autonomic nervous system, but its effects on the higher centers are different. Atropine is a stimulant on the central nervous system, whereas scopolamine is a depressant.

Scopolamine is encountered as an ingredient in formulations classified as excepted preparations. The following table indicates the drug/scopolamine minimum ratio found in these preparations:

Drug	Drug/Scopolamine Ratio
Amobarbital	1/0.05 with 13.3 dehydrocholic acid
Butabarbital	1/0.1

Also see **HYOSCINE**.

Toxicology–Pharmacology: Scopolamine is one of the major alkaloids occurring in several solanaceous plants, including the genera *Atropa* (belladonna) and *Datura*, many species of which are native to the southwestern United States. Pharmacologically, scopolamine is a cholinergic blocking agent, antagonizing the effects of the parasympathetic nervous system. Many actions are similar to those of atropine. It dilates the pupils, and inhibits salivary and respiratory tract secretions. It normally causes drowsiness, lack of attentiveness, mental disorientation, apathy, amnesia, and sleep. The extractives of the plant *Datura* are used in some localities as hallucinogenic agents.

It is also effective as a preventative for motion sickness. Toxic symptoms may range from complete disorientation to an active delirium. In three cases of nonfatal scopolamine poisoning, all three developed dizziness, blurred vision, muscular weakness, and difficulty in maintaining their equilibrium. They had fixed, dilated pupils, and were delirious to unconscious when admitted to the emergency room (Kaplan *et al.*, 1974).

▶ **SECOBARBITAL**
Schedule II

or

Schedule III. The Controlled Substances Act states that Schedule III will apply unless listed in another schedule. Any material, compound, mixture, or preparation that contains any quantity of secobarbital having a potential for abuse associated with a depressant effect on the central nervous system, and that contains, in addition to secobarbital, one or more active medicinal ingredients that are not scheduled substances will fall in Schedule III. Also, any suppository dosage approved by the Food and Drug Administration that contains secobarbital falls into Schedule III. Thus, any of the Schedule III preparations are subject to the excepted substance clause in Schedule III.

Synonyms: Quinalbarbitone, meballymal, 5-allyl-5-(1-methylbutyl) barbituric acid.

Pharmaceutical Preparations

Schedule II

S.B.P.^{R} (Lemmon)—Tablet: white, scored, containing 50 mg sodium secobarbital, 30 mg sodium butabarbital, and 15 mg sodium phenobarbital

Seco-B^R (Fleming)—Capsule: maroon and gray, containing 100 mg secobarbital

Seconal^R (Lilly)—Elixir: each 5 ml containing 22 mg secobarbital. Ampules: each 1 ml containing 50 mg sodium secobarbital. Capsules, orange, containing sodium secobarbital: "f72," 30 mg; "f42," 50 mg; "F40," 100 mg.

Tuinal^R (Lilly)—See **AMOBARBITAL.**

Schedule III

S.B.P.^{R} Plus (Lemmon)—Tablet: orange, scored, containing 50 mg sodium secobarbital, 30 mg sodium butabarbital, 15 mg sodium phenobarbital, and 2.5 mg homatropine methylbromide

Seconal^R (Lilly)—Suppositories, containing sodium secobarbital: "517," 30 mg; "514," 60 mg; "505," 120 mg; "511," 200 mg

Also see Chapter 6.

Biochemistry: The major metabolites of secobarbital are the two diastereoisomers of hydroxysecobarbital, and secodiol, which have been isolated from

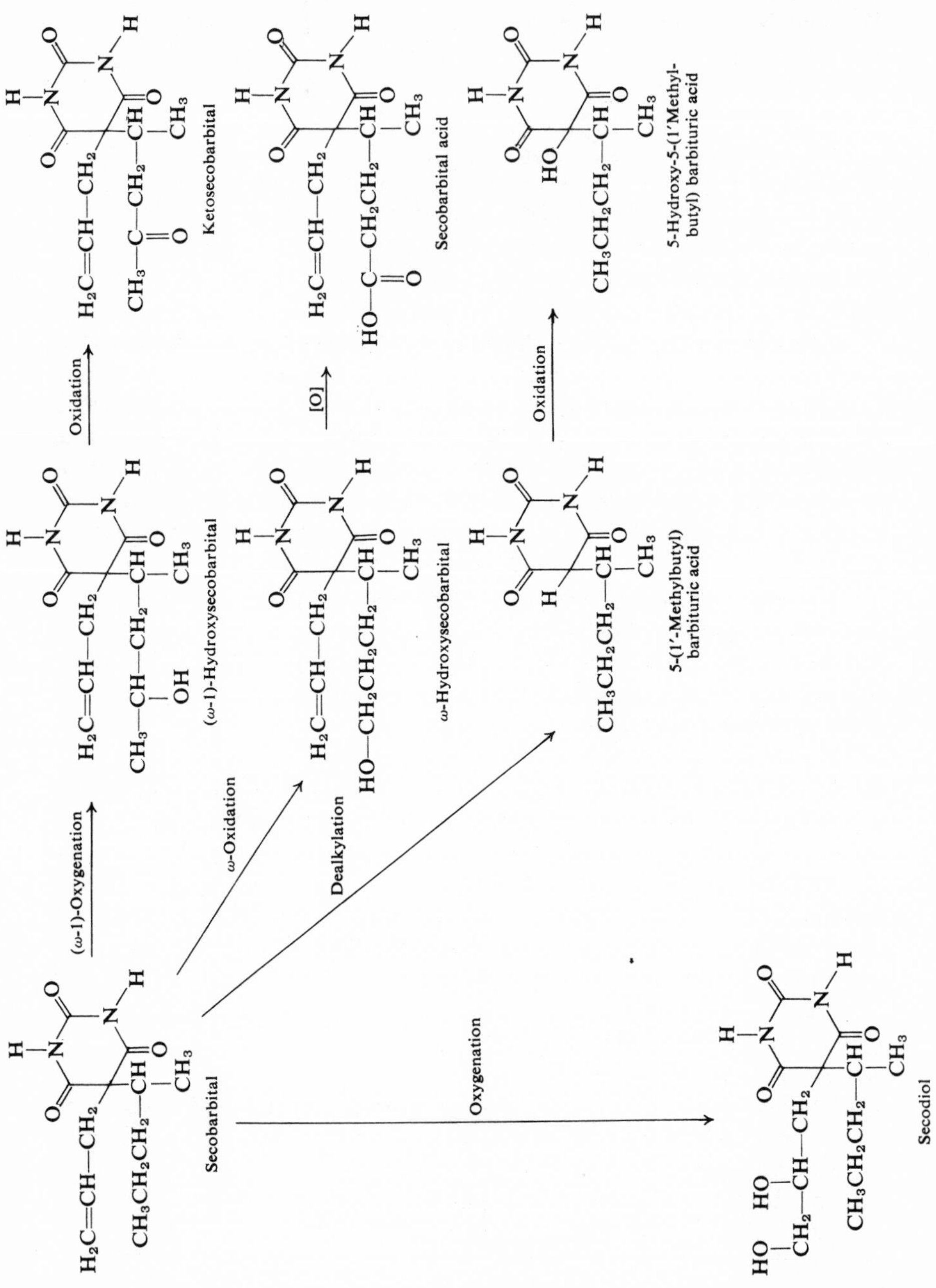
(ω-1)-Oxygenation
ω-Oxidation
Dealkylation
Oxygenation
Oxidation
[O]
Oxidation
Secobarbital
(ω-1)-Hydroxysecobarbital
ω-Hydroxysecobarbital
5-(1'-Methylbutyl) barbituric acid
Ketosecobarbital
Secobarbital acid
5-Hydroxy-5-(1'Methylbutyl) barbituric acid
Secodiol

human urine in about 50 percent of the administered dose (Waddell, 1962, 1963, 1965). Only 5 percent of the dose was excreted unchanged. In addition, 5-(1'-methylbutyl) barbituric acid has been identified (Cochin and Daly, 1963). The latter substance can also be formed by spontaneous atmospheric oxidation of 5-(1'-methylbutyl) barbituric acid.

Microsomal studies have shown that secobarbital is metabolized by (ω-1)-oxidation to hydroxysecobarbital and by ω-oxidation to secobarbital acid. The (ω-1)-oxidation is catalyzed by $NADPH_2$-dependent microsomal enzymes. (ω-1)- and ω-hydroxysecobarbital are oxidized to ketosecobarbital and secobarbital acid, respectively, in the soluble fraction of the liver (Waddell, 1965).

Secodiol has also been shown to be a metabolite of secobarbital (Niyogi, 1964).

Toxicology–Pharmacology: Secobarbital is a short-acting barbiturate. It is used for short-term sedation and hypnosis with a very rapid onset of effects. Depending on dosage, it will produce responses ranging from mild sedation to profound hypnosis. The usual hypnotic dose of secobarbital is 100 mg to be taken at bedtime. For sedation, 15–50 mg may be given three or four times a day.

In cases of acute poisoning, it may begin as a mild state (person is comatose, but responds to painful stimuli), proceed to a moderate stage (person does not respond to painful stimuli), and then to severe poisoning (person does not respond to painful stimuli, and supportive measures for maintenance of blood pressure and respiration are required).

Simultaneous ingestion of other sedative drugs or tranquilizers, narcotics, and especially alcohol, gives rise to dangerous potentiation of the toxic effects of barbiturates. Under these conditions, doses of hypnotics that are in themselves not dangerous may cause fatal poisoning.

After administration of hypnotic doses of 244 mg to six adult subjects, maximum blood concentrations at 3 hours were 0.18–0.22 mg/dl (Clifford et al., 1974). Secobarbital has a plasma half-life of about 1.2 days (Fazekas et al., 1956).

Lethal concentrations of secobarbital range from about 1.00 to 7.40 mg/dl, with the great majority being from 1.50 to 3.30 mg/dl (Cimbura et al., 1972; Baselt and Cravey, 1977).

▶ **SODIUM NITRITE**
Noncontrolled Substance
Encountered in Excepted Substances

$$NaNO_2$$

General Comments: Inclusion of sodium nitrite in the *U.S. Pharmacopeia* is for its use as an antidote to cyanide poisoning. The basis for this use is that it converts hemoglobin to methemoglobin, which has a powerful affinity for cyanide, forming cyanmethemoglobin. The cyanide is therefore prevented from interfering with the enzyme, cytochrome oxidase, which is how cyanide acts as a poison.

Toxicity from sodium nitrite is due to methemoglobin formation, and subsequent anoxia. After toxic doses, breathing becomes rapid and dyspneic. The mucous membranes acquire a slate color, and convulsions may occur.

Sodium nitrite also has pharmacological actions on smooth muscles. It produces a marked fall of blood pressure and an increase in pulse rate. Sodium nitrite is found in phenobarbital preparations classified as excepted preparations with a minimum phenobarbital/sodium nitrite ratio of 1/4.

▶ **SULFONDIETHYLMETHANE**
Schedule III

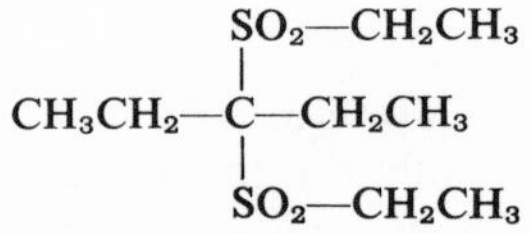

$$CH_3CH_2-\underset{\underset{SO_2-CH_2CH_3}{|}}{\overset{\overset{SO_2-CH_2CH_3}{|}}{C}}-CH_2CH_3$$

Synonym: 3,3-Bis(ethylsulfonyl)pentane.
Pharmaceutical Preparations: Sulfondiethylmethane is not found in pharmaceutical preparations sold in the United States.
General Comments: None.
Biochemistry: See Toxicology–Pharmacology below.
Toxicology–Pharmacology: Sulfondiethylmethane is a hypnotic drug. The effects caused by accumulation make sulfondiethylmethane (as well as sulfonethylmethane and sulfonmethane) one of the most dangerous of the hypnotics. It may lead to the destruction of hemoglobin in the blood.

▶ **SULFONETHYLMETHANE**
Schedule II

$$CH_3CH_2-\underset{\underset{SO_2-CH_2CH_3}{|}}{\overset{\overset{SO_2-CH_2CH_3}{|}}{C}}-CH_3$$

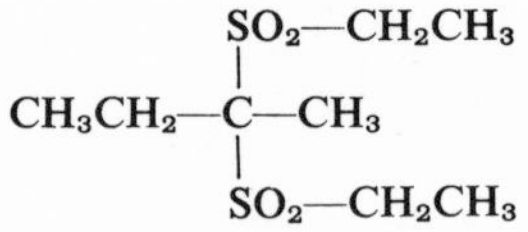

Synonym: 2,2-Bis(ethylsulfonyl) butane.

Pharmaceutical Preparations: Sulfonethylmethane is not found in pharmaceutical preparations sold in the United States.
General Comments: None.
Biochemistry: See **SULFONDIETHYLMETHANE.**
Toxicology–Pharmacology: See **SULFONDIETHYLMETHANE.**

▶ **SULFONMETHANE**
Schedule III

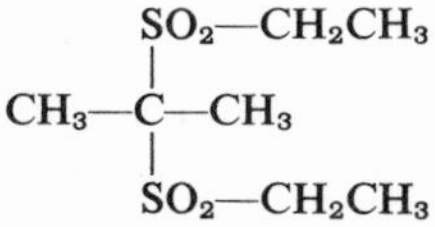

$$CH_3-\underset{\underset{SO_2-CH_2CH_3}{|}}{\overset{\overset{SO_2-CH_2CH_3}{|}}{C}}-CH_3$$

Synonyms: Sulfonal, 2,2-bis(ethylsulfonyl)propane.
Pharmaceutical Preparations: Sulfonmethane is not found in pharmaceutical preparations sold in the United States.
General Comments: None.
Biochemistry: See **SULFONDIETHYLMETHANE.**
Toxicology–Pharmacology: See **SULFONDIETHYLMETHANE.**

▶ **TETRAHYDROCANNABINOL**
Schedule I

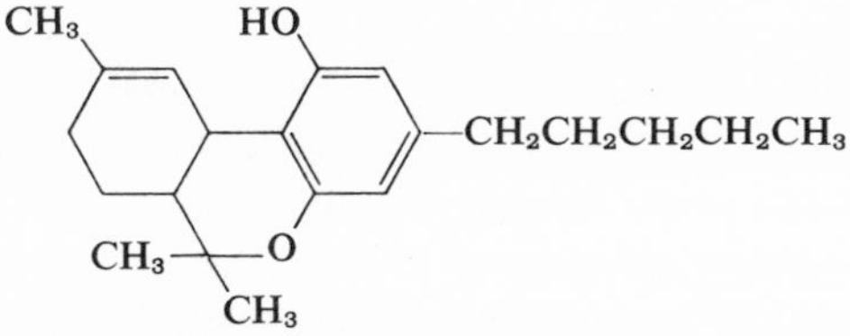

General Comments: The Controlled Substances Act includes "any material, compound, mixture, or preparation which contains any quantity of tetrahydrocannabinols (other than marijuana) and synthetic equivalents of the substances contained in the plant, or in the resinous extractives of *Cannabis*, or synthetic substances, derivatives, and their isomers with similar chemical structure and pharmacological activity such as the following: delta-1-*cis* or -*trans*-tetrahydrocannabinol, and their optical isomers; delta-6-*cis* or -*trans*-tetrahydrocannabinol, and their optical isomers; delta-3,4-*cis* or -*trans*-tetrahydrocannabinol, and its optical isomers."

Since the nomenclature of these substances is not internationally standardized, compounds of these structures, regardless of numerical designation of atomic positions, are covered.

Pharmaceutical Preparations: Tetrahydrocannabinol is not found in any pharmaceutical preparations sold in the United States.

General Comment: See **MARIJUANA.**

Biochemistry: Hashish is controlled under tetrahydrocannabinol. Tetrahydrocannabinol, commonly referred to as THC, was isolated almost simultaneously from *Cannabis* by two teams of investigators. One group viewed it as a substituted monoterpene derivative and assigned the name delta-1-3,4-*trans*-tetrahydrocannabinol. The other group applied dibenzopyran nomenclature, resulting in the designation delta-9-*trans*-tetrahydrocannabinol. Both names are found in the literature, but the former has been more widely accepted.

Other constituents isolated from *Cannabis* include cannabidiol, cannabinol, cannabidiolic acid, cannabichromene, cannabigerol, and delta-1,6-tetrahydrocannabinol. The tetrahydrocannabinols possess euphoric activity, cannabinol being weakly active; cannabichromene and cannabidiolic acid are sedative principles. THC has been found to be more potent when smoked than when taken orally. (For further discussion, see **MARIJUANA.**)

Toxicology–Pharmacology: Isomers of tetrahycrocannabinol have been found to be the chief pharmacologically active component of the marijuana plant, *Cannabis sativa*. The *levo*-Δ^9-*trans* tetrahydrocannabinol is the primary natural isomer, although small amounts of Δ^8-tetrahydrocannabinol also occur. The classic effects obtained from use of marijuana can also be elicited by administering tetrahydrocannabinol. Typically, these effects include the physiological effects of increase in heart rate and reddening of the conjunctivae of the eyes. A slight lowering of or no effect on blood pressure may occur. The most prominent effects are the psychic and perceptual changes. These include euphoria, sleepiness, alteration of time sense, decreased discrimination in the sense of hearing, dizziness, and visual distortions. Depersonalization, difficulty in concentrating and thinking, and dreamlike states are prominent. Increased jocularity and hunger, sometimes ravenous desire for sweets, are often reported.

The effects of tetrahydrocannabinol, when smoked, usually begin within seconds to a few minutes, and last for 2–3 hours. After oral ingestion of marijuana extracts, the absorption may be delayed for much longer periods of time, and the effects may persist for 24 hours or longer.

High doses of tetrahydrocannabinol may lead to psychotomimetic effects, anxiety states, delirium, hallucinations of sight, hearing, taste, and smell, and delusions of persecution. Recent literature indicates that tetrahydrocannabinol does not induce *de novo* psychosis, although in some individuals predisposed to mental illness, a psychotic reaction may be precipitated.

Plasma concentrations of tetrahydrocannabinol after smoking reached 67 ng/ml in one subject after smoking 10 mg of THC, but body redistribution effects a rapid decline to very low concentrations within an hour (Galanter *et al.*, 1972; Soares and Gross, 1976). The metabolite, 11-nor-carboxy-Δ^9-tetrahydrocannabinol, persists for a longer period in the plasma, and may be detected in urine for up to 48 hours (Soares and Gross, 1976).

Tetrahydrocannabinol and related substances have a very low acute toxicity. No substantiated deaths in humans have appeared in the literature from use of marijuana or tetrahydrocannabinol. Due to the depressant component of the drug, synergism may occur when taken in the presence of other depressant drugs, such as alcohol.

▶ THEBACON
Schedule I

Synonyms: Acetylhydrocodone, acetyldihydrocodeinone, acetyldemethyldihydrothebaine, diacodon, dihydrocodeinone enol acetate, 6-acetoxy-4,5-epoxy-3-methyloxy-*N*-methylmorphin-6-ene.

Pharmaceutical Preparations: Thebacon is not found in any pharmaceutical preparations sold in the United States.

General Comment: Thebacon is a semisynthetic narcotic analgesic that has no accepted medicinal value in the United States.

Biochemistry: Unknown.

Toxicology–Pharmacology: Unknown.

▶ THEBAINE
Schedule II

Synonyms: Paramorphine, 3,6-dimethoxy-4,5-epoxy-*N*-methylmorphin-6,8-diene.

Pharmaceutical Preparations: Thebaine is not frequently found in pharmaceutical preparations sold in the United States.

General Comments: None.

Biochemistry: Thebaine is the least abundant among the hydrophenanthrene alkaloids in *Papaver somniferum*, and it is of little medicinal value itself. However, in 1967, an Iranian chemist discovered that *Papaver bracteatum*, which does not contain opium and grows wild in some parts of the Middle East, has as its major alkaloid thebaine. When a practical synthesis of codeine from thebaine was developed, thebaine became a medicinally valuable substance (Barber and Rapoport, 1975, 1976).

Morphine, the base for heroin, cannot be efficiently obtained from thebaine. Therefore, *P. bracteatum* will probably not enter the illicit drug market.

Toxicology–Pharmacology: Thebaine is one of the principal alkaloids of opium, present from 0.5 to 2 percent in raw opium. It induces seizures at relatively low doses, and is essentially devoid of narcotic actions. However, it can be converted through simple chemical modification into chemicals with narcotic analgesic activity.

▶ **THEOBROMINE**
Noncontrolled Substance
Encountered in Excepted Substances

General Comments: Theobromine is an alkaloid found in the plant *Theobroma cacao* Linne (Family Sterculicaceae). It is closely related to other xanthine derivatives such as theophylline and caffeine. On the central nervous system, caffeine is the most powerful stimulant, theophylline is less stimulating, and theobromine is least so. It is found in formulations containing phenobarbital that are classified as excepted preparations. In such preparations, the minimum phenobarbital/theobromine ratio is 1/10.

Toxicology–Pharmacology: Theobromine is closely related to the xanthines caffeine and theophylline in structure and pharmacological actions. Theobromine has the least central stimulant effect of these three. Its primary actions are to stimulate the heart muscle and to effect a relaxation of the bronchial musculature. It may therefore be useful in the treatment of bronchial asthma. Theobromine, as the other xanthines, has diuretic actions.

Theobromine has been used as its soluble salts, theobromine sodium salicylate, theobromine sodium acetate, and theobromine calcium salicylate, as a diuretic, a myocardial stimulant, and a dilator of coronary or peripheral arteries.

Doses of theobromine range from 300 to 500 mg, three or four times a day. Theobromine is metabolized by demethylation, mainly to 7-methyl xanthine, together with some 3-methyl xanthine. The 7-methyl xanthine derivative is further oxidized to 7-methyl uric acid (Clarke, 1969).

▶ **THEOPHYLLINE**
Noncontrolled Substance
Encountered in Excepted Substances

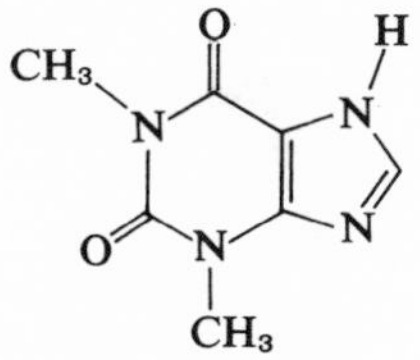

General Comments: Theophylline is a xanthine derivative related to theobromine and caffeine. It has been encountered in various formulations classified as excepted preparations. The following table shows the minimum drug/theophylline ratio in such preparations:

Drug	Drug/Theophylline Ratio
Allobarbital	1/6.25 (with 0.5 stramonium extract and 0.5 ephedrine)
Cyclophentenylallybarbituric acid	1/4 (with 0.75 ephedrine)
Phenobarbital	1/16.25 (with 4 benzylephedrine)
Phenobarbital	1/3.7 (with 0.74 ephedrine)

Toxicology–Pharmacology: Theophylline is a xanthine compound, isomeric with theobromine. It occurs naturally in tea leaves, but is prepared commercially by synthesis. Theophylline is the most potent of the three xanthines in relaxing arteries and smooth muscle, and has only a slight stimulant effect on the central nervous system. It also acts as a diuretic and increases cardiac output.

The primary usefulness of theophylline is in the treatment of bronchial asthma. It is also useful in paroxysmal dyspnea secondary to acute left ventricular strain, and possibly in angina pectoris and coronary artery disease. The most widely used form of theophylline is the ethylene diamine salt, aminophylline, which is better absorbed than theophylline. Other more soluble forms include theophylline sodium acetate, theophylline sodium glycinate, theophylline monoethanolamine, and diphylline [7-(2,3-dihydroxy-propyl)theophylline].

The plasma half-life averages 3.6 hours in children (range, 1.5–9.5 hours) and 4.5 hours in adults (range, 3.0–9.5 hours). Factors such as cigarette smoking and long-term theophylline use can shorten half-lives (Davis, 1976). Toxic symptoms occurring with blood concentrations above 2.0 mg/dl include nausea and vomiting, delirium, convulsions, coma, and cardiac arrest.

In a fatality reported from overdose of theophylline, a blood concentration of 6.30 mg/dl was reported, and the liver had 27.5 mg/100 g (Loveland, 1974). A 72-year-old man with impaired theophylline degradation had convulsions when the level was 8.6 mg/dl (Jacobs and Senior, 1974).

▶ **THIALBARBITAL**
Schedule III

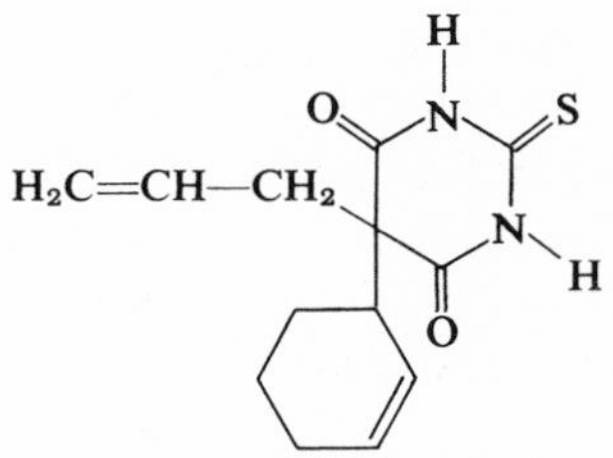

Synonyms: Thialbarbitone, thiohexallymal, 5-allyl-5-cyclohex-2'-enyl-2-thio-barbituric acid.
Pharmaceutical Preparations: Thialbarbital is not found in any pharmaceutical preparations sold in the United States.
General Comment: Thialbarbital is a barbiturate that is controlled under Schedule III of the Controlled Substances Act as a "derivative of barbituric acid."
Biochemistry: Thialbarbital is metabolized by desulfuration to give the 5-allyl-5-(2'-cyclohexenyl)barbituric acid, and by oxidation to give ketothialbarbital. When administered to rabbits, thialbarbital is slowly excreted in the urine as a mixture of the unchanged thiobarbiturate (allylcyclohexenyl barbituric acid), ketothialbarbital, and thiourea (Raventos, 1954; Carrington and Raventos, 1946).

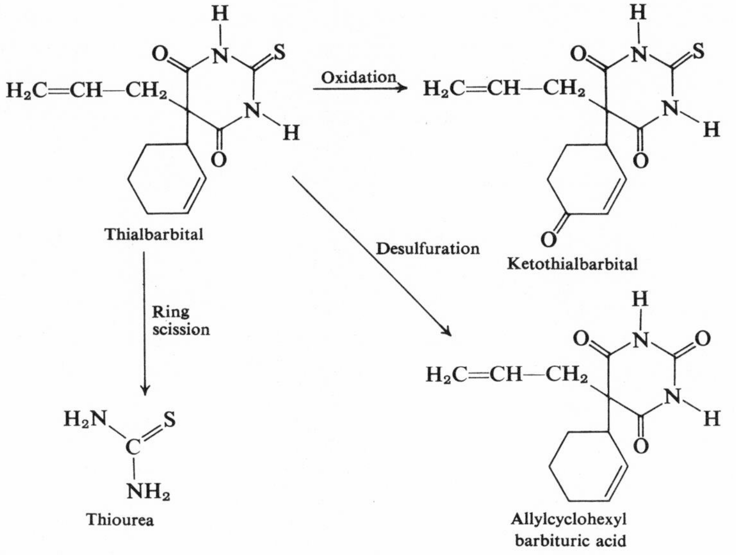

Toxicology–Pharmacology: Thialbarbital is an ultra-short-acting thiobarbiturate with actions similar to thiamylal. It is reported to give rise to less respiratory depression than other intravenously administered barbiturates.

It may be used for rapid induction of short-term anesthesia, for minor surgical procedures, or as an adjunct to longer-acting anesthesia. Thialbarbital has a half-life in the plasma of 7 hours (Matthew, 1971).

▶ **THIAMYLAL**
Schedule III

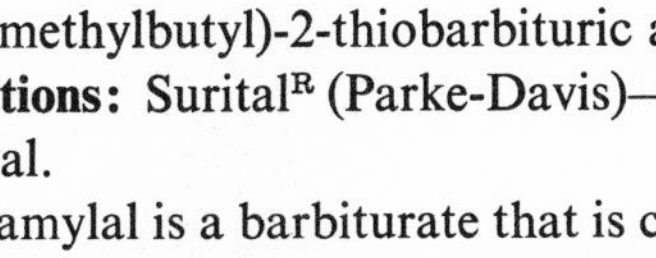

Synonym: 5-Allyl-5-(1-methylbutyl)-2-thiobarbituric acid.
Pharmaceutical Preparations: Surital[R] (Parke-Davis)—Vials or ampules containing sodium thiamylal.
General Comment: Thiamylal is a barbiturate that is controlled under Schedule III of the Controlled Substances Act as a "derivative of barbituric acid."
Biochemistry: As with other thiobarbiturates, thiamylal is metabolized by simultaneous desulfuration and oxidation of the 5-alkyl substituents. Six metabolites have been identified and are shown on page 394 (Tsukamoto *et al.*, 1963).

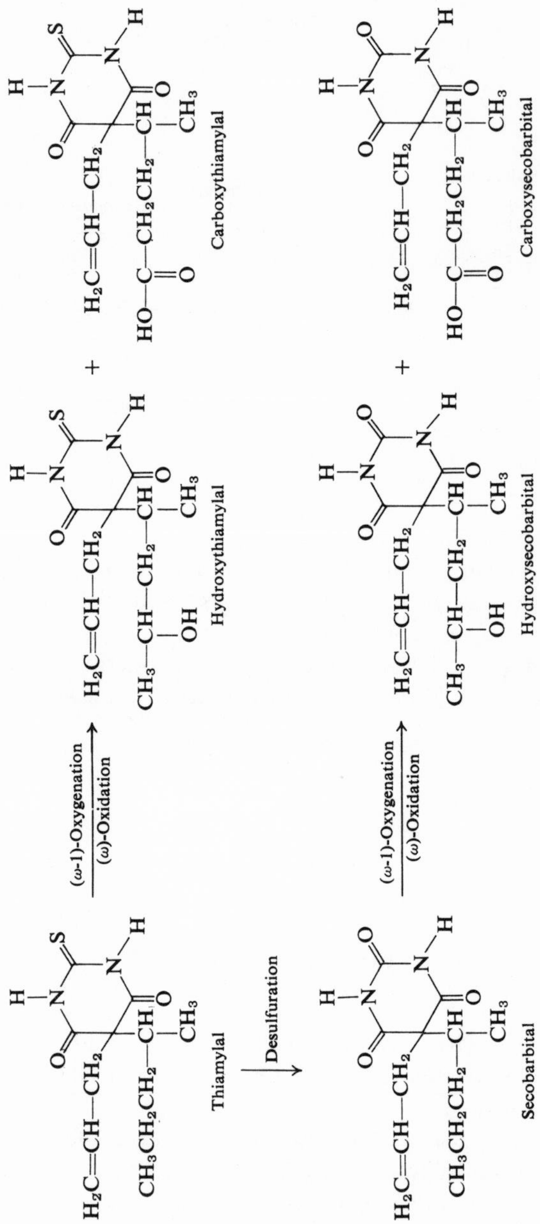

Thiamylal

Carboxythiamylal

Hydroxythiamylal

$(\omega-1)$-Oxygenation
(ω)-Oxidation

Desulfuration

Secobarbital

Carboxysecobarbital

Hydroxysecobarbital

$(\omega-1)$-Oxygenation
(ω)-Oxidation

Toxicology–Pharmacology: Thiamylal is an ultra-short-acting thiobarbiturate. It is used for rapid induction of anesthesia of short duration, or as an adjunct to other agents.

Thiamylal is metabolized by desulfuration and oxidation of the 5-allyl substituents. Six compounds have been characterized from the urine (Matthew, 1971).

▶ **1-[1-(2-THIENYL)-CYCLOHEXYL]-PIPERIDINE**
Schedule I

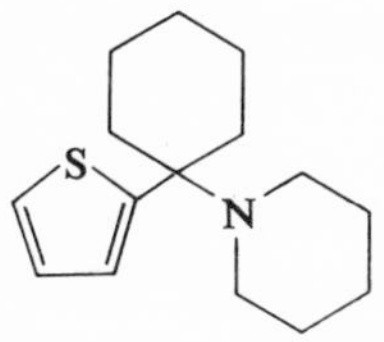

Synonyms: None found.
Pharmaceutical Preparations: 1-[1-(2-Thienyl)-cyclohexyl]-piperidine is not found in any pharmaceutical preparations sold in the United States.
General Comments: 1-[1-(2-Thienyl)-cyclohexyl]-piperidine is the thiophene analogue of phencyclidine. It is similar to phencyclidine in activity, both quantitatively and qualitatively.
Biochemistry: Unknown.
Toxicology–Pharmacology: Unknown.

▶ **THIOPENTAL**
Schedule III

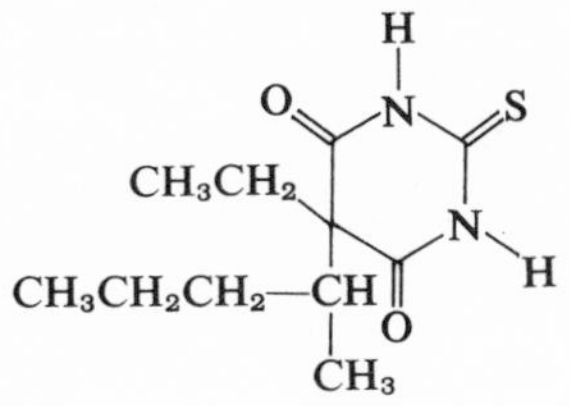

Synonyms: Thiopentone, pentothiobarbital, thiomebumal, 5-ethyl-5-(1-methylbutyl)-2-thiobarbituric acid.

Pharmaceutical Preparations: Thiopental is not frequently found in pharmaceutical preparations sold in the United States (except for hospitals).

General Comment: Thiopental is a barbiturate that is controlled in Schedule III of the Controlled Substances Act as a "derivative of barbituric acid." ·

Biochemistry: Thiopental is the 2-sulfur analogue of pentobarbital. The metabolism of theopental is of major importance in the rapid reduction of blood levels of the drug, which limits the duration of its action.

Thiopental is almost completely metabolized by oxidation of the 5-substituent, producing thiopentalcarboxylic acid, and desulfuration, producing pentobarbital and its metabolites (Mark *et al.*, 1965) and are shown on page 397.

Toxicology–Pharmacology: Thiopental, most commonly used as the sodium salt or sodium thiopental, is an ultra-short-acting thiobarbiturate used intravenously as an anesthetic. It is widely employed for induction of general anesthesia, for maintenance of anesthesia in conjunction with other agents, and as the sole anesthetic agent in minor operative or diagnostic procedures. It may also be used for the immediate control of certain convulsive states.

The primary action is to depress the central nervous system, leading to the hypnotic state of general anesthesia when given intravenously. It also depresses respiration when given rapidly or in large doses. This can be controlled by artificial respiration and administration of oxygen and carbon dioxide.

Thiopental is not metabolized predominantly in the liver, as most other barbiturates are, but is broken down in the body generally. Only about 0.3 percent of a dose of thiopental is excreted as such by man (Brodie *et al.*, 1950). The half-life of thiopental is estimated to be 8 hours (Brodie, 1952). The short duration of action of the thiobarbiturates is believed to be attributed to the rapid rate of distribution in various tissues, especially muscle and fat. Within 30 minutes after a single dose, 90 percent of the maximum concentration in the brain may be redistributed to other tissues, and the patient may awaken. The fatty tissues may accumulate concentrations six to twelve times greater than the plasma.

Deaths from overdose of thiopental have occurred from careless administration along with other depressant drugs for short-term anesthesia in dental surgery, and overdoses have been reported after intravenous self-infusion (Backer *et al.*, 1975).

It is estimated that a plasma concentration of 0.80 mg/dl is necessary for induction of coma, and that peak plasma levels in anesthesia are 3.0–5.0 mg/dl. Fatalities from overdose have resulted with blood concentrations of 14.1–28.5 mg/dl (Backer *et al.*, 1975).

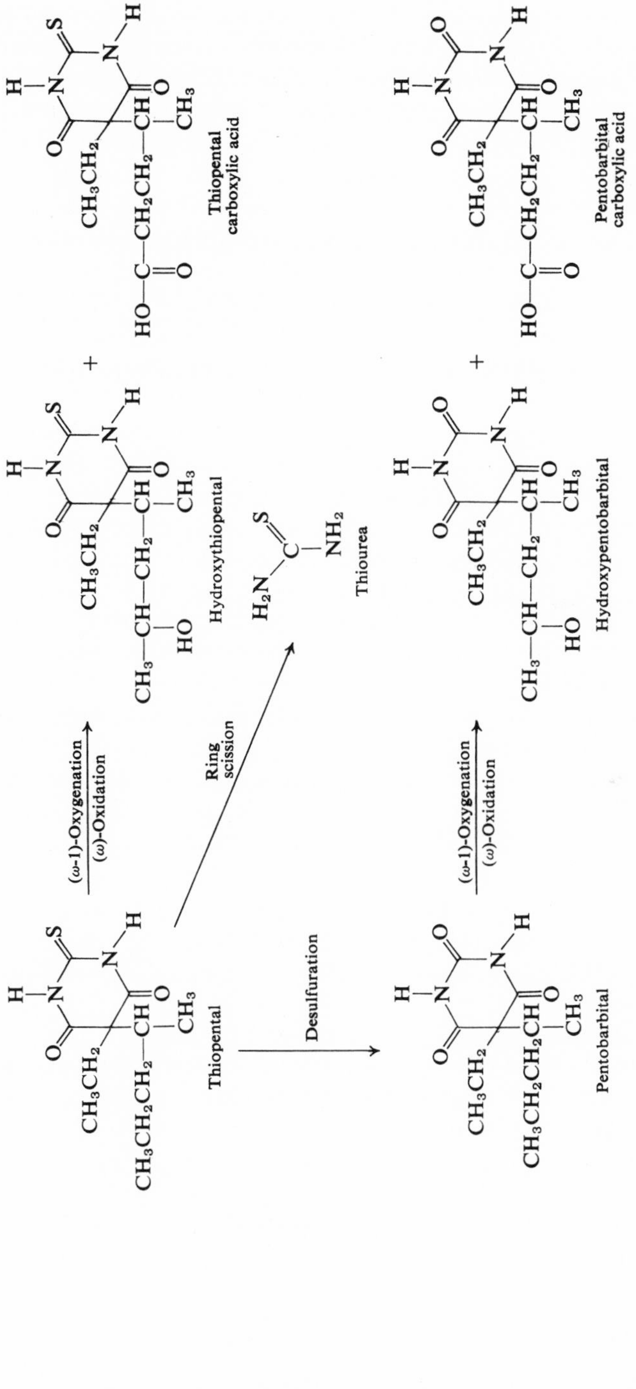
Thiopental
(ω-1)-Oxygenation
(ω)-Oxidation
Hydroxythiopental
+
Thiopental carboxylic acid
Ring scission
Thiourea
Desulfuration
Pentobarbital
(ω-1)-Oxygenation
(ω)-Oxidation
Hydroxypentobarbital
+
Pentobarbital carboxylic acid

▶ **THIOPROPAZATE**
Dangerous Drug

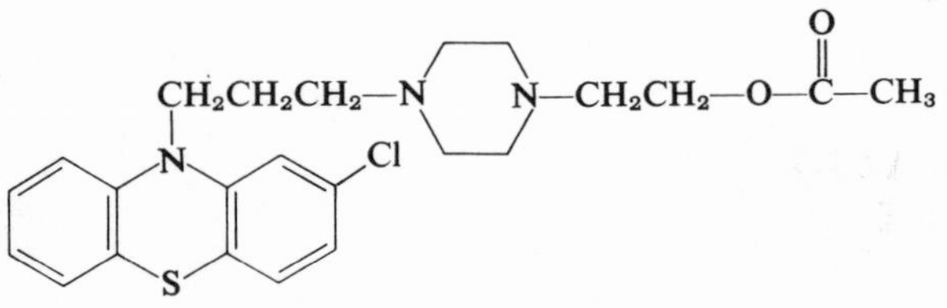

Synonym: 10-[3-[4-(-Acetoxyethyl)piperazin-1-yl]propyl]-2-chloro-phenothi-
azine.

Pharmaceutical Preparations: Thiopropazate is not found in pharmaceutical
preparations sold in the United States.

General Comment: Thiopropazate is a phenothiazine tranquilizer, and as
such is classified in this text as a Dangerous Drug.

Biochemistry: Unknown.

Toxicology–Pharmacology: Thiopropazate is structurally related to the
piperazine group of phenothiazines such as prochlorperazine and perphenazine. It is used in the management of psychoses in which agitation, tension,
and aggressiveness predominate.

The untoward effects and toxicity are similar to those for chlorpromazine.

▶ **THIOPROPERAZINE**
Dangerous Drug

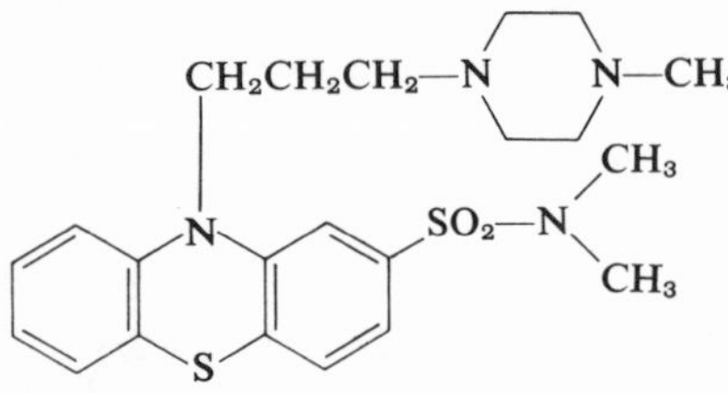

Synonym: *N,N*-dimethyl-10-[3-(4-methylpiperazine-1-yl)propyl]phenothia-
zine-2-sulfonamide.

Pharmaceutical Preparations: Thioproperazine is not found in any pharmaceutical preparations sold in the United States.

General Comment: Thioproperazine is a phenothiazine tranquilizer, and as
such is classified in this text as a Dangerous Drug.

Biochemistry: Similar to that of thiothixene.

Toxicology–Pharmacology: Thioproperazine is a psychotherapeutic agent,
related to the piperazine group of substituted phenothiazines. It is similar in

actions to chlorpromazine, but is effective in smaller doses. It is used in the management of psychoses in which agitation, tension, and aggressiveness predominate.

▶ **THIORIDAZINE**
Dangerous Drug

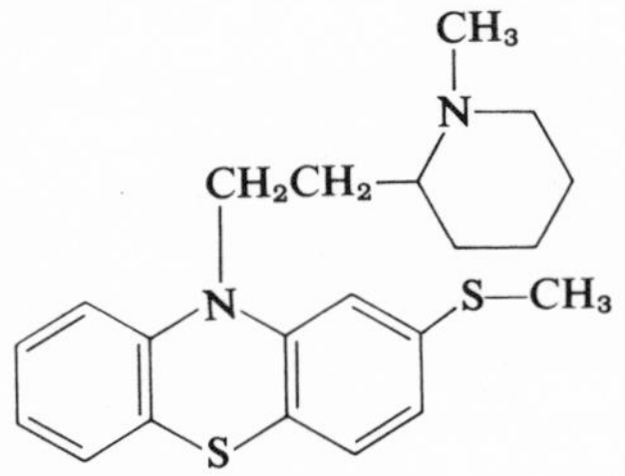

Synonym: 10-[2-(1-Methylpiperid-2-yl)ethyl]-2-methylthiophenothiazine.
Pharmaceutical Preparations: Mellaril^R (Sandoz)—Tablets, containing thioridazine hydrochloride: 10, 15, 25, 50, 100, 150, or 200 mg. Concentrate: containing thioridazine hydrochloride, each 1 ml containing 30 or 100 mg.
General Comment: Thioridazine is a phenothiazine tranquilizer, and as such is classified in this text as a Dangerous Drug.
Biochemistry: Thioridazine in its metabolism undergoes oxidative N-demethylation, oxidation of both sulfur atoms to sulfoxide and sulfone, and formation of glucuronides of hydroxylated derivatives (Zehnder et al., 1962).
Toxicology–Pharmacology: Thioridazine is a piperidyl-type phenothiazine tranquilizer having sedative and behavioral effects similar to those of chlorpromazine. It is useful in the management of a variety of psychopathological conditions, including anxiety and tension states, acute and chronic psychoneuroses, schizophrenia, and manic psychoses. It is also sometimes used in the management of the alcohol withdrawal syndrome, intractable pain, and senility.

Thioridazine is given for mild to moderately severe emotional disturbances in dose ranges of from 10 to 25 mg, three to four times daily. In psychiatric patients, it may be given in dosages of 50–100 mg, three to four times a day, and in severely disturbed patients, up to 600 mg per day may be required.

Therapeutic blood concentrations of thioridazine have been reported at 0.20–0.23 mg/dl in patients on chronic therapy (Viukari and Salmines, 1973). After a 100-mg single dose of thioridazine, serum concentrations of 0.006–0.051 mg/dl were reported 1.75 hours after administration (Martensson and Ross, 1977).

In overdoses from thioridazine, blood concentrations may be from 0.20 to 2.00 mg/dl. One fatality after ingestion of 3 g thioridazine was reported, in which the blood concentration was found to be 1.80 mg/dl (Joubert and Olivier, 1974).

THIOTHIXENE
Dangerous Drug

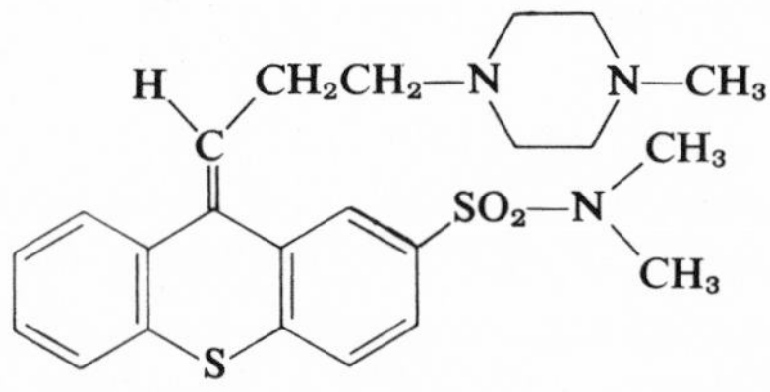

Synonym: *cis*-2-Dimethylsulfamoyl-9-[3-(4-methylpiperazin-1-yl)propylidene] thiazanthen.

Pharmaceutical Preparations: Navane^R (Roerig)—Capsules, containing thiothixene hydrochloride: 1, 2, 5, or 10 mg. Concentrate: each ml containing 5 mg thiothixene. Vial: each 1 ml containing 2 mg thiothixene.

General Comment: Thiothixene is a tranquilizer, and as such is classified in this text as a Dangerous Drug.

Biochemistry: Thiothixene is a thioxanthene-$\Delta^{9,\gamma}$-propylamino derivative that is approximately equipotent with the corresponding phenothiazine, thioproperazine. The metabolism of thiothixene also resembles the metabolism of thioproperazine. The metabolic reactions that thiothixene undergoes are oxidative N-demethylation and sulfoxidation (Huus and Khan, 1967).

Toxicology–Pharmacology: Thiothixene is a thioxanthene derivative resembling the piperazine group of phenothiazine derivatives in pharmacological characteristics. It has tranquilizing and antiemetic actions primarily, and to a lesser degree hypotensive and spasmolytic effects.

It is used in the treatment of chronic schizophrenia patients, and is generally used for similar purposes as are the phenothiazines. The thioxanthene derivatives are slightly less potent than the corresponding phenothiazine derivatives, however.

After chronic daily doses of thiothixene of 20–60 mg, plasma concentrations were 0.001 mg/dl after 2 hours. After 8 hours, the average plasma concentration was 0.007 mg/dl (Hobbs *et al.*, 1974).

► **THIPHENAMIL**
Noncontrolled Substance
Encountered in Excepted Substances

General Comments: Thiphenamil is encountered in formulations containing phenobarbital that are classified as excepted preparations. In such preparations, the minimum phenobarbital/thiphenamil ratio found is 1/6.25.
Toxicology–Pharmacology: Thiphenamil is a synthetic antimuscarinic drug pharmacologically used as a substitute for the belladonna alkaloids. It is used primarily to treat gastrointestinal disorders, such as peptic ulcer or hypermotility, by antagonizing the actions of the cholinergic nervous system.

► **TOCAMPHYL**
Noncontrolled Substance
Encountered in Excepted Substances

General Comments: Tocamphyl is a choleretic drug, which is a drug that stimulates the liver to increase the output of bile. It is encountered in formulations containing phenobarbital and promatropine that are classified as excepted preparations. The minimum phenobarbital/tocamphyl/promatropine ratio encountered in such preparations is 1/9.37/0.028.

TRANYLCYPROMINE
Dangerous Drug

Synonyms: Transamine, *trans*-(+)-2-phenylcyclopropylamine.

Pharmaceutical Preparations: Parnate^R (Smith Kline & French)—Tablet: containing 10 mg tranylcypromine sulfate

General Comments: Tranylcypromine is an antidepressant-monoamine oxidase (MAO) inhibitor that is classified in this text as a Dangerous Drug under the "legend drug" provision since all pharmaceutical preparations containing tranylcypromine require a prescription and bear the label "Caution: Federal law prohibits dispensing without a prescription."

Tranylcypromine was removed from the United States market at one time due to reports of headache, increased blood pressure, and cerebrovascular accidents. However, later it was returned to the market with additional labeling requirements.

Biochemistry: MAO is an enzyme that catalyzes the following reaction:

$$R\text{---}CH_2\text{---}NH_2 + O_2 + H_2O \xrightarrow{\text{MAO}} R\text{---}C\!\!\begin{matrix} O \\ \diagup\!\!\diagdown \\ H \end{matrix} + NH_3 + H_2O_2$$

There are specific structural requirements necessary for this reaction to take place. Among the substrates for MAO are phenylethylamine, tyramine, catecholamines, and tryptophan derivatives. However, if the amine has a methyl group on the α carbon, the oxidation will not take place. Amphetamine, methamphetamine, and ephedrine are such examples.

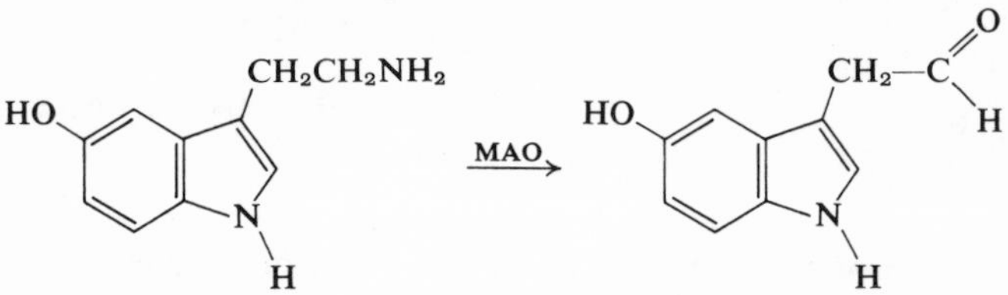

Serotonin   5-Hydroxyindoleacetaldehyde

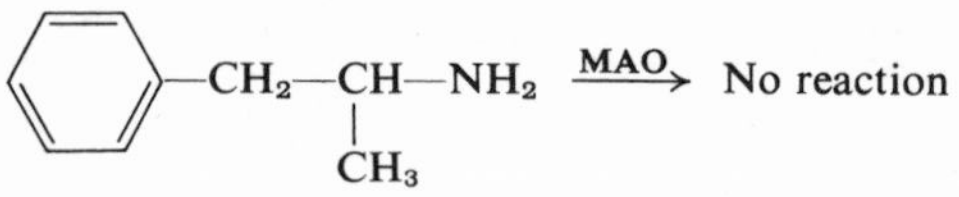

Amphetamine

This reaction can be prevented by blocking MAO. Several drugs can inhibit this enzyme in addition to tranylcypromine. These include nialamine, iproniazid, and pargyline. The effects of MAO inhibition include augmentation of the central effects of monoamines and potentiation and prolongation of the effects of adrenergic agents on blood pressure and smooth muscle, as well as antidepressant effects (Goldberg, L. I., 1964).

Toxicology–Pharmacology: Tranylcypromine is a MAO inhibitor used for the treatment of severe mental depression. By inhibiting the effects of monoamine oxidase, which aids in the degradation of adrenaline and other catecholamines, tranylcypromine increases the concentration of adrenaline, noradrenaline, and serotonin throughout the nervous system. This action is believed to be responsible for the antidepressant actions. Since the toxic actions of the MAO inhibitors are frequent and can be severe, they are recommended for use only in patients who do not respond well to other forms of therapy.

The most severe toxic reaction occurring from tranylcypromine and the MAO inhibitors is the occurrence of hypertensive crisis. This may be precipitated by the use of a variety of other drugs or the consumption of certain foods containing tyramine by patients being treated with tranylcypromine. These include chianti wine, certain cheeses, chicken livers, sour cream, figs, and others. Death or paralysis from intracranial bleeding may result (Espir and Mitchell, 1963).

A fatality has been reported as the result of a massive cerebral hemorrhage, when 25 mg of methamphetamine was given to a patient being treated with tranylcypromine (Mason, 1962).

▶ **TRICYCLAMOL**
Noncontrolled Substance
Encountered in Excepted Substances

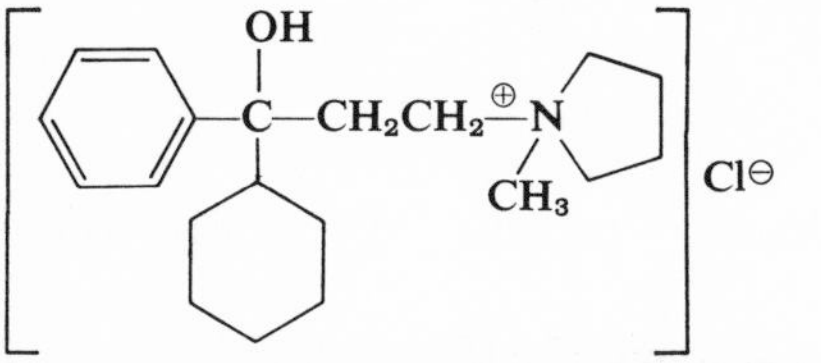

General Comments: Tricyclamol, also called procyclidine, is a synthetic antiparkinsonism drug. It is structurally and pharmacologically related to cycrimine and trihexyphenidyl. It is encountered in several formulations classified as excepted preparations. The following table indicates the minimum drug/ tricyclamol ratios encountered in such preparations:

Drug	Drug/Tricyclamol Ratio
Amobarbital	1/3.125
Phenobarbital	1/3.125

▶ **TRIDIHEXETHYL CHLORIDE**
Noncontrolled Substance
Encountered in Excepted Substances

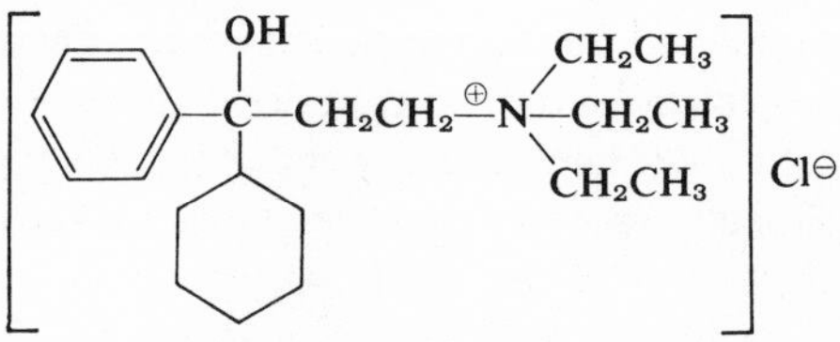

General Comments: Tridihexethyl chloride is encountered in formulations containing meprobamate that are classified as excepted preparations. The minimum meprobamate/tridihexethyl chloride found in such preparations is 1/0.06.

Toxicology–Pharmacology: Tridihexethyl chloride is a quaternary ammonium anticholinergic drug. It is used as adjunctive therapy in the treatment of peptic ulcer. It may also be used in treatment of irritable bowel syndromes, and in neurogenic bowel disturbances.

▶ **TRIFLUOPERAZINE**
Dangerous Drug

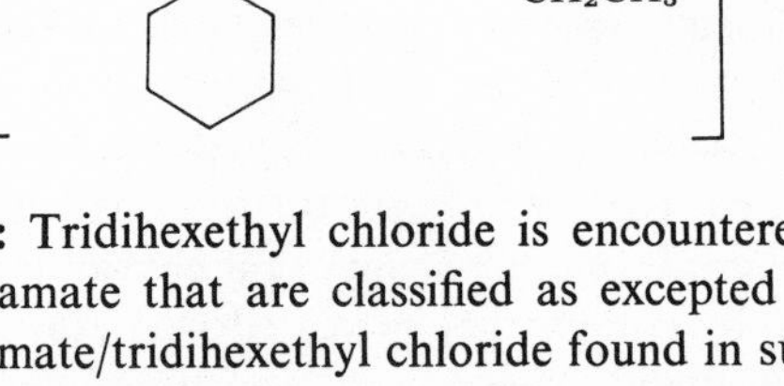

Synonym: 10-[3(4-Methylpiperazin-1-yl)propyl]-2-trifluoromethylphenothiazine.

Pharmaceutical Preparations: Stelazine[R] (Smith Kline & French)—Tablets, containing trifluoperazine hydrochloride: 1, 2, 5, or 10 mg

General Comment: Trifluoperazine is a phenothiazine tranquilizer, and as such is classified in this text as a Dangerous Drug.

Biochemistry: Trifluoperazine has two important factors that enhance potency for neuroleptic activity. These are the trifluoromethyl group in position 2 and the piperazine group on the side chain. Thus, trifluoperazine is one of the most potent compounds among prochlorperazine, perphenazine, and fluphenazine.

Toxicology–Pharmacology: Trifluoperazine is a psychotherapeutic agent of the piperazine group of phenothiazines. Its actions are similar to those of chlorpromazine, but it is considerably more potent than chlorpromazine. Its hypotensive actions and sympatholytic effects are substantially less than those of chlorpromazine. Its antiemetic effects are greater than those of chlorpromazine.

It is effective in relieving agitation and tension in selected psychosomatic patients. It exerts an overall calming effect in chronic psychotics, and good results have been obtained in schizophrenia, manic–depressive psychoses, chronic brain syndromes, and senile psychoses.

Untoward effects may occur with larger doses, and include extrapyramidal symptoms, such as spasm of neck muscles, rigidity of back muscles, and swallowing difficulty. Other depressant medications may potentiate the depressant actions of trifluoperazine, and alcohol and other sedative hypnotic drugs may result in fatal central nervous system depression.

In four cases of overdose with trifluoperazine, the serum concentrations ranged from 0.12 to 0.31 mg/dl (Tompsett, 1968).

▶ **TRIFLUPROMAZINE**
Dangerous Drug

Synonyms: 10-[3-(Dimethylamino)propyl]-2-(trifluoromethyl)phenothiazine, fluopromazine.
Pharmaceutical Preparations: Vesprin^R (Squibb)—Vials, containing triflupromazine hydrochloride: each 1 ml containing 10 or 20 mg. Tablets, containing triflupromazine hydrochloride: 10 or 25 mg. Suspension: each 1 ml containing 10 mg triflupromazine hydrochloride.
General Comment: Triflupromazine is a phenothiazine tranquilizer, and as such is classified in this text as a Dangerous Drug.
Biochemistry: Similar to that of chlorpromazine.
Toxicology–Pharmacology: Triflupromazine is a substituted phenothiazine, which is structurally and pharmacologically similar to chlorpromazine. It is, however, effective in smaller doses than chlorpromazine. It is used to control psychotic symptoms in schizophrenia, manic states, and psychoses associated with brain disease. It is also of value as an antiemetic, in treatment of the alcohol withdrawal syndrome, and as a general tranquilizer for inducing sedation.

Dosage of triflupromazine varies from 20–30 mg/dl in nausea and vomiting to 100–150 mg/dl in more severe mental disorders and behavioral problems.

▶ **TRIHEXYPHENIDYL**
Noncontrolled Substance

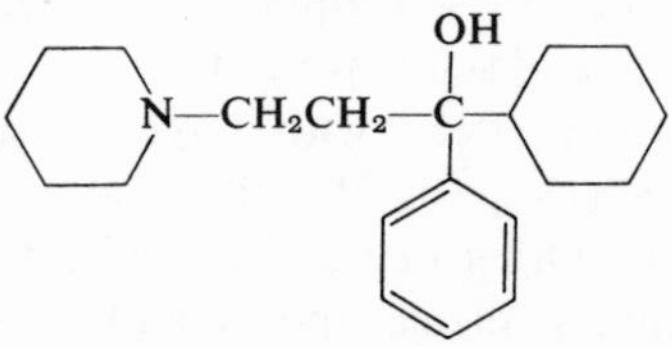

Toxicology–Pharmacology: Trihexyphenidyl acts principally as an antispasmodic on smooth muscles, and as an inhibitory agent to the parasympathetic nervous system. Its actions are similar to those of atropine, although less potent.

It is used primarily in treatment of various forms of parkinsonism. Adverse effects include dryness of the mouth, blurring of vision, dizziness, nausea, or nervousness.

Therapeutic blood concentrations of trihexyphenidyl are less than 0.10 mg/dl.

In one case of ingestion of four 20-mg tablets of trihexyphenidyl, followed by death by drowning, a blood concentration of trihexyphenidyl was 0.003 mg/dl (Kopjak and Jennison, 1976).

▶ **TRIMEPERIDINE**
Schedule I

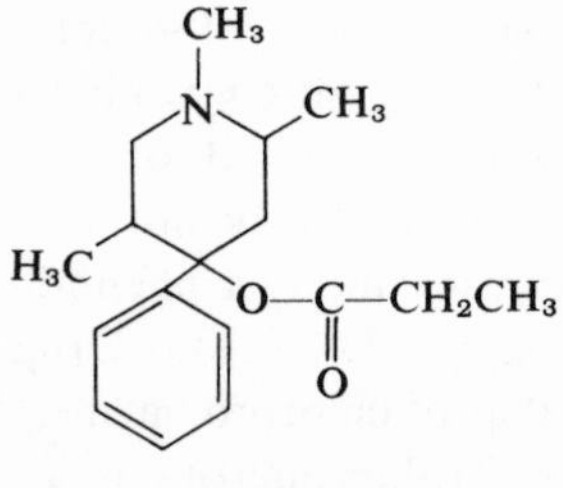

Synonyms: Trimethylmeperidine, 1,2,5-trimethyl-4-phenyl-4-propionyloxy-piperidine.

Pharmaceutical Preparations: Trimeperidine is not found in any pharmaceutical preparations sold in the United States.

General Comment: Trimeperidine is a synthetic narcotic analgesic that has no accepted medicinal value in the United States.

Biochemistry: Trimeperidine is the α-2,5-dimethyl derivative of prodine, and was developed in the U.S.S.R. in 1961 (Nazarov, 1962). A stereoisomer of trimeperidine, isopromedol, has been used clinically (Eddy *et al.*, 1957).
Toxicology–Pharmacology: Unknown.

▶ **TRIMEPRAZINE**
Dangerous Drug

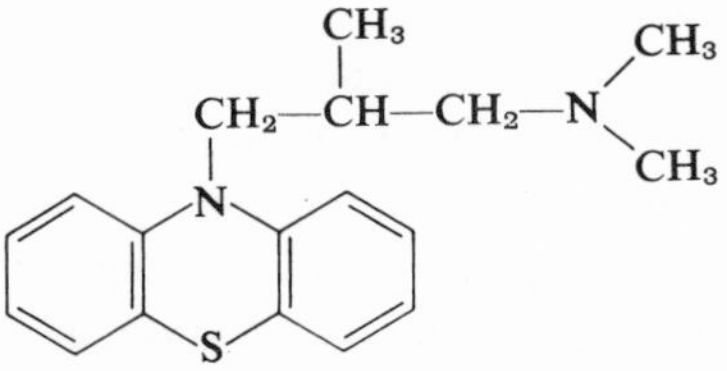

Synonym: ($\pm$)-10-[3-(Dimethylamino)-2-methylpropyl]phenothiazine.
Pharmaceutical Preparations: Temaril[R] (Smith Kline & French)—Tablet: containing 2.5 mg trimeprazine tartrate. Syrup: each 5 ml containing 2.5 mg trimeprazine tartrate. Capsule: containing 5 mg trimeprazine tartrate.
General Comment: Trimeprazine is a phenothiazine tranquilizer, and as such is classified in this text as a Dangerous Drug.
Biochemistry: The introduction of a 2-methyl substituent into the propylene bridge enhances antihistaminic and antipruritic properties. The optical isomers in the isobutyl derivatives have significantly different potencies. The *levo*-isomer of trimeprazine is many times more effective than the *dextro*-isomer (Gordon *et al.*, 1963).
Toxicology–Pharmacology: Trimeprazine is a substituted phenothiazine related to promazine. It has moderate anticonvulsant and antiemetic properties, and is a potent antihistaminic agent. It also has antipruritic actions (relieves itching).

Undesirable side effects include drowsiness and dizziness. Other central nervous system depressants may be potentiated in their action by trimeprazine.

▶ **3,4,5-TRIMETHOXYAMPHETAMINE**
Schedule I

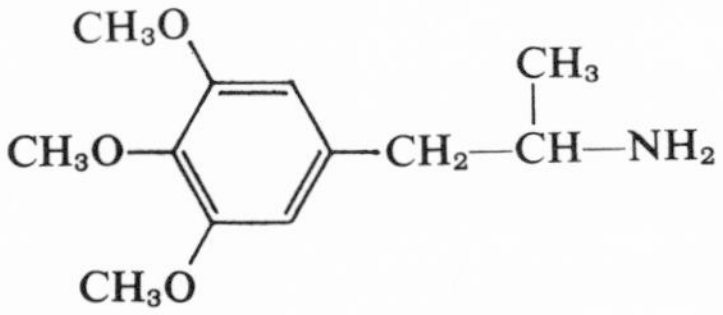

Synonyms: TMA, α-methyl-3,4,5-trimethoxyphenethylamine, trimethoxyamphetamine.

Pharmaceutical Preparations: 3,4,5-Trimethoxyamphetamine is not found in any pharmaceutical preparations sold in the United States.

General Comment: 3,4,5-Trimethoxyamphetamine has no accepted medicinal value in the United States.

Biochemistry: Similar to that of mescaline.

Toxicology–Pharmacology: Trimethoxyamphetamine is the α-methyl homologue of mescaline. Doses of 0.8–2 mg/kg produce fairly vivid hallucinations similar to those produced by mescaline. At higher doses (2.8–3.5 mg/kg), dramatic and dangerous psychotropic responses may occur. The initial effects, occurring about 2 hours after ingestion, are mescaline-like, but between 3 and 5 hours after ingestion, anger, hostility, and megalomaniac euphoria may dominate the person's thoughts and conversation. During this later period, provocation of the person may precipitate violence.

▶ **TROLNITRATE**
Noncontrolled Substance
Encountered in Excepted Substances

$$O_2N-O-CH_2CH_2 \diagdown \quad \diagup CH_2CH_2-O-NO_2$$
$$N$$
$$|$$
$$CH_2CH_2-O-NO_2$$

General Comments: Trolnitrate is an organic nitrate vasodilator. It is encountered in formulations containing butabarbital that are classified as excepted preparations. The minimum butabarbital/trolnitrate ratio found in such preparations is 1/0.12.

Toxicology–Pharmacology: Trolnitrate is an organic nitrate having persisting vasodilating actions on smooth muscles. It is of value in treatment of patients with angina pectoris, as the vasodilating actions increase the blood supply to the heart. It is used prophylactically, and is of little value in treating attacks, due to its delayed onset of action, in contrast to rapid-acting vasodilators such as nitroglycerin or amyl nitrite.

The usual daily dose for prophylactic treatment of angina pectoris is 8–16 mg. No significant effect occurs before the third day of treatment.

▶ **TYBAMATE**
Dangerous Drug

$$\begin{array}{ccccc} & O & & CH_3 & & O \\ & || & & | & & || \\ H_2N-C-O-CH_2-&C-CH_2-O-&C-NH-CH_2CH_2CH_2CH_3 \\ & & | & & \\ & & CH_2CH_2CH_3 & & \end{array}$$

Synonyms: 2-(Hydroxymethyl)-2-methylpentylbutylcarbamate carbamate, 2-butycarbamoyloxymethyl-2-carbamoyloxymethylpentane.

Pharmaceutical Preparations: Tybatran[R] (Robins)—Capsules, green, one-piece, containing tybamate: 125, 250, or 350 mg.

General Comment: Tybamate is pharmacologically classified as a tranquilizer, and as such is classified in this text as a Dangerous Drug.

Biochemistry: Tybamate is the *N*-butyl derivative of meprobamate, being slightly less potent in anticonvulsant tests (Surber *et al.*, 1959). However, it does antagonize the pressor effect of serotonin and the EEG activation caused by lysergic acid diethylamide, which meprobamate does not. In addition, unlike meprobamate, convulsions do not follow its withdrawal from chronic use (Colmore and Moore, 1967).

Toxicology–Pharmacology: Tybamate is a carbamate tranquilizer with actions similar to those of meprobamate. It exerts a taming effect on wild or aggressive animals, and has a centrally mediated muscle-relaxant action. It is effective in the treatment of anxiety, tension, agitation, and depression in psychoneuroses and behavioral disorders.

Administration of phenothiazines or other central nervous system depressants simultaneously may induce seizures. Additive actions may occur when given in combination with other sedative or depressant medications.

In one case of detection of tybamate in blood, 0.5 mg/dl was found after arrest of a motor-vehicle driver (Finkle, 1969b).

▶ **VINBARBITAL**
Schedule III

Synonyms: Vinbarbitone, butenemal, 5-ethyl-5-(1-methylbut-1-enyl)barbituric acid.

Pharmaceutical Preparations: Vinbarbital is not found in any pharmaceutical preparations sold in the United States.

General Comment: Vinbarbital is a barbiturate that is listed under Schedule III of the Controlled Substances Act as a "derivative of barbituric acid."

Biochemistry: Similar to that of cyclobarbital.

Toxicology–Pharmacology: Vinbarbital is an intermediate-acting barbiturate. It has been used in the past as a sedative and hypnotic; however, over the past ten years, it has declined in use. It is no longer marketed in any dosage form by its original producer. Its pharmacological effects are similar to those of amobarbital.

▶ **YOHIMBINE**
Dangerous Drug

Synonyms: Aphrodine, corymine, quebrachine.

Pharmaceutical Preparations: Andro Medicone[R] (Medicone)—Tablet: containing 5.4 mg thyroid, 1.0 mg strychnine sulfate, and 5.4 mg yohimbine hydrochloride

General Comment: Yohimbine is classified in this text as a Dangerous Drug under the legend drug provision because the pharmaceutical preparations containing yohimbine bear the label "Caution: Federal law prohibits dispensing without a prescription."

Biochemistry: Similar to that of reserpine.

Toxicology–Pharmacology: Yohimbine is the principal alkaloid of the bark of the yohimbe tree, *Pausinystalia yohimbe* (*Corynanthe yohimbi*) (Family Rubiaceae). Yohimbine produces a competitive α-adrenergic blockade of limited duration. This effect is of primary value in alleviating hypertension, by its vasodilating action.

    It has little central nervous system actions. It produces diuresis, probably by antagonizing the release of antidiuretic hormone (ADH). Yohimbine has been promoted as an aphrodisiac, but there is little convincing evidence for its effectiveness. This drug has no current therapeutic applications.

Bibliography and References

BIBLIOGRAPHY

The general publications listed below are recommended to the reader having an interest in or a need for further information in the field of forensic toxicology.

Baker, E. C., Levine, J. M., Huff, B. B., Levitus, I. M., Caruso, E. H., Clark, J. M., Brogeler, E. B., Oakley, G. L., Paterniti, F. E., Ross, M., and Cece, J. W., eds., 1976, *Physicians' Desk Reference*, 30th ed., Medical Economics, Oradell, New Jersey.

Clarke, E. G. C., ed., 1969, *Isolation and Identification of Drugs*, The Pharmaceutical Press, London.

Code of Federal Regulations, 21, Food and Drugs, Part 1300 to End, 1974, Published by Office of the Federal Register, National Archives and Records Service, U.S. Government Printing Office.

The United States Pharmacopeia, 1975, 19th revision Committee of Revision, United States Pharmacopeial Convention, Inc., U.S.P. Inc., Rockville, Maryland.

Gleason, M. N., Gosselin, R. E., Hodge, H. C., and Smith, R. P., 1969, *Clinical Toxicology of Commercial Products*, 3rd ed., Williams and Wilkins, Baltimore.

Goldstein, A., Aronow, L., and Kalman, S. M., 1974, *Principles of Drug Action: The Basis of Pharmacology*, Wiley, New York.

Goodman, L. S., and Gilman, A., eds., 1970, *The Pharmacological Basis of Therapeutics*, 4th ed., Macmillan, New York.

Martin, E. W., 1971, *Hazards of Medication*, Lippincott, Philadelphia.

Osol, A., and Pratt, R., 1973, *The United States Dispensatory*, 27th ed. Lippincott, Philadelphia.

Rossoff, I. S., 1974, *Handbook of Veterinary Drugs*, Springer, New York.

Stecher, P. G., Windholz, M., Leahy, D. S., Bolton, D. M., and Eaton, L. G., eds., 1968, *The Merck Index*, Merck & Co., Rahway, New Jersey.

REFERENCES

Abbott Pharmaceutical Co., 1976, Product information files.

Abood, L. G., Ostfeld, A. M., and Biel, J. H., 1959, *Arch. Intern. Pharmacodyn.* **120**: 186.

Adams, R., Pease, D. C., Cain, C. K., and Clark, J. H., 1940, *J. Am. Chem. Soc.* **62**: 2402.

Afifi, A.-H. M., and Way, E. L., 1967, *J. Pharm. Sci.* **56**:720.

Aghajanian, G. K., and Bing, O. H. L., 1964, *Clin. Pharmacol. Ther.* **5**:611–614.

Algeri, E. J., and McBay, A. J., 1956, *Science* **123**:183.

Allgen, L. G., Hellström, L., and Sant'Orp, C. J., 1963, *Acta Psychiatr. Scand. Suppl.* **169**:39, 366.

Anderson, L. C., 1974, *Bot. Mus. Leafl. Harv. Univ.* **24**:29.

Anlage, H. J., 1973, Smith, Kline, and French Laboratories, Philadelphia, Personal communication.

Avis, K. E., 1975, Parenteral preparations, in: *Remington's Pharmaceutical Sciences* John E. Hoover, Mng. ed., Vol. 15, pp. 1461–1487, Mack Publishing Co., Easton, Pennsylvania.

Avison, W. P., and Morrison, A. L., 1950, *J. Chem. Soc.* 1469.

Axelrod, J., 1958, *J. Pharmacol.* **124**:9.

Backer, R. C., Caplan, Y. H., and Duncan, C. E., 1975, *Clin. Toxicol.* **8**(3):283–287.

Bailey, D. N., and Jatlow, P. I., 1973, *Clin. Toxicol.* **6**(4):563–569.

Barber, R. B., and Rapoport, H., 1975, *J. Med. Chem.* **18**(11):1074.

Barber, R. B., and Rapoport, H., 1976, *J. Med. Chem.* **19**(10):1175.

Barnhill, M. T., Jones, J. K., Mills, T., Slighton, G. L., and Walker, B. A., 1974, *Bull. IAFT* **10**(1):19.

Barowsky, H., and Schwartz, S. A., 1962, *J. Am. Med. Assoc.* **180**:1058.

Baselt, R. C., and Cravey, R. H., 1977, *J. Anal. Toxicol.* **1**(2):81–103.

Baselt, R. C., Wright, J. A., Turner, J. E., and Cravey, R. H., 1975a, *Arch. Toxicol.* **34**:145.

Baselt, R. C., Wright, J. A., and Cravey, R. H., 1975b, *Clin. Chem.* **21**:44.

Beckett, A. H., Casy, A. F., Harper, N. J., and Phillips, P. M., 1956, *J. Pharmacol.* **8**:860.

Beckett, A. H., Brookes, L. G., and Shenoy, E. V. B., 1969, *J. Pharm. Pharmacol.* **21**: 1515–1565.

Bennett, W. H., Singer, I., Coggins, C. J., *J. Am. Med. Assoc.*, **230**:1544–1553 (1974).

Benson, W. M., Stefko, P. L., and Randall, L. O., 1953, *J. Pharmacol. Exp. Ther.* **109**: 189.

Bentley, K. W., and Cardwell, H. M. E., 1955, *J. Chem. Soc.* **325**:2.

Berger, F. M., 1954, *J. Pharmacol. Exp. Ther.* **112**:413.

Berger, F. M., Douglas, J. F., Kletzkiu, M., Ludwig, G. J., and Margolin, S., 1961, *J. Pharmacol. Exp. Ther.* **134**:356.

Berkowitz, B. A., Asling, J. H., Shnider, S. M., and Way, E. L., 1969, *Clin. Pharmacol. Ther.* **10**:320.

Beyer, K. H., and Sadie, V. W., 1969, *Arzneim.-Forsch.* **19**(12):1929–1931.

Biel, J. H., *et al.*, 1961, *J. Med. Chem.* **26**:4096.

Biltz, H., 1908, *Berichte* **41**:1379.

Bilzer, W., and Gundert, R. V., 1973, *Eur. J. Clin. Pharmacol.* **6**:268.

Blair, A. M. J. N., and Stephenson, R. P., 1960, *Br. J. Pharmacol.* **15**:247.

Bock, G., and Sherwin, A. L., 1971, *Clin. Chim. Acta* **34**:97–103.

Bockmühl, M., and Ehrhart, G., 1948, *Ann. Chem. Liebigs*, **561**:52.

Boissier, J. R., Dumont, C., and Ratouis, R., 1967, *Therapie* **22**:129.

Booker, R. N., and Pohland, A., 1975, *J. Med. Chem.* **18**:266.

Borkowski, T., and Dluzniewaska, A., 1976, *Bull. IAFT* **12**(3):7.

Bösche, J., Reibel, J., and Schmidt, G., 1969, *Arch. Toxicol.* **25**:65–75.

Boszormenyi, Z., and Szara, S., 1958, *J. Ment. Sci.* **104**:445–453.

Braithwaite, R. A., Goulding, R., Thean, G., Bailey, V., and Coppen, A., 1972, *Lancet* **June 17**: 7764.

Brilmayer, H., and Loennecken, S. J., 1962, *Arch. Intern. Pharmacodyn.* **136**:137.

Brodie, B. B., 1952, *Fed. Proc.* **11**:632.

Brodie, B. B., Lief, P. A., and Poet, R., 1948, *J. Pharmacol. Exp. Ther.* **94**:359.

Brodie, B. B., *et al.*, 1950, *J. Pharmacol.* **98**:85.

Bruce, R. B., Pitts, J. E., Pinchbeck, J., and Newman, J., 1965, *J. Med. Chem.* **8**:157.

Bush, M. T., Berry, G., and Hume, A., 1966, *Clin. Pharmacol. Ther.* **7**:373.

Butler, T. C., 1956, *J. Am. Pharm. Assoc. Sci.* **116**:326.

Butler, T. C., and Waddall, W. J., 1958, *Neurology* **8**:106.

Campbell, D. B., and Moore, B. W. R., 1969, *Lancet* **7633**:1307.

Carrington, H. C., and Raventos, J., 1946, *Br. J. Pharmacol.* **1**:215.

Casy, A. F., and Hassan, M. M. A., 1967, *J. Pharm. Pharmacol.* **19**:114.

Cerletti, A., 1959, in: *Neuropsychopharmacology* (P. B. Bradley, P. Deniker, and T. C. Rodoves, eds.), Elsevier, Amsterdam.

Charalampous, K. D., Orengo, A., Walker, D. E., and Kinross-Wright, J., 1964, *J. Pharmacol. Exp. Ther.* **145**:242.

Charpentier, T., 1950, U.S. Patent 2,519,886 (1950); U.S. Patent 2,530,451.

Chen, G., and Bass, P., 1964, *Arch. Intern. Pharmacodyn.* **152**:115.

Cherniack, R. M., and Young, G., 1964, *Ann. Intern. Med.* **60**:631.

Chess, D., and Yonkman, F. F., 1946, *Proc. Soc. Exp. Biol. Med.* **61**:127.

Cimbura, G., Garry, E. M., and Diagle, J., 1972, *J. Forensic Sci.* **17**(4):640–644.

Clark, T., 1973, *Tex. Med.* **69**, 74.

Clarke, E. G. C., ed., 1969, *Isolation and Identification of Drugs*, The Pharmaceutical Press, London.

Clifford, J. M., Cookson, J. H., and Wickham, P. E., 1974, *Clin. Pharmacol. Ther.* **16**:376.

Cochin, J., and Daly, J. W., 1963, *J. Pharmacol. Exp. Ther.* **139**:154.

Collard, J., 1971, *Arzneim.-Forsch.* **21**(7a):1091–1095.

Colmore, J. P., and Moore, J. D., 1967, *J. Clin. Pharmacol.* **7**:319.

Condouris, G. A., and Bonnycastle, D. D., 1961, *Am. J. Med. Sci.* **242**:574.

Conney, A. H., Trovsof, N., and Burns, J. J., 1960, *J. Pharmacol. Exp. Ther.* **128**: 333.

Cravey, R. H., and Baselt, R. C., 1968, *J. Forensic Sci.* **13**(4):532–561.

Cravey, R. H., and Reed, D., 1970, *J. Forensic Sci.* **10**(2):109–112.

Cummins, L. M., Martin, Y. C., and Scherfling, E. E., 1971, *J. Pharm. Sci.* **60**:261.

Curry, A. S., 1955, *J. Pharm. Pharmacol.* **7**:1072.

Curry, S. H., Riddall, D., and Gordon, J. S., 1971, *Clin. Pharmacol. Ther.* **12**:849–859.

Davis, W. J., 1976, *Drug Therapy*, pp. 175–185.

Degerholm, D., Harrison, A., Leiderman, T., and Sterner, N., 1964, *Chem. Abstr.* **60**: 3945.

Delay, J., Deniker, T., and Harl, J. M., 1952, *Ann. Med. Psychol. Fr.* **110**:112.

De Silva, J. A. F., and D'Arconte, L., 1969, *J. Forensic Sci.* **14**(2):184–204.

De Silva, J. A. F., and Strojny, N., 1971, *J. Pharm. Sci.* **60**(9):1303–1314.

Di Carlo, F. J., Viace, J. P., Epps, J. E., and Haynes, L. J., 1970, *Clin. Pharm. Ther.* **11**:890.

DiMaio, V. J. M., and Garriott, J. C., 1974, *Forensic Sci.* **3**:275–278.

DiMaio, V. J. M., and Garriott, J. C., 1977a, *Forensic Sci. Gaz.* **8**:1–2.

DiMaio, V. J. M., and Garriott, J. C., 1977b, *J. Forensic Sci.* **22**(1):152–158.

DiMaio, V. J. M., and Garriott, J. C., 1978, *Forensic Sci.* (accepted for publication).

Domino, E. F., 1964, *Int. Rev. Neurobiol.* **6**:303–347.

Douglas, J. F., Ludwig, B. J., Ginsberg, T., and Berger, F. M., 1962, *J. Pharmacol. Exp. Ther.* **136**:5.

Eddy, N. B., and Mary, E. L., 1973, *Science* **181**:407–414.

Eddy, N. B., Halbach, H., and Braenden, O. J., 1957, *Bull. WHO* **17**:569.

Eisleb, O., and Schaumann, O., 1939, *Dtsch. Med. Wochenschr.* **65**:967.

Espir, M. L. E., and Mitchell, L., 1963, *Lancet*, 639.

Fabig, H. D., and Hawkins, J. R., 1956, *Science* **123**:886–887.

Fatteh, A., 1972, *J. Am. Med. Assoc.* **219**(6):756–757.

Fazekas, J. F., Goldbaum, L. R., Koppanyi, T., and Shea, J. G., 1956, *Am. J. Med. Sci.* **231**:531.

Finkle, B. S., 1969a, *Bull. IAFT* **6**(4):5.

Finkle, B. S., 1969b, *Bull. IAFT* **6**(3):4.

Fischer, R., 1958, *Rev. Canad. Bio.*, **17**:389–409.

Fisk, M. S., Johnson, N. M., and Horning, E. C., 1955, *J. Am. Chem. Soc.* **77**:5892.

Fleischer, M. R., and Campbell, D. B., 1969, *Lancet* **2**:1306.

Flintan, P., and Keele, C. A., 1954, *Br. J. Pharmacol.* **9**:106.

Fretwurst, F., Halberkann, J., and Reiche, F., 1932, *Muench. Med. Wochenschr.* **79**:1429.

Frey, H. H., Sudendey, F., and Krause, D., 1959, *Arzneim.-Forsch.* **9**:294.

Galanter, M., Wyatt, R. J., Lemberber, L., Weingarter, H., Vaughan, T. B., and Roth, W. T., 1972, *Science* **176**:934.

Gaoni, Y., and Mechoulam, R., 1964, *J. Am. Chem. Soc.* **86**:1646.

Garland, W. A., Hsiao, K. C., Pantuck, E. V., and Conney, A. H., 1977, *J. Pharm. Sci.* **66**:340.

Garriott, J. C., 1977, Case files of the Dallas County Medical Examiner's Office.

Garriott, J. C., 1977, Unpublished data.

Garriott, J. C., and Latman, N., 1976, *J. Forensic Sci.* **21**:398.

Garriott, J. C., Sturner, W. Q., and Mason, M. F., 1973, *Clin. Toxicol.* **6**(2):163–173.

Gates, M., and Shepard, M. S., 1962, *J. Am. Chem. Soc.* **84**:4125.

Gianelly, R., *et al.*, 1967, *N. Engl. J. Med.* **277**(2):1215–1219.

Gibson, J. T., 1976, in: *Medication Law and Behavior*, pp. 59–61, Wiley-Interscience, Wiley, New York.

Glazko, A. J., Dill, W. A., Young, R. M., Smith, T. C., and Ogilvie, R. E., 1974, *Clin. Pharmacol. Ther.* **16**(6):1067–1076.

Gleason, M. N., Grosselin, R. E., Hodge, H. C., and Smith, R. P., 1969, *Clinical Toxicology of Commercial Products*, 3rd ed., Williams and Wilkins, Baltimore.

Goldberg, L. I., 1964, *J. Am. Med. Assoc.* **190**:456.

Goldberg, W. M., and Chakrabarti, S. G., 1964, *Can. Med. Assoc. J.* **91**:991.

Goodman, L. S., and Gilman, A. (eds.), 1970, *The Pharmacological Basis of Therapeutics*, 4th ed., Macmillan, New York.

Gordon, M., Cook, L., Tedeschi, D. H., and Tedeschi, R. E., 1963, *Arzneim.-Forsch.* **13**:318.

Goto, K., Yamasaki, H., Yamamoto, I., and Ohno, H., 1957, *Proc. Jpn. Acad.* **33**:660.

Graves, M. H., and Schwartz, G., 1974 *Bull. IAFT* **10**(2):10.

Hafliger, F., and Schindler, W., 1951, U.S. Patent 2,554,736.

Hall, A. P., Czerwinski, A. W., Madonia, E. C., and Evenson, K. L., 1973, *Clin. Pharmacol. Ther.* **14**:580.

Hansen, A. R., Kennedy, K. A., Ambre, J. J., and Fischer, L. J., 1975, *N. Engl. J. Med.* **292**(5):250–252.

Hansen, C. E., and Larsen, N. E., 1974, *Psychopharmacologia* **37**:31.

Harper, N. J., Simmonds, A. B., Wakoma, W. T., Hall, G. H., and Vallance, D. K., 1966, *J. Pharm. Pharmacol.* **18**:150.

Hine, C. H., and Pasi, A., 1972, *Clin. Toxicol.* **5**(3):307–315.

Hirsh, H. L., 1977, *Case Comment* **82**:14–19.

Hobbs, D. C., Welch, W. M., and Short, M. J., 1974, *Clin. Pharmacol. Ther.* **16**:473.

Hofmann, A., 1961, *J. Exp. Med.* **V**(2):31–51.

Hofmann, A., 1963, *Bot. Mus. Leafl. Harv. Univ.* **20**:194–212.

Hofmann, A., 1975, *LSD: A Total Study* (D. V. Siva Sankar, ed.), pp. 107–115, PJD Publications, Westbury, New York.

Hollister, L. E., and Kanter, S. L., 1965, *Clin. Pharmacol. Ther.* **6**:5.

Hucker, H. B., 1962, *Pharmacologist* **4**:171.

Hundt, H. D. L., Clark, E. G., and Muller, F. O., 1975, *J. Pharm. Sci.* **64**:1041.

Huus, I., and Khan, A. R., 1967, *Acta Pharmacol. Toxicol.* **25**:397.

Inturresi, C. E., and Verebely, K., 1972, *Clin. Pharmacol. Ther.* **13**:633.

Isbell, H., and Fraser, H. F., 1950, *Pharmacol. Rev.* **2**:355.

Jacobs, M. H., and Senior, R. M., 1974, *Am. Rev. Respir. Dis.* **110**:342–345.

Janssen, P. A. J., 1956, *J. Am. Chem. Soc.* **78**:3862.

Janssen, P. A. J., 1960, in: *Synthetic Analgesics*, Part I, Pergamon, New York.

Janssen, P. A. J., 1967, in: *Psychopharmacological Agents* (M. Gordon, ed.), Vol. II, p. 199, Academic Press, New York and London.

Janssen, P. A. J., and Jageneau, A. H., 1957, *J. Pharm. Pharmacol.* **9**:381.

Janssen, P. A. J., Niemeyeers, C. J. E., and Schellekins, K. H. L., 1965, *Arzneim.-Forsch* **15**:1196.

Jones, J. K., 1973, Georgia Crime Laboratory, Personal Communications.

Joshi, B. C., Chignell, C. F., and May, E. L., 1965, *J. Med. Chem.* **8**:694.

Joubert, P., and Olivier, J., 1974, *Clin. Toxicol.*, **7**(2):133–138.

Kapadia, G. J., and Fales, H. M., 1968, *Chem. Commun.* **1968**:1688.

Kaplan, M. M., Register, D. C., Bierman, A. H., and Risacher, R. L., 1974, *Clin. Toxicol.* **7**(5):509–512.

Karim, A., Ranney, R. E., Evensen, K. L., and Clark, M. L., 1972, *Clin. Pharmacol. Ther.* **13**(3):407–419.

Karreman, G., Isenberg, I., and Szent-Györggi, A., 1959, *Science* **130**:1191.

Keberle, H., Riess, W., and Hoffmann, K., 1963, *Arch. Intern. Pharmacodyn.* **142**:117.

Kersh, E. J., 1973, *Chest* **63**(1):112–114.

King, A. G., 1956, *Am. J. Obstet. Gynecol.* **71**:1001.

Klock, J. C., Boerner, J., and Becker, C., 1973, *Clin. Toxicol.* **8**(2):191–209.

Knowles, J. A., and Ruelius, H. W., 1972, *Arzneim.-Forsch.* **22**:687.

Knowles, J. A., Corner, W. H., and Ruelius, H. W., 1971, *Arzneim.-Forsch.* **21**(7a): 1055–1059.

Koe, B. K., and Pinson, R., Jr., 1964, *J. Med. Chem.* **7**:635.

Koechlin, B. F., and D'Arconte, L., 1963, *Anal. Biochem.* **5**:195–207.

Koechlin, B. F., Schwartz, M. A., Krol, G., and Oberhausli, W., 1965, *J. Pharmacol. Exp. Ther.* **148**(3):399–411.

Kopjack, L., and Jennison, T. A., 1976, *Bull. IAFT* **12**(1):12.

Kuhn, R., 1957, *Schweiz. Med. Wochenschr.* **87**:1135.

Kuntzman, R., Ikeda, M., Jacobson, M., and Conney, A. H., 1967, *J. Pharmacol. Exp. Ther.* **157**:220.

Lebish, P., Finkle, B. S., and Brackett, J. W., 1970, *Clin. Chem.* **16**:195.

Lewin, L., 1928, *Arch. Exp. Path. Pharmakol.* **129**:133–149.

Lewis, W. H., and Elvin-Lewis, M. P. F., 1977, *Medical Botany*, pp. 412–413, John Wiley, New York.

Liden, C. B., Lovejoy, F. H., and Costello, C. E., 1975, *J. Am. Med. Assoc.* **234**(5): 513–516.

Loew, G. H., and Jester, J. R., 1975, *J. Med. Chem.* **18**:1051.

Lous, P., 1954, *Acta Pharmacol. (Copenhagen)* **10**:147.

Loveland, M. R., 1974, *Bull. IAFT* **10**(1):16.

Lowry, W. T., 1976, *J. Forensic Sci.* **21**:453.

Lowry, W. T., and Barklow, J. P., Jr., 1976, *J. Forensic Sci.* **21**:416–421.

Lucas, R. A., 1963, *Prog. Med. Chem.* **3**:146.

Ludwig, B. J., and Piech, E. C., 1951, *J. Am. Chem. Soc.* **73**:5779.

Lundberg, G., *et al.*, 1977, *J. Forensic Sci.* **22**:402.

Lundstrom, J., and Agurell, S., 1968, *J. Chromatogr.* **36**:105.

Maes, R., Hodnett, N., Landesman, H., Kananen, G., Finkle, B., and Sunshine, I., 1969, *J. Forensic Sci.* **14**(2):235–254.

March, J., 1968, *Advanced Organic Chemistry: Reactions, Mechanisms, and Structure*, pp. 71–124, McGraw-Hill, New York.

Mark, L. C., Brand, L., Kamvyssi, S., Button, R. C., Perel, J. M., Landrau, M. A., and Dayton, P. G., 1965, *Nature (London)* **206**:1117.

Marsden, P., and Sheldon, J., 1972, *Br. Med. J.* **1**(5802):730.

Marsh, D. F., 1955. *Fed. Proc.* **14**:366.

Martensson, E., and Ross, B. E., 1977, *Eur. J. Clin. Pharmacol.* **6**:181.

Mason, A., 1962, *Lancet*, 1073.

Matthew, H., 1971, *Acute Barbiturate Poisoning*, p. 29, Excerpta Medica, Amsterdam.

May, E. L., and Sargent, L. J., 1965, in: *Analgetics* (S. de Stevens, ed.), Vol. 5, pp. 171–172, Academic Press, New York.

Maynert, E. W., 1965, *J. Pharmacol. Exp. Ther.* **150**:118.

Maynert, E. W., and Van Dyke, H. B., 1950, *J. Pharmacol. Exp. Ther.* **98**:180.

McLaughlin, J. L., and Paul, A. G., 1966, *Lloydia* **19**:315.

McMahon, R. E., 1959, *J. Org. Chem.* **24**:1834.

McMahon, R. E., Marshall, F. J., Culp, H. W., and Miller, W. M., 1963, *Biochem. Pharmacol.* **12**:1207.

McMahon, R. E., Culp, H. W., and Marshall, F. J., 1965, *J. Pharmacol. Exp. Therap.* **149**:436.

Merritt, H. H., and Putnam, T. J., 1938, *Arch. Neurol. Psychiatry* **39**:1003.

Mikailova, D., Roser, A., Testa, B., and Beckett, A. H., 1974, *J. Pharm. Pharmacol.* **26**:711–721.

Milberg, R. M., Rinehart, K. L., Sprague, R. L., and Sleator, E. K., 1975, *Biomed. Mass Spectrum* **2**:2.

Mills, D. H., 1965, *J. Am. Med. Assoc.* **192**:116–118.

Morris, R. N., Gunderson, C. A., Babcock, S. W., and Zaroslinski, J. F., 1972, *Clin. Pharmacol. Ther.* **13**:719.

Musto, D., 1968, *J. Am. Med. Assoc.* **204**:27.

Nash, F., Bennett, I. F., Bopp, R. J., Brunson, M. D., and Sullivan, H. R., 1975, *J. Pharm. Sci.* **6**(3):129–133.

Nazarov, I. N., 1962, *Chem. Abstr.* **56**:8682.

Niyogi, S. K., 1964, *Nature (London)* **202**:1225.

Norheim, G., 1973, *J. Forensic Sci. Soc.* **13**:187.

Parker, K. D., Elliott, H. W., Wright, J. A., Nomof, N., and Hine, C. H., 1970, *Clin. Toxicol.* **3**(12):131–145.

Pascarelli, E. F., 1973, *J. Am. Med. Assoc.* **224**(11):1512–1514.

Patterson, S., and Peat, M. A., 1976, *Bull. IAFT* **12**(2):25.

Peat, M. A., and Sengupta, A., 1977, *J. Forensic Sci.* **9**:21–22.

Peets, E. A., Jackson, M., and Symchowiecz, S., 1972, *J. Pharmacol. Exp. Ther.* **180**(2): 464–474.

Pennes, H. H., and Hoch, P. H., 1957, *Am. J. Psychiatry* **113**:887.

Peters, J. M., 1967, *J. Clin. Pharmacol.* **7**:131–141.

Plaa, G. L., and Hine, C. H., 1960, *Arch. Intern. Pharmacodyn.* **128**:375.

Plummer, A. J., Barrett, W. E., and Rugledge, R. A., 1954, *Fed. Proc.* **13**:395.

Poldinger, W., 1964, *Schweiz. Arch. Neurol. Psychiatr.* **94**:440.

Poole, J. W., and Gardocki, J. F., 1963, *J. Pharm. Sci.* **52**:486.

Popovic, K., Stanulovic, D., and Stanulovic, M., 1973, *Clin. Tox.*, **6**:585–598.

Price, K., 1974, *Bull. IAFT* **10**(1):12.

Quinn, G. P., Cohn, M. M., Reid, M. B., *et al.*, 1967, *Clin. Pharmacol. Ther.* **8**:369.

Randall, L. O., Ilieu, W., and Brandman, O., 1956, *Arch. Intern. Pharmacodyn.* **106**:388.

Ratcliff, B. A., 1974, Editorial, *Clin. Toxicol.* **7**(4):409–411.

Raven, P. H., 1974, *Lloydia* **37**:321.

Raventos, J., 1954, *J. Pharm. Pharmacol.* **6**:217.

Reider, V. J., 1965, *Arzneim.-Forsch.* **15**:1134.

Reynolds, P. C., 1976, *Clin. Toxicol.* **9**(4):547–552.

Rheinstein, P. H., 1976, *J. Legal Med.* **4**:22–24.

Robinson, A. E., and Williams, F. M., 1971, *J. Pharm. Pharmacol.* **23**:353.

Robinson, D. W., Cimbura, G., Fenwick, J., 1973, *Bull. IAFT.* **9**:13–14.

Roche, 1975, Product information files.

Roszkowski, A. P., 1960, *J. Pharmacol. Exp. Ther.* **129**:75.

Rowland, M., and Beckett, A. H., 1966, *Arzneim.-Forsch.* **11a**:1369.

Sawhney, S. N., 1970, in: *Medicinal Chemistry*, Pt. 2, p. 869, Wiley, New York.

Schatz, F., and John, A., 1966, *Arzneim.-Forsch.* **16**:866.

Schaumann, O., 1949, *Pharmazie* **4**:364.

Schlittler, E., and Bein, H. J., 1967, in: *Antihypertensive Agents* (E. Schlittler, ed.), pp. 191–221, Academic Press, New York.

Schmidt, A. M., Whitehorn, W. V., and Martin, E. W., 1976, *FDA Drug Bull.*

Schnider, O., and Grussner, A., 1951, *Helv. Chim. Acta* **34**:2211.

Schrappe, O., 1971, *Arzneim.-Forsch.* **21**(7a):1079–1082.

Schultes, R. E., and Hofmann, A., 1973, *The Botany and Chemistry of Hallucinogens*, p. 81, Charles C. Thomas, Springfield, Illinois.

Schultes, R. E., Klein, W. M., Plowman, T., and Lockwood, T. E., 1974, *Bot. Mus. Leafl. Harv. Univ.* **23**:337.

Schwartz, M. A., and Postma, E., 1970, *J. Pharm. Sci.* **59**:1800.

Schwartz, M. A., Postma, E., and Gaut, Z., 1971, *J. Pharm. Sci.* **60**(10):1500–1503.

Schwartz, M. A., Covino, B. G., Narang, R. M., *et al.*, 1974, *Am. Heart J.* **88**(6):721–723.

Segaloff, A., Baggard, B., Carriere, B. T., and Rongone, E. L., 1965, *Steroids*, Suppl. I.

Seth, P. K., and Parmar, S. S., 1965, *Can. J. Physiol. Pharmacol.* **43**:1019.

Shih, A. P., Robinson, K., and An, W. Y. W., 1976, *Eur. J. Pharmacol.* **9**:451.

Shimkin, P. M., and Shaiviz, S. A., 1966, Oxazepam poisoning in a child, *J. Am. Med. Assoc.* **196**:662.

Shulgin, A. T., 1964, *Nature (London)* **201**:1120–1121.

Simpson, G. M., and Salim, T., 1965, *Current Ther. Res.* **7**:661.

Small, E., 1972, *Can. J. Bot.* **50**:1947.

Small, L. F., and Rapoport, H., 1947, *J. Org. Chem.* **12**:284.

Smits, S. E., 1974, *Res. Commun. Chem. Pathol. Pharmacol.* **8**:575.

Smythies, J. R., Bradley, R. J., and Johnston, V. S., 1967, *Nature (London)* **216**:128.

Snyder, S. H., and Merril, C. R., 1965, *Proc. Natl. Acad. Sci. U.S.A.* **54**:258.

Snyder, S. H., Faillace, L., and Hollister, L., 1967, *Science* **158**:669–670.

Soares, J. R., and Gross, S. J., 1976, *Life Sci.* **19**: 1711–1718.

Spath, E., 1920, *Monatschr. Chem.* **41**:297.

Speck, L. B., 1957, *J. Pharmacol. Exp. Ther.* **119**:78–84.

Stambough, J. E., Wainer, I. W., Sanstead, J. K., and Hemphill, D. M., 1976, *J. Clin. Pharmacol.* **16**:245.

Stearn, W. T., 1974, *Bot. Mus. Leafl. Harv. Univ.* **23**:325.

Stein, L., 1964, *Fed. Proc.* **23**:836.

Stein, L., and Berger, D., 1971, *Arzneim.-Forsch.* **21**(7a):1075–1079.

Sternbach, L. H., 1971, *Angew. Chem.* **10**:34.

Sturner, W. Q., and Garriott, J. C., 1973, *J. Am. Med. Assoc.* **223**:1125–1130.

Surber, W., Wagner-Jauregg, T., and Haring, M., 1959, *Arzneim.-Forsch.* **9**:143.

Surrey, A. R., Webb, W. G., and Gesler, R. M., 1958, *J. Am. Chem. Soc.* **80**:517.

Taylor, P. A., and Egan, L. P., 1964, *Finnegan Spectra* **4**(3).

Tenckhoff, H., Sherrand, D. J., Hickmann, R. O., and Ladd, K. L., 1968, *Am. J. Dis. Child.* **116**:422.

Toki, K., Toki, S., and Tsukamoto, H., 1963, *J. Biochem.* **53**:43.

Tompsett, S. L., 1968, *Acta Pharmacol. Toxicol.* **26**:298.

Tsukamoto, H., Takabatake, E., and Ariyoshi, T., 1955, *Pharm. Bull. (Tokyo)* **3**:459.

Tsukamoto, H., Yoshimura, H., Ide, H., and Mitsui, S., 1963, *Chem. Pharm. Bull.* **11**: 429.

The United States Pharmacopeia, 1975, 19th revision (Committee of Revision, United States Pharmacopeial Convention, Inc.), U.S.P. Inc., Rockville, Maryland.

Van Dyke, C., Barashi, P. G., Jatlow, P., and Byck, R., 1976, *Science* **191**:859.

Veath, R. M., Alder, T. K., and Way, E. L., 1964, *J. Pharmacol. Exp. Ther.* **145**:11.

Verebely, K., and Inturresi, C. G., 1973, *J. Chromatogr.* **75**:195.

Vesell, G. S., and Passananti, G. T., 1971, *Clin. Chem.* **17**:851.

Viala, A., Carro, J. P., *et al.*, 1969, *Ann. Pharm. Fr.* **27**:511–518.

Viukari, N. M. A., and Salmines, P., 1973, *Lancet*, 127.

Waddell, W. J., 1962, *Fed. Proc.* **21**:182.

Waddell, W. J., 1963, *Fed. Proc.* **22**:480.

Waddell, W. J., 1965, *J. Pharmacol. Exp. Ther.* **149**:23.

Waggoner, W. C., Gagliardi, V. J., and Lund, M. H., 1973, *Clin. Toxicol.* **6**(3):317–323.

Walls, H. C., 1976, *Bull. IAFT* **12**(3):7.

Wassermann, A. J., and Richardson, D. W., 1963, *Clin. Pharmacol. Ther.* **4**:321.

Welles, J. S., McMahon, R. E., and Doran, W. J., 1963, *J. Pharmacol. Exp. Ther.* **137**: 166.

Widdop, B., 1970, *J. Chromatogr.* **47**:485–486.

Williams, R. T., 1959, *Detoxication Mechanisms*, Vol. 2, p. 593, Chapman and Hall, London.

Winek, C. L., Davis, E. R., Collom, W. D., and Shanor, S. P., 1974, *Clin. Toxicol.* **7**(2): 129–132.

Winter, L., Calman, H. I., Caruso, W. A., and Post, A., 1973, *Current Ther. Res.* **15**(7): 383–390.

Wiseman, E. H., Schreiber, E. C., and Pinson, R., Jr., 1964, *Biochem. Pharmacol.* **13**: 1421.

Witiak, D. T., 1970, in: *Medicinal Chemistry*, Part II, p. 1653, Wiley, New York.

Woods, J. H., and Tessel, R. E., 1974, *Science* **185**(4156):1067–1068.

Woods, L. A., McMahon, F. G., and Severs, M. H., 1951, *J. Pharmacol. Exp. Ther.* **101**: 200.

Wright, W. B., Brabauder, H. J., and Hardy, R. A., 1959, *J. Am. Chem. Soc.* **81**:1518.

Zbinden, G., and Randall, L. Q., 1967, *Advances in Pharmacology*, Vol. 5 (S. Garrattini and P. A. Shore, eds.), p. 213, Academic Press, New York.

Zbinden, G., Bagdon, R. E., Keith, G. F., Phillips, R. D., and Randall, L. O., 1961, *Toxicol. Appl. Pharmacol.* **3**: 619–637.

Zehnder, K., Kalberer, K., Kreis, W., and Rutschmann, J., 1962, *Biochem. Pharmacol.* **11**:535.

Zirkle, C. L., and Kaiser, C., 1970, in: *Medicinal Chemistry*, Part II (A. Burger, ed.), p. 1447, Wiley-Interscience, New York.

Index